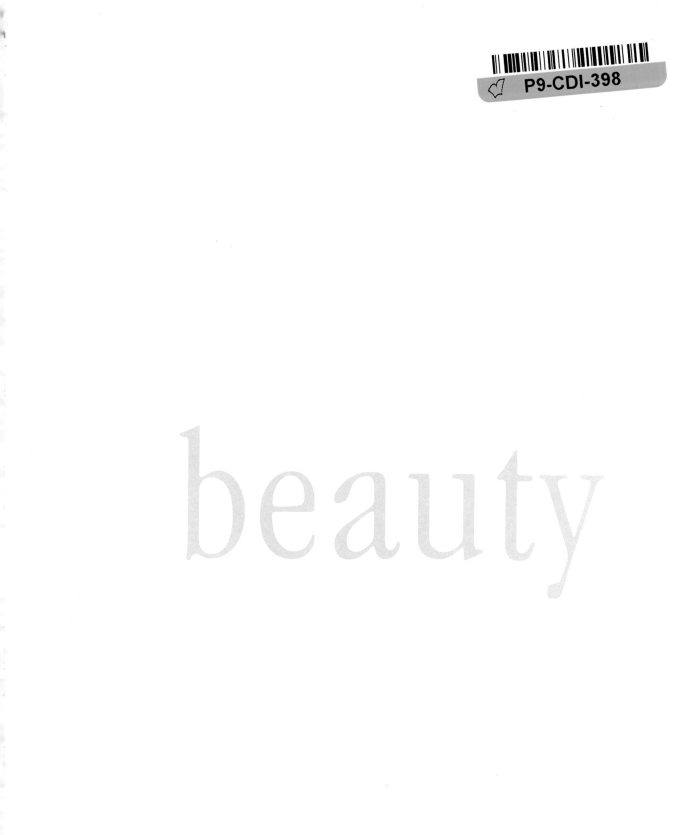

beauty

illustrations by anja kroencke

beauty

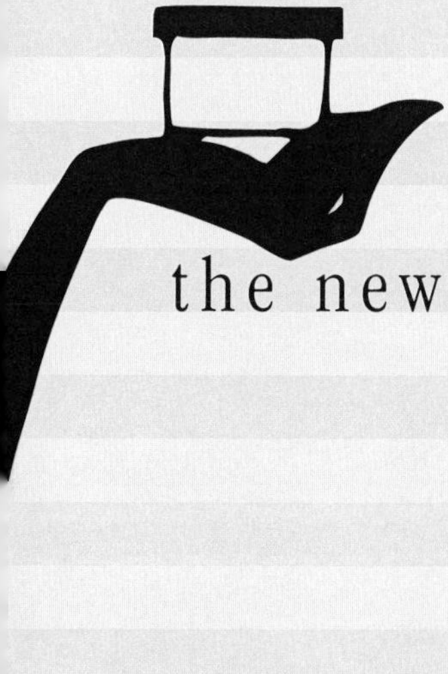

the new basics by **rona berg**

photography by deborah jaffe

WORKMAN PUBLISHING • NEW YORK

Copyright © 2001 by Rona Berg

Illustrations copyright © 2001 by Anja Kroencke

Photography © 2001 by Deborah Jaffe

Design by Paul Hanson and Elizabeth Johnsboen

Library of Congress Cataloging-in-Publication Data
Berg, Rona.
Beauty : the new basics / by Rona Berg ; illustrations by Anja Kroencke ;
photographs by Deborah Jaffe.
p. cm.
Includes index.
ISBN 0-7611-0186-1
1. Beauty, Personal. I. Title.
RA778.B473 2000
646.7'2—dc21   00-043631

Workman books are available at special discounts
when purchased in bulk for premiums and sales promotions
as well as for fund-raising or educational use.
Special editions or book excerpts can also be created to specification.
For details, contact the Special Sales Director at the address below.

Workman Publishing Company, Inc.
708 Broadway
New York, NY 10003-9555
www.workman.com

Printed in the U.S.A.

First printing January 2001

10 9 8 7 6 5 4 3

D EDICATED TO MY BREATHTAKING,

BEAUTIFUL GRANDMOTHER, LILLIAN BERG,

WHO TAUGHT ME THAT TRUE BEAUTY LIES WITHIN—

BUT A LITTLE LIPSTICK DOESN'T HURT, AND

YOU MAY AS WELL PUT ON SOME POWDER,

STAND UP STRAIGHT, AND DAZZLE 'EM

WHILE YOU'RE AT IT.

T O MY BELOVED BRUCE AND SOPHIE,

WHO SHARE THE BEAUTY OF LIFE WITH ME.

A ND TO MY PARENTS, ALAN AND SHEILA BERG,

WHO NEVER CEASE TO AMAZE ME.

CONTENTS

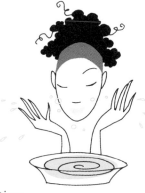
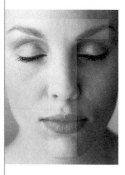

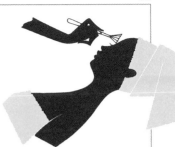

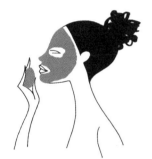

PART TWO # hair

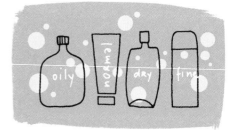

HAIRCARE · *183*

HAIR COLOR · *207*

HAIRCUTS & -STYLES · *227*

BEAUTY TIME LINE: HAIR · *262*

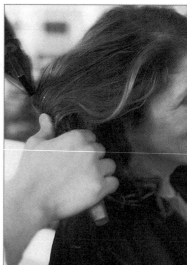

PART THREE # the body

BATH & BODY · *269*

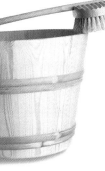

HANDS & FEET · *293*

THE SPA · *315*

BEAUTY TIME LINE: THE BODY · *330*

GLOSSARY · *335*

APPENDICES · *347*

INDEX · *389*

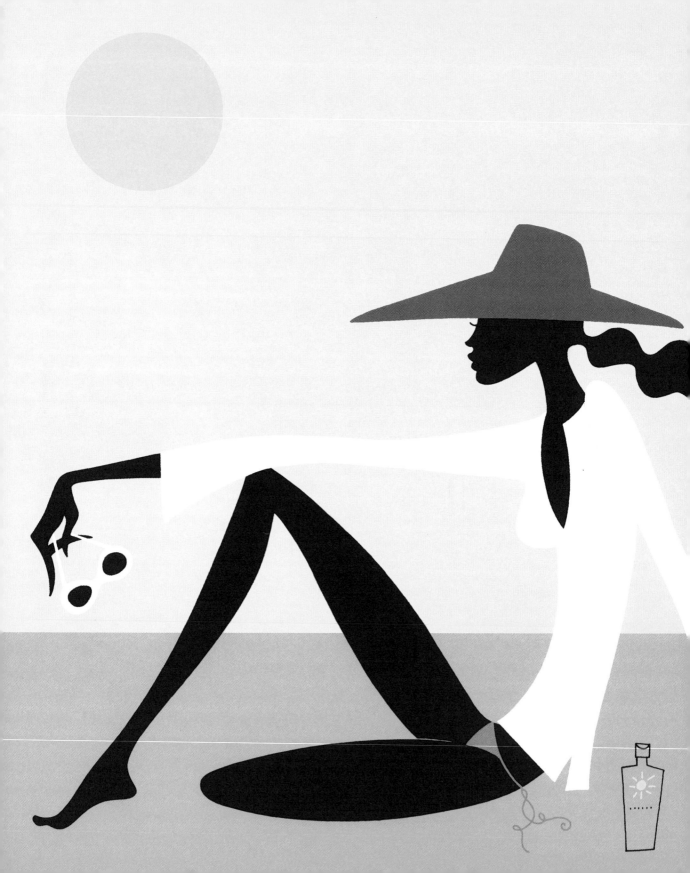

introduction

What is beauty? Does anyone really know? We search for it and make art to try to capture its essence. We share in the pleasure of it, and when it seems absent from our daily lives, we long for it. We thrive on it—and are often willing to suffer for it. Beauty is personal and political. It is elusive and eternal. It is many things: strength, confidence, passion, grace—a sense of style, a turn of head, a state of mind. In truth, no one can say exactly what beauty is, but one thing is certain: Every woman wants it.

As a fashion editor and beauty writer for the past 15 years, I've investigated and reported on the stuff that beauty's made of; and as a woman, I've consumed it. I've attended hundreds of product launches, press conferences, and industry debuts. Truckloads of products have crossed my desk. Not only have I sampled virtually every hair mask, cleanser, powder, and detoxifying body treatment in existence, I've analyzed each one.

I've covered the industry from a few unusual perspectives: scribbling notes as I lay half-naked on massage tables or in scented aromatherapy baths. Backstage at fashion shows in Paris, Milan, and New York, where I watched the bare-faced, ponytailed Kate Moss and Christy Turlington arrive in jeans and T-shirts, and emerge, hours later, like painted butterflies. I've soaked up tricks and tips from the pros, and I've absorbed everyone's behind-the-scenes beauty secrets. I share the best of them in this book: how Bobbi Brown gives Moss's skin such a dewy glow (baby oil), how Frédéric Fekkai adds volume to Claudia Schiffer's hair (StiffStuff), what makes Naomi Campbell's lashes look so long (Maybelline Great Lash). I've interviewed cosmetic chemists, industry executives, top dermatologists, leading plastic surgeons, and aestheticians, and seen that there's a lot of good products out there—and plenty of brilliant spin.

Like many women, you've probably left a cosmetics counter dazed, dizzy, and suddenly $150 poorer. You got home and wondered: *What is all this?* And so I've cut through the hype to create a book that's jam-packed with everything you'll need to become not only an informed consumer but an expert on how to attain head-to-toe beauty through gentle, healthy means.

You'll learn about ingredients so you can decode a cosmetics label and enough about skin cells, hair follicles, and oil glands so you understand the effect of products on your body. We all want to know whether status brands like Chanel and Estée Lauder are really better than cheaper, mass-market brands like Revlon and Maybelline, or whether Avon's inexpensive alpha-hydroxy acids measure up to Elizabeth Arden's pricier ones. What do makeup artists and hairstylists know that we don't? In the real world, women need simple, straightforward, real information, and the kinds of shortcuts, tips, and techniques that you'll find in this book. The less intimidated you are, the more fun you'll have exploring the realm of beauty.

As most mothers know, almost as soon as little girls are old enough to look in the mirror, they get together with friends and "style" their hair, paint their nails, and rub fire-engine-red Crayolas on their lips. Hopefully this book will bring back some of that liberating sense of play you felt when you first experimented with makeup as a child. Applying makeup can be immensely satisfying once you have the confidence to play in your paint box. The right stuff and the attitude behind its use can transform you into a more confident, more beautiful version of yourself.

Unlike most authors of beauty books, I am not a makeup artist, aesthetician, or hairstylist. I have no products to sell, though I do recommend what I believe to be the best across a broad spectrum, from blush to body scrubs and for all skin colors and types. I've evaluated products on overall quality, healthfulness of ingredients, effectiveness, and sensory appeal.

When *ELLE* magazine premiered in 1985, I found myself editing the hottest fashion and beauty magazine launch in history, at a time when standards of beauty were radically changing in America. In the 1970s, leggy blondes like Cheryl Tiegs and Christie Brinkley were the main models. But changing demographics over the next decades helped African American, Latin, and Asian models transform traditional Western standards of what is beautiful. Images of full-figured women in magazines broke through a barrier for women of all sizes. Now, every woman can see a gorgeous reflection of herself—and this book reflects that, too.

It's been a long struggle. I'm reminded of a striking photo by Horst, the renowned fashion photographer. "Electric Beauty" depicts a woman with a heat mask on her face, an electric nail buffer in her hand, her legs in a bucket of suds, and her body encircled by cords. She is bound, gagged, and about to be electrocuted by her own beauty regimen. I'd like to believe that Horst's view of the lengths women go for beauty is passé, and if this book accomplishes one thing, I hope it will help women realize that cosmetics exist to empower —not enslave them.

These days, most women prefer to seek out beauty by less risky, gentler, more pleasurable means. We want to reveal, not conceal, our natural beauty and let our true selves shine through. After all, beauty begins in the brain, and what makes us truly beautiful is born well below the surface: a gleam in our eye, an ear-to-ear grin, a bounce in our step. But sometimes a little powder or a little paint doesn't hurt—just a little, of course. So dig in, play around, and, most of all, enjoy.

PART ONE **the face**

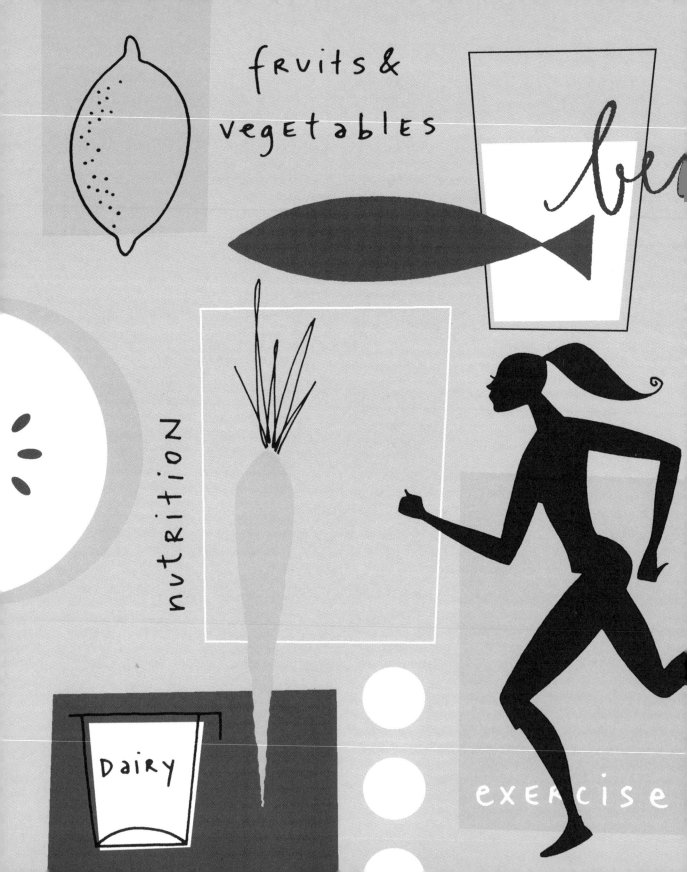

fruits &
vegetables

nutrition

Dairy

exercise

uty basics

Secrets are the essence of the beauty business.

—KENNEDY FRASER, *Scenes from the Fashionable World*

The world of beauty is a mad, funny, seductive world. Misguided in some ways, misleading in others, it's also a source of great pleasure to a great many women. Let's face it, we all use cosmetics (even the least vain among us), and some of us are pretty passionate about it. Why else would American women spend almost $25 billion each year on beauty products alone? We search for that perfect powder, pomade, or lipstick, the one that's going to make us look gorgeous, the one we hope will change our lives. And the beauty industry is happy to oblige—with a battalion of products that promise everything from eternal youth to enhanced sensuality, or what Revlon founder Charles Revson called "hope in a jar."

The beauty industry does exploit women's insecurities, and yet, more often than not, it also helps us achieve what we want: to feel more beautiful. Any woman who has mastered a trick of light and shadow that makes her eyes sparkle or discovered a slick of gel that smooths her spiraling tendrils understands that beauty is not necessarily what we are born with, but what we can learn to create: the sleight-of-hand stuff that dreams are made of.

As a beauty journalist, I've attended literally thousands of new-product launches over the years. Each product claimed to be "revolutionary," "breakthrough," or "350 percent more effective." Confronted with all the hype, how do you know which ones to choose? It seems that just when you've got a grip on alpha-hydroxy acids, along come the betas. Like most women, you're probably happy to spend money on beauty aids that really work—but how do you know which ones do?

Every once in a while, I have the fantasy that somewhere on the outskirts of Geneva, Paris, or maybe even Bayonne, New Jersey, there's a huge cosmetics manufacturing plant. There, every beauty product on today's market is scooped out of three creamy white vats (dry/normal/oil-free), poured into jars of varying size and design, and slapped with pretty labels, which is basically what differentiates a $3.95 tube of Nivea from an $85 jar of Creme de la Mer. (Both, by the way, are good-quality moisturizers.)

There is some truth to my fantasy: At least a third of the cost of beauty products goes into packaging and advertising. Ever since beauty divas Elizabeth Arden and Helena Rubinstein opened the first salons and pioneered the sale of exclusive cosmetics, competition has been fierce. Copycat manufacturers steal ideas from each other so quickly that often the only difference between one product and the next is a paler shade of blue. Sure, marketing claims are misleading and advertising images set an impossible standard. But the industry has also developed sublime and truly effective products that are well worth your time and attention.

Recent advances in technology have resulted in protective makeup that looks naturally healthy, styling aids that actually improve the condition of your hair, and skincare products that correct rather than camouflage.

To navigate the vast and complex realm of beauty, all you really have to do is gain some basic knowledge of beauty products and ingredients and ask the right questions. (This book will help you know what to ask and where to find the answers.) And then use your good sense. Remember, when it comes to beauty, Everything Is Simpler Than It Seems. With a healthy dose of skepticism, a commitment to simplifying your regimen, a good attitude, and intelligent choices, you can cut through the hype and find what you need to look and feel great. Are you ready for that?

Smart Shopping

When you walk into a store that is brimming with hundreds of beauty products and tools, from moisturizers and revitalizing masks to eyelash curlers and tweezers, it's easy to let sheer product overload short-circuit your self-confidence. Those bulging shelves are intimidating to consumers, and they're intended to be. The idea is, the more insecure you feel, the more you'll buy blind.

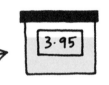

So do a little homework before you shop for cosmetics. That way, you won't present yourself as defenseless prey to the impeccably groomed woman behind the cosmetics counter, and you'll avoid a $38 impulse buy that is destined to join the drawerful waiting at home.

Smart shopping for cosmetics should be easy for anyone who knows how to shop for groceries. The guidelines are the same: Know what you want, buy only what you need, don't shop when you're feeling desperate (hungry), comparison shop, and read the labels.

Prep Online

Before you buy anything, it's helpful—and fun—to do a bit of prep work online. You'll zero in on products, prices, colors, and small "boutique brands" and save time in the long run. In many cases, you can order online as well (see page 6). But be aware that although Websites try, technology isn't always able to provide perfect color matches. So check out each company's return policy in advance.

Try Before You Buy

Don't ever let yourself be intimidated or bullied at the cosmetics counter. Remember two things: (1) you don't have to buy anything at all, and (2) you know more than you think you do.

For instance, you know that you don't want to go out and spend $32.50 on an antioxidant mois-

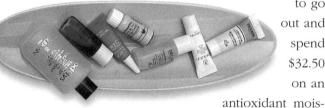

turizer unless it will work. So before you buy anything, walk up to the counter with confidence and ask for a sample. (Whoever said nothing in life is free obviously hasn't shopped for cosmetics lately.) Cosmetics companies are prepared to give away free beauty booty (especially Kiehl's), and they regularly supply department stores with cute little doll-sized tubes of makeup, skincare, fragrance, and more—which are yours for the asking. (And

WHAT PRICE BEAUTY?

What does it actually cost to make the stuff? Well, in most cases, not much. The actual cost of the average cosmetic product is about 10 percent of what you pay at retail whether you're shopping at Saks or Sav-On Drugs. Some ingredients (like squalene and shea butter) do cost more than others (like mineral oil), which is another reason to learn how to read a label—so that you can gauge value.

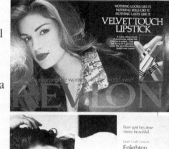

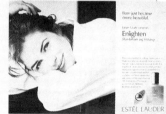

Let's say your favorite up-market skin cream costs $30 in a department store. Subtract $15 right away (it's what the store pays the cosmetic company). So, the company books a profit of $15. But how much of that goes into making the lotion or cream? Around $3. Gross profit for the company? $12.

The rising cost of advertising: In 1974, Lauren Hutton signed a $100,000 contract as the first spokesmodel for Revlon. Sixteen years later, Revlon signed Cindy Crawford (above, top) to a $4 million, four-year deal. And in 1995, Elizabeth Hurley became the new "face" of Estée Lauder for a reported $10 million.

But the bucks don't stop there. Though the beauty industry has extremely high gross margins, their net margins are not so high. Out of that profit, the company subtracts substantial costs for—you guessed it—advertising and marketing.

What about a mass market product at a drugstore level? Basically the same equation applies. If a product costs you $10, the drugstore pays the manufacturer about $5.50. The cost of the product, however, including packaging, container, and contents, will rarely exceed $1.25.

CYBER BEAUTY

Surf's up! If the sea of beauty Websites is too daunting to navigate on your own, here are some good destinations.

ADVICE AND CHAT

On the Net, of course, *everyone* is an expert. Some of the more engaging and opinionated beauty buffs can be found at these sites:

www.beautybuzz.com A fun site . . . with a conscience. In addition to beauty-relevant links, reviews, recommendations, and a lively message board, there's info about causes like HIV awareness and the Americans with Disabilities Act. Look great and do good!

www.beautyguru.com BeautyGuru's well-designed site serves up detailed product reviews, friendly counsel, and extensive links to other beauty-related sites.

www.i-iman.com On the Internet domain of the Somalian supermodel, you can find tips and techniques from the goddess herself, with special attention paid to the beauty concerns of women of color. There's also plenty of info about Iman's terrific, affordable cosmetics and skincare line. Check out the outrageous graphics.

"E-ZINES"/"E-TAIL"

If you can't stand cosmetics counters and salespeople—or if you just don't have the time—these sites offer an easy way to shop.

www.beauty.com An attractively designed site offering expert advice (from makeup guru Kevyn Aucoin and hairstylist Sally Hershberger) and a selection of first-rate products.

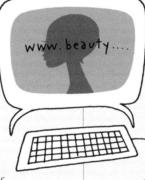

www.beautybuys.com A discount shop, featuring bargains on cosmetic lines from Cover Girl to Clinique, and hard-to-find haircare lines.

www.beautycafe.com Beauty Cafe is especially strong on botanical-based goods.

www.beautyjungle.com One of Beautyjungle's best features is that it carries both boutique and mass-market brands, so you can buy your Revlon lipstick *and* your Karin Herzog Vit-A-Kombi moisturizer here.

www.bellisima.com This tasteful site carries cosmetics, haircare, and skincare by top-shelf brands, including Bumble and bumble, Molton Brown, Philip B., and Mon Jardinet.

www.blissworld.com The Internet home of New York City's trendy Bliss day spa. A user-friendly site from which to purchase upscale products from Creme de la Mer, Shu Uemura, YonKa, and more.

www.ibeauty.com High-end beauty advice from former *Vogue* beauty diva Shirley Lord, a stable of pricey products, and a solid city-by-city resource list for services like facials, body wraps, eyebrow shaping, and electrolysis.

HONORABLE MENTIONS

Some of the most informative and user-friendly cosmetics company sites are: www.aveda.com, www.clinique.com, www.neutrogena.com, and www.smashbox.com.

don't worry about getting "something for nothing." Women spent $6.2 billion on cosmetics at department stores last year—so companies can afford to give a little away.) You won't find every product available at all times, but you're likely to discover something that will interest you. If you run into a reluctant salesperson, tell her you have sensitive skin and really need to try products out before you buy them. Watch how quickly she'll come through for you.

Most samples provide a week's supply, which is time enough to tell whether you like the results. Once you know that a product works for you, you'll feel a lot better about spending money on it.

And if you do end up dropping a wad of cash on something that doesn't live up to its claims, by all means return it. You're not the first to do so, and you certainly won't be the last. Even drugstore chains like CVS, Rite Aid, and Walgreens offer refunds and take products back as a matter of policy.

Go for a Professional Consultation

Good skincare—along with a healthy diet and exercise—is basic to beauty. So at least once, treat yourself to a professional consultation and a facial, just to learn the ropes, along with some guidelines about caring for your skin. A professional consultation is a great way to arm yourself with useful information about your personal beauty needs. If you know more, you'll be less likely to leave the cosmetics

counter dazed, $150 poorer, and wondering what you're going to do with all that stuff. If you can't afford to pay full price for a professional, find a salon or day spa that offers a discount on "trainee night." (See appendix C, page 361.)

Know When to Splurge

No one wants to feel ripped off. That's why it's important to know when it pays to splurge. Throughout this book, I'll tell you which products are worth spending money on and which aren't. For example, it's worth spending money on skincare, foundation, and powder. Quality brands of face powder are pressed more compactly than cheaper versions, which means that they last longer. On the other hand, it's not worth it to spend more on sunblock, lip or eye pencils, or mascara. Top makeup artists agree that Maybelline Great Lash, at $5.98, is still tops. And if you are under 35, don't waste your money on alpha-hydroxy acids (see page 31). There's plenty of time for that later.

Remember, you don't need to buy a company's entire line. How many women dress in Calvin Klein from head to toe? Not only would it be really pricey to do so, but it also wouldn't be much fun. Just as you mix and match your wardrobe, you can choose products from different companies that work best for you. If you don't like night cream or clarifying lotion, don't get talked into buying it because a saleswoman with beautiful skin tells you that you need a company's entire regimen in order for any single product to work. You don't.

Use Your Senses

It's important to use common sense when you shop, but you should incorporate your other senses, too. The realm of beauty is a sensory realm, and sometimes indulging yourself is what it's all about. A jewel-encrusted compact may cost triple what you usually pay, but if you powder your nose in public and that extra touch of elegance pleases you, why not go for it—as long as it doesn't eat up your entire paycheck. A lipstick may be the exact replica of a cheaper model, except that it smells like violets, and that fact alone may make it worth an extra $9. Beauty, after all, is in the details. Cosmetics companies spend millions of dollars refining the nuances of texture, fragrance, and packaging, and you may as well take advantage of their efforts.

Never settle for second best or "good enough." Make sure that you really like the feel and smell of a product. If, for example, you like the way a product works but don't like its smell, keep sampling and reading ingredients labels (more on that follows) until you find a comparable product with a scent that pleases you. Beauty products should not only help you look good, they're supposed to make you feel good, too.

Cracking the Cosmetic Code

You read food ingredients labels, don't you? After all, it's the only way to compare the value between products and to know which foods to avoid. Similarly, on beauty products, the ingredients label is the only part of the packaging that has useful information. It will alert you to any potentially irritating ingredients, such as citrus oils or propylparaben, and whether a product contains pore-clogging ingredients like cocoa butter or lanolin. You'll also know when you're getting less than you bargained for: for example, when the $27 moisturizer you bought at Nordstrom has exactly the same ingredients as the one that sells for $4.29 at Cosmetics Plus, minus the stylish packaging.

You don't need to be a chemist to master a few common catchphrases and be able to decode a label (see facing page). As on food labels, ingredients that make up the largest percentage of a product are listed first. Past the halfway point, the amount of any ingredient listed is negligible. If a product lists collagen, royal jelly, or aloe vera on its label but doesn't require refrigeration, don't waste your money: either the amount is minuscule, or it has been pasteurized past the point of effectiveness.

Cosmetics companies jealously guard their secret ingredients from competitors for as long as they can. Occasionally, the Food and Drug Administration (FDA) grants a company "trade secret status," which means those secret ingredients don't have to appear on the label. If you have a history of sensitivity to cosmetics, when you see the phrase ". . . and other ingredients,"

HOW TO READ A LABEL

It's important to acquaint yourself with some of the most common chemical ingredients listed on cosmetics labels so you can avoid those that irritate your skin and can compare labels from product to product. Below are ingredients listed on a typical drugstore moisturizer. They are listed in descending order. Here's how to decipher them.

DERMATOLOGIST TESTED	Means a dermatologist was within five miles of the plant and may or may not have looked on the product.
FRAGRANCE-FREE	Does not mean no fragrance added—only means no perceptible fragrance.
ACTIVE INGREDIENT: OCTYL METHOXYCINNAMATE	A sunscreen. The reason it's listed separately is because it makes a medical claim to protect against sun damage.
INGREDIENTS: TRIPLE PURIFIED WATER	The average moisturizer contains 65 percent water.
MINERAL OIL ISOPROPYL PALMITATE	Emollients to be avoided if you have oily skin; can clog pores.
PROPYLENE GLYCOL	Humectant that binds water to the skin, often used in oil-free moisturizers.
GLYCERYL STEARATE SE CAPRYLIC/CAPRIC TRIGLYCERIDE SODIUM DIHYDROXYCETYL PHOSPHATE CETEARYL ALCOHOL STEARIC ACID	Emulsifiers—keep the oil and water from separating and give a rich, smooth texture.
TOCOPHERYL ACETATE (VITAMIN E) ALOE EXTRACT	Bonus ingredients—hyped on the label but the amount is so small, it's window dressing.
SIMETHICONE	An emollient derived from silicone—softens skin and adds "slip" to the product.
BENZOPHENONE-3	Common ingredient in sunscreens. Helps prevent product from breaking down in sunlight. Can cause hives.
ISOPROPYL MYRISTATE	An emollient that can be comedogenic. Its use is contested by consumer advocates who claim it may be carcinogenic.
CARBOMER	A thickener—usually 1 percent of total, so use it as a marker. Any ingredients that follow are less than 1 percent.
TRIETHANOLAMINE	An ammonia derivative that's harsh on the skin
PHENOXYETHANOL	A coal-tar ingredient, a suspected carcinogen; that's why it's for external use only. Often added for fragrance.
METHYLPARABEN, ETHYLPARABEN, PROPYLPARABEN, BUTYLPARABEN	The parabens are the most common synthetic preservatives used today. Any beauty product that contains water needs preservatives.

WHO OWNS WHAT?
TWO COSMETIC FAMILY TREES

Do you ever think there's not much difference between one cosmetic product and the next other than the name/image, the packaging, and the cost? Well, here's a look at all the companies owned by two of the cosmetics giants—Estée Lauder and L'Oréal. Kind of makes you wonder who else is left.

I guess the assumption with a company like Estée Lauder is that you graduate as you get older from, for example, Origins and Prescriptives to Clinique and Estée Lauder, the same way you're supposed to graduate from *YM* to *Glamour,* and eventually to *Vogue.*

M·A·C

JO MALONE

ARAMIS, INC.

AVEDA CORP.

STILA MAKEUP

JANE COSMETICS

PRESCRIPTIVES, INC.

ESTÉE LAUDER COSMETICS

BOBBI BROWN ESSENTIALS

CLINIQUE LABORATORIES, INC.

DONNA KARAN BEAUTY PRODUCTS

CREME DE LA MER FACIAL TREATMENT LINE

ORIGINS NATURAL RESOURCES COSMETICS

L'ORÉAL COSMETICS

L'ORÉAL PARIS

BIOTHERM

GIORGIO ARMANI PARFUMS

HELENA RUBINSTEIN

KIEHL'S

LABORATOIRES GARNIER

LANCÔME PARIS

MAYBELLINE

RALPH LAUREN PARFUMS

REDKEN 5TH AVENUE NYC

VICHY

SOFT SHEEN PRODUCTS, INC.

Estée Lauder, Inc.

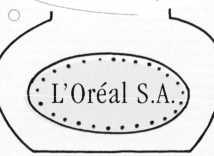

L'Oréal S.A.

beware. There's no way to guess what surprises you may be in for.

Cutting Through the Hype

Unfortunately, most of us pay more attention to the marketing claims than to the ingredients. Slick marketing lingo, like a fickle suitor, is designed to promise and seduce—to overstate the qualities of the product, but just enough so that the company's claims won't get it in trouble with the FDA. The bottom line is, if something sounds too good to be true, it usually is. For example, no product will "close your pores" or "erase wrinkles" as many claim on their labels. Nothing short of cosmetic dermatology or surgery will "erase wrinkles." And if your pores close, your skin can't breathe, and you'll suffocate. However, clean and unclogged pores look smaller, which is what you really want anyway.

The claims "fragrance-free," "natural," and "hypoallergenic" mean absolutely nothing in the beauty biz. Most skincare products smell bad in the lab, because they're loaded with chemicals and raw ingredients. So manufacturers do scent them—not to make them smell good, but just to make them *not* smell bad. So "fragrance-free" only means free of all perceptible fragrance. And the FDA has never spelled out exactly what "hypoallergenic" means. As a result, some companies test their products for allergic reactions, but many do not. The most misleading claim (and my personal favorite) is "dermatologist-tested"—which means that there was a dermatologist within a 5- or 10-mile radius of the testing center who may or may not have looked at the product.

How Do They Get Away with It? Beauty and the FDA

When you pull a cosmetic product off the drugstore shelf, you probably assume that it's been tested, monitored, and regulated for safety and effectiveness. Well, it may or may not have been. Since the FDA spends only about one percent of its budget to monitor the entire beauty industry, the industry has remained largely "self-regulated." In other words, while in theory there are industry standards to uphold and truth-in-advertising rules to adhere to, in actual practice cosmetics manufacturers are free to say and do almost anything to sell their products.

Under the less-than-watchful eye of the FDA, cosmetics companies can use just about

A BRIEF HISTORY OF COSMETICS
AND THE FDA: THE RULES OF THE GAME

Cosmetics manufacturers have always been vigorously opposed to outside regulation. In 1906, the government finally passed the Pure Food and Drug Act, which restricted the false marketing of cosmetics. But the legislation was far from comprehensive. Though U.S. companies could no longer claim that their products were made in Paris, the ingredients in cosmetics were left unregulated.

The turning point came in the 1930s, with the publication of two sensational books—*100,000 Guinea Pigs* and *American Chamber of Horrors*—that were harshly critical of the beauty industry. In the aftermath of their publication, a New York senator named Royo Copeland crusaded to amend the 1906 act to include cosmetics, but he couldn't beat the powerful cosmetics lobby. However, when several women suffered serious cosmetics-related injuries—blindings caused by "Lash Lure," an eyelash dye, and poisoning by "Koremlu," a popular depilatory laced with rat poison (thalium acetate)—Congress approved the Food, Drug and Cosmetic Act (the FD&C Act) in 1938.

The FD&C Act expanded the 1906 act by restricting the use of adulterated, dangerous, or impure substances and exaggerated, misleading, and adulterated claims by cosmetics manufacturers. It also established legal definitions for cosmetics.

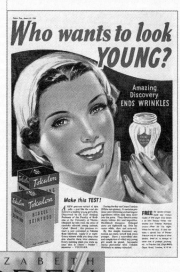

Cosmetics, according to the FD&C Act, are "articles intended to be applied to the human body for cleansing, beautifying, promoting attractiveness, or altering the appearance without affecting the body's structure or functions."

Another restrictive piece of legislation was passed in 1960: the Color Additive Amendment requires that coloring ingredients be tested for safety and approved by the FDA. And in 1973, the Fair Packaging and Labeling Act (FPLA) mandated that cosmetic ingredients in products for home use be listed on the outer label, in decreasing order according to the amount used in the product (just like food ingredients listings). The name and address of the manufacturer must also be listed, along with the product weight.

REVOLTING INGREDIENTS

The following organic ingredients, though not for the squeamish, are still in use in everyday products. They are just not hyped the way they once were. Nowadays, "cruelty-free" products—especially plant derivatives—have relegated them to some dark, dank corner of the lab and the label. Here are some of the more revolting things we're putting on our faces today.

Human placenta. The protein-rich lining of the womb, expelled after birth, was first used in cosmetics in the 1940s. Because of its hormone content, manufacturers claimed that placental material would stimulate tissue growth and eradicate wrinkles. When the FDA challenged these claims, manufacturers changed their pitch, but still claimed that placenta was an aid to aging skin.

Animal amniotic liquid. The fluid that surrounds and protects a cow or ox fetus, touted as a valuable source of protein and vitamins, is used in moisturizers and shampoos.

Fish scales. Used in some glittery eye shadow.

"Live" sheep cells. Used in antiaging skin treatments.

Beetle carapace. The shell of a beetle is the source of "carmine," a common ingredient in red lipsticks.

Cattle, ox, or swine brain cells. Used in moisturizers.

any ingredient on the planet. Barring certain prohibited color additives and the obviously forbidden "poisonous or putrid ingredients," only a few—10, actually—are explicitly prohibited for use in cosmetics. And unless a company makes a drug claim for its product (for example, that it will "cure, prevent or mitigate a disease"), just about any fancy verbal footwork will fly. Cosmetics companies are not required to test for product safety, report adverse reactions, register with the FDA, or release their formulas to the FDA. But many do so voluntarily. They want your repeat business, after all, and it's in their interest to avoid using ingredients that could turn out to be irritating or harmful. They have to be fairly responsible about regulating themselves if they don't want the government to step in and do it for them.

But as far as I'm concerned, it makes good sense to always assume that cosmetic chemicals are harsher than the claims suggest. Many peevish little skin problems—blackheads, dermatitis, rashes, cosmetic acne—can be traced back to bad beauty product choices. Over the long term, your body responds best to gentle care, anyway. So until truth in advertising—and consumer safety—is better enforced, a healthy dose of skepticism is not only reasonable but required.

Beauty from the Inside Out

The minute you begin to take better care of yourself—developing and sticking to a regimen, becoming more discerning about what you put on your skin and a more sophisticated consumer—you will not only look better but feel better, too. "A good appearance is part of good health," says Dr. Ellen Gendler, a New York City dermatologist. "It's more than a cosmetic concept," she continues, "it's a wellness concept."

As more women work toward achieving beauty from the inside out and focus on the importance of a healthy diet and exercise, we have changed our dependence on products that work only on the outside. A generation or two ago, the beauty industry sold powders and paints to create the illusion of beauty. A spackling of makeup was intended to transform or conceal whatever wreckage lay hidden below. Now, in the age of health and fitness, women prefer to reveal—not conceal—the results of a healthy lifestyle. Makeup is sheerer, lighter, and

Tip Don't use testers at a cosmetics counter. If you must test makeup, do it on the back of your hand or on your fingertips, and use a fresh applicator like a cotton ball or a Q-tip. In a store, the preservatives don't have time to kill bacteria after each use.

more streamlined than ever. No one has time for elaborate beauty rituals anymore. Any regimen that's too complicated is doomed. According to Gina Kolata, writing in *The New York Times,* "Somehow, that loosely defined word 'health' and that loaded word 'beauty' are so intricately entwined that many of us confuse them, consciously or subconsciously, in our incessant dream of perfect health—or is it perfect beauty?" And does it really matter where one leaves off and the other begins?

Beauty products are only a small part of the beauty equation. Granted, using the right stuff—and developing an informed approach to it—can transform you into a more confident, more beautiful version of yourself. But more important than any particular product is the mind-set behind its use. Simplicity, elegance, self-confidence, common sense, and good health are the cornerstones of beauty.

Your health is the very best "beauty aid" you will ever have. Looking good depends on taking good care of your body—from the inside out. And your body will respond best to intelligent, gentle, and consistent care. There are "quick fixes" when you need them, and they are liberally sprinkled throughout this book. But remember, it is a lifetime of good care that will yield a lifetime of healthy good looks. And that's something you can't buy in a bottle.

SPREAD THE WORD

If you do experience an adverse reaction to a product, report your experience to the FDA. Write to the Food and Drug Administration Center for Food Safety and Applied Nutrition, Office of Colors and Cosmetics, 200 C Street, S.W., Washington, DC, 20204. Or call the FDA Consumer Complaint Coordinator in your state; to obtain the telephone number of the coordinator in your area, call 800-270-8869. To reach the FDA via the Internet, log on to its Website at www.fda.gov.

The FDA—and most reputable cosmetics companies—are highly responsive to consumer complaints. If the FDA receives a cluster of complaints concerning one product or a type of product, it will investigate, so taking the time to make a complaint *can* make a difference.

10 Steps to Real Beauty

There are lots of good books that can help you learn how to create and maintain a healthy diet (see appendix F, page 381). This section is not intended to be a comprehensive guide to nutrition; rather, it focuses on points directly related to healthy skin, hair, and nails. Keep these basics in mind as you learn to achieve a glow from the inside out.

1. Eat a diet rich in fresh fruits and vegetables. Five daily servings of each is the recommended requirement. There's no substitute for the vitamins and minerals in food, and you'll give your body what it needs only if you're conscientious about eating healthy, unprocessed, non–junk food. Fruits and vegetables provide necessary substances called phytochemicals, which you can't get from nutritional supplements. They lower cholesterol, flush out carcinogens, boost the immune system, and reduce the effects of aging.

2. Take a high-quality multiple vitamin every day, "not as a substitute for food, but as a supplement," says nutritionist David Schardt of the Center for Science and the Public Interest. Vitamin A stimulates healthy cell growth, Vitamin C helps oxygen flow to the skin, and Vitamin E helps fight acne. B vitamins aid the production of collagen in the skin and are essential for healthy hair. Vitamin B_2 (riboflavin) in particular helps prevent oily skin and strengthens the nails. Biotin can help prevent scaly skin and dermatitis and helps the body process protein, which is what your skin, hair, and nails are made of. The minerals included in most multivitamin supplements are also important. Zinc promotes healthy skin and hair; selenium preserves the elasticity of the skin. Your body needs to process these nutrients through digestion. A moisturizer loaded with Vitamin C, magnesium, and ginkgo biloba may sound healthy, but it won't make up for a nutritional deficiency. You can't feed your skin on the outside what it's missing on the inside.

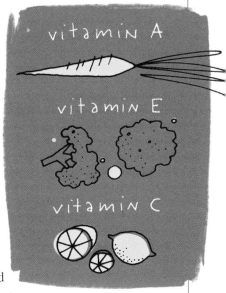

EAT COLOR

Eat orange foods (carrots, pumpkins, dried apricots) that are rich in beta-carotene; eat leafy greens that are rich in Vitamin E; and eat yellow foods (grapefruit, lemons) for Vitamin C. White foods like dairy, eggs, and fish are an important source of Vitamin A. And drink raw fruit and vegetable juices daily. Raw food gives your body the enzymes it needs to maintain good health. Enzymes—whose chemical names always end in the suffix "-ase"—affect the synthesis of skin lipids as well as the skin's support structure of collagen and elastin.

SKIN VITAMINS:

VITAMIN	WHAT IT DOES INTERNALLY	BEST FOOD SOURCES
A	Necessary for normal growth, development, and renewal of skin cells; keeps skin tissue, red blood cells, and immune system healthy; antioxidant	Egg yolks, milk and other dairy products, fish oil, margarine, liver
B	Necessary for protein metabolism; building red blood cells; immune function; hormone synthesis; venous system function	Poultry, fish, whole grains, dried beans, bananas, meat, dairy products, leafy green vegetables
C	Necessary for collagen production; not synthesized by body and needs to be provided by food; neutralizes free radicals	Citrus fruits, broccoli, cabbage, tomatoes, fortified cereals, berries, melon, peppers, potatoes
D	Necessary for development of skin cells; promotes calcium absorption	Egg yolks, salmon, liver, herring, fortified milk
E	Necessary for growth of healthy tissue; an extremely stable antioxidant	Wheat germ, nuts, vegetable oil, green leafy vegetables, whole grains
F	An essential fatty acid that is a building block of the surface skin	Flaxseed oil, evening primrose oil, blackcurrants, safflower oil, borage seed oil, linolenic acid
K	Helps promote blood clotting	Green leafy vegetables

feed your face and body, too

WHAT IT DOES TOPICALLY	HOW IT'S LABELED
Evens out skin tone; diminishes fine lines; enhances epidermal turnover; may make skin more elastic; used in prescription drugs to treat acne and psoriasis; may stimulate renewal of skin cells	Retinol, retinyl acetate, retinyl proprionate, retinyl palmitate; also known as Retin-A, Renova
Regulates oil secretion and prevents extreme oiliness; decreases tendency toward blemishes; prevents scaly skin and dermatitis; may aid in collagen formation	Biotin, niacin, PABA
Helps heal scar tissue, cuts, and bruises; protects against UVA/UVB rays and may stimulate collagen production	L-ascorbic acid, magnesium ascorbyl, ascorbyl palmitate, phosphate
Moisturizes and conditions skin; may encourage normal tissue development; used in over-the-counter medications to treat eczema, dry skin, and diaper rash; used in prescription drugs to treat psoriasis	Ergocalciferol
Conditions and moisturizes skin; inhibits free-radical damage; helps heal burns, inflammation, cuts, and irritation; may minimize formation of scars; protects against UV damage; improves skin tone; enhances moisture retention; should not be taken before surgery because it inhibits absorption of Vitamin K, which helps blood coagulation and reduces bruising	Tocopheryl linoleate, tocopheryl acetate, alpha tocopheryl, alpha tocopherol
Helps maintain barrier function of the skin; treatment for acne; moisturizes skin	Lineolic acid
Reduces bruising; may help relieve dark circles under eyes; treats actinic purpura in aged skin, and may help make broken capillaries fade	Vitamin K

BEAUTY VITAMINS

Cosmetics companies now market "beauty" vitamin pills with special blends of Vitamins C, E, A, and B that target hair, skin, and nails. Forget about them. Not only are they more expensive than a generic or health-food-store multiple vitamin, but you may be getting too much of one nutrient and not enough of another. If you already take a daily multiple vitamin and then take a "skin-enhancing" vitamin on top of it, you could easily ingest too much zinc or Vitamin A, which can build up to dangerous levels in the body. Taking excessive amounts of some vitamins can also lead to depletion of other vitamins or minerals. And if you replace your daily multiple vitamin with beauty vitamins, you could miss out on other important nutrients that are crucial for good health.

buyer beware

3. Fat—in moderation—is a well-kept but invaluable beauty secret. Fat helps your body (and skin) utilize protein. This isn't to say that you should load up on cholesterol-raising saturated animal fats. You shouldn't. But your body does need unsaturated fats—from vegetable oils like olive, corn, safflower, or canola —every day. These "good fats" keep hair soft and skin supple. So don't deprive yourself of that vinaigrette on your salad—a tablespoon of olive oil, a squeeze of lemon, a dab of Dijon mustard—it's good for you. Enjoy it!

4. Drink at least eight glasses of water each day. The best way to keep your skin hydrated is to moisturize from the inside out. Since the human body, like the earth, is

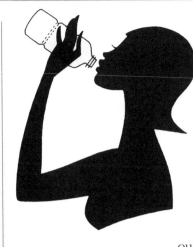

made up of approximately 70 percent water and water accounts for 70 percent of our skin weight, it makes sense that we need to continuously replenish our precious bodily fluid and keep our cells hydrated. P.S.: Coffee, soda, caffeinated teas, and caffeine-enhanced water don't count. In fact, they will actually dehydrate your body.

5. Exercise. Daily exercise will get your blood flowing and stimulate the oxygen flow to feed the skin. The minimum amount of aerobic exercise necessary to maintain good health is 20 minutes, three times a week. Avoid taking shallow, quick breaths; try to breathe deeply and from the diaphragm.

6. Don't drink too much coffee, tea, or alcohol. Enjoy your vices in moderation, but don't overdo it. All three of these liquids are diuretics that dehydrate the body and sap it of Vitamin B, which helps keep nails hard, hair thick, and skin luminous. A deficiency of Vitamin B can result in dry, thin skin.

7. **Don't smoke.** If you won't quit for health reasons, maybe vanity will motivate you. It's been scientifically proven that smoking wreaks havoc on your skin, and nicotine-stained teeth are hardly attractive. Smoking (and drinking) depletes the body of Vitamin B and damages the capillary walls, which deprives the skin cells of oxygen. The elastin fibers, which keep skin supple, thicken and fragment in smokers' skin, much like skin that's been overexposed to sunlight. Smoking also stunts the growth of collagen, and loss of collagen can lead to wrinkles.

Nicotine retards cell growth in the skin and reduces the blood supply, which also slows healing. Both tar and nicotine cause artificial aging of the skin, much like the sun does. If you spend unprotected time in the sun, your skin ages at three times the normal rate. If you smoke, you age it at four times the normal rate. The combination factors out to 12 times normal. Who needs that?

8. **Use sun protection every day,** all year round, rain or shine, and follow the skincare regimen in this book. Conscientious use of sunscreen will prevent up to 90 percent of the skin damage caused by ultraviolet rays.

9. **Get your fair share of shut-eye.** The term "beauty sleep" is no joke, and everyone needs it. Lack of sleep can dehydrate the skin and cause flaky patches, pale or ashy skin, brittle nails, and hair loss—not to mention puffiness around the eyes.

10. **Laugh. Relax. Enjoy life.** As the poet William Blake wrote, "Exuberance is Beauty." Words to live by!

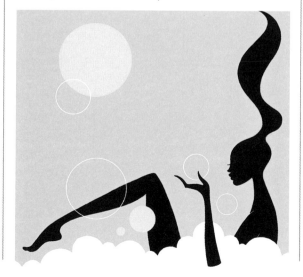

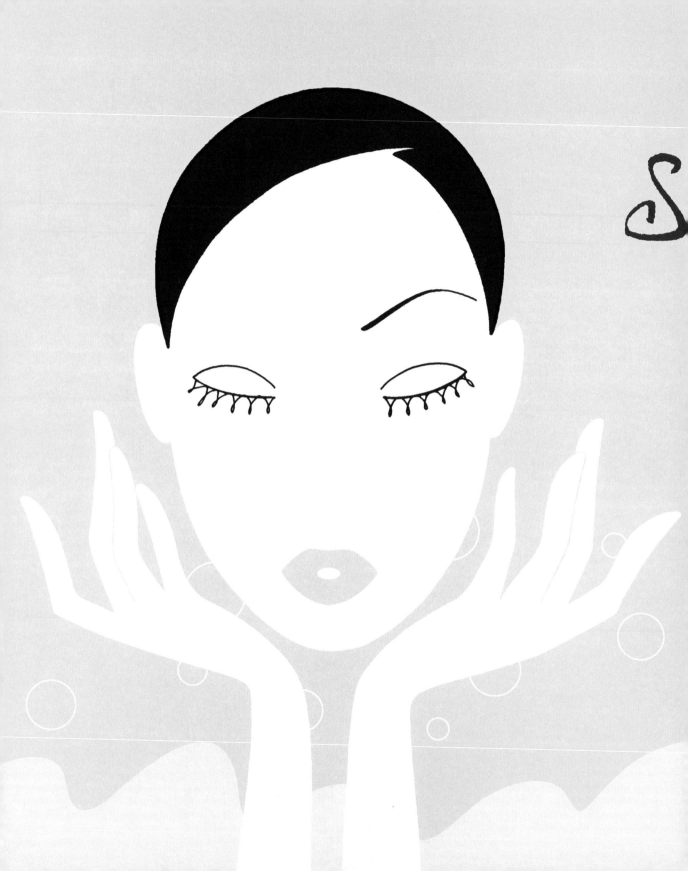

CHAPTER TWO

skincare

If you take care of your skin,
your "complexion" will take care of itself.

—HELENA RUBINSTEIN

The skin holds no secrets. If the eyes are the mirror of the soul, the skin is the body's lie detector. When something isn't right internally—if you're stressed out, eating poorly, overtired, sick—it will show up on your face. While other organs of the body lie sealed in, protected, and shrouded in mystery, the skin, as the Chinese say, is always "open to inspection by others." It's the first thing people notice about us. In traditional Chinese medicine, the skin is considered a diagnostic. Because it is connected to all the bodily systems, it tells the world not only about our emotional state but about the health of our circulation, hormone balance, and nervous system.

The skin is an intricate structure that depends on a complex chain of elaborate, integral chemical processes. It's the largest organ in the body, totaling one-sixth of our body weight. It breathes, excretes, absorbs, and protects. Rich in nerve endings and touch receptors, the skin transmits exquisite sensations of pleasure and pain to the brain, which, over time, are etched into the map of our faces. Our skin reveals the quality of our lives and reflects the passage of time through sun damage, gravity, and genetically determined signs of aging. Yet most of us don't treat the skin with the respect and gentle care that such a responsive organ deserves.

But there's nothing like a little healthy vanity to motivate you. When stress overstimulates the oil glands and your skin begins to break out or flake, you'll want to fix it. And once you realize how easy it is to maintain good skin, you'll be inspired to keep it that way.

The good news is that the minute you begin to take care of your skin—keep it clean, nourish it, and pamper it a bit—it will respond with gratitude. Nothing takes the place of good, gentle, consistent, balanced care. The simple skincare regimen described in this chapter will help you understand your skin, recognize what

ABOUT FACE

▨ Breakouts on one side of your face could mean that your phone is dirty.

▨ Chin breakouts? Stop touching it or resting it on your hands.

▨ Forehead breakouts? Keep your bangs clean.

▨ Make sure your pillowcase is always clean.

▨ As Grandma always said, keep your hands off your face!

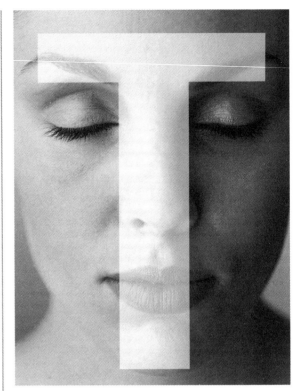

The T-Zone: There are more oil glands in the nose, chin, and forehead than anywhere else. Most women have oiliness in the T-Zone.

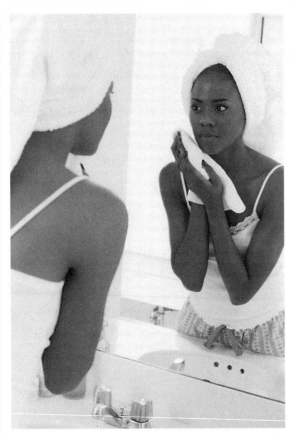

Your skin should come with a warning label: Handle with care. Anyone can have great skin if they treat it as gently as possible, care for it consistently, keep it clean, and pat it—don't rub!—dry.

products can and can't do, and help you avoid major beauty pitfalls along the way. Because even with the best or most expensive products, you can overmoisturize the skin in an attempt to beat dryness, irritate the skin trying to combat acne, and make oily skin even oilier by overdrying it.

What Skin Type Are You?

Knowing your skin type can help you minimize irritation and cosmetics-related acne. So, before you begin, give yourself the quick

SKIN TYPES AT A GLANCE

Your skin type is determined by how much—or how little—oil your skin produces. And what determines that? Genes, diet, stress level, medication, even your skincare regimen and the products you choose. The amount of oil your skin produces naturally will determine the amount of oil you need in your products.

OILY	Shiny skin, enlarged pores, prone to blackheads and blemishes, some tightness.
COMBINATION/ NORMAL	Medium pores, smooth and even texture, good circulation, healthy color, may tend toward dryness on the cheeks, may be oily in T-Zone.
SENSITIVE	Thin, delicate, fine pores. Flushes easily, prone to broken capillaries, frequently allergic, can be rashy.
DRY	Feels tight, especially after cleansing; fine wrinkles, flaking, red patches. In women of color, appears ashy or dull from dead skin buildup.
AGING OR SUN-DAMAGED	Feels tight, visible wrinkles, slack skin tone—especially around cheeks and jawline—leathery texture, broken capillaries.

skin-type test below so you'll know the right products to use.

Wash your face with a nonmoisturizing soap like Neutrogena and pat dry. Take a few pieces of rice paper or lens-cleaning tissue paper, and press them on different spots on your face. If your skin is oily, the paper will stick, pick up oily spots, and become translucent. If the paper doesn't stick and leaves no oily spots, your skin is dry. If it sticks in the T-Zone (forehead, nose, and chin) but not on the cheeks, your skin is combination (or normal). Most women (about 70 percent)

have combination or normal skin.

You can expect your skin to change at various points throughout your life, so recheck your skin type periodically and fine-tune your regimen in different climates and at different times of the year. (For example, most women need less moisturizer in the summer, when the oil glands are more active.) However, this does not mean you need to run out and buy separate products for the oily and dry areas of your face, for day and night, or for travel across time zones. Not at all. The beauty of a good skincare regimen lies in its simplicity.

Basic Four-Step Regimen

"If it takes more than two minutes, I'm not going to do it," Donna Karan once told me, and most women share that sentiment about their daily skincare regimen. But if you want healthy, beautiful skin, there are four things you must do regularly: cleanse, exfoliate, moisturize, and apply sun protection—even if it takes as long as three or even four minutes!

■ STEP 1

Cleanse

The best way to cleanse your face is the gentlest way: use a rinse-off cleanser and forget about soap. "Soap," a French cosmetics executive once told me, "should only ever touch your skin from the neck down." When it comes to caring for the face, I'm with the French. Unlike soaps, cleansers remove makeup and dirt, but leave the skin feeling silky and supple.

When you wash your face, you want to do two things: dissolve the dirt and oil on the surface of the skin and normalize your skin condition. Cleansers basically consist of oil, water, and surfactants. The oil dissolves the oil on the face; the surfactants dissolve everything else; and water washes it all away. Some cleansers contain lots of oil; others have none. If you use a cleanser that's too rich for your skin, it can clog your pores; if it's too drying, it can irritate your skin. So choosing the right one is

Not too hot and not too cold; make sure the water temperature's just right.

Splashing cool water on your face will jazz up your circulation.

Massage your cleanser around your face in circular motions, and rinse, rinse, rinse again.

important. Here's where knowing your skin type comes into play.

If your skin is normal or dry, you need a more emollient cleanser. Look for a milky or creamy cleanser with plant oils like sweet almond oil or jojoba. If your skin is oily, you need a cleanser that will control some of the excess oil. Look for "lite" humectants like glycerine or butylene or polyethylene glycol used as substitutes for oil. If your skin is really oily, a foaming gel or an oil-free cleanser, especially one with citrus, will cut through the oil.

It is important to clean your face thoroughly, but overly aggressive cleansing strips the skin's surface lipids. If you lose those, your skin loses its natural protection and can become dry and irritated—even if you have oily skin.

Most women with normal skin should use a cleanser at night to remove makeup, cellular debris, and the grime of the day. In the morning, however, plain old lukewarm water is all you need to get rid of any overnight oil buildup. If you apply moisturizer overnight (see page 40), you'll need a cleanser in the morning, too.

Don't be lazy about washing your face at night. If you fall into bed with your makeup on at the end of an evening, you may look

Some women with extremely dry skin— mainly Europeans—prefer tissue-off cleansers for general use, because they do not contain water. "In Europe," says Thierry, makeup director for Yves Saint Laurent, "women thought, for ages, that water was bad for the skin. In France, some women still think water dries the skin. That's why I use a tissue-off cleanser on myself and the fashion models."

How To: cleanse gently

1. Wash your face in warm—not hot!—water to loosen clogged pores and stimulate blood circulation to the skin.

2. Wet the face, then squeeze a dime-sized dab of cleanser into your palm, rub your hands together, and gently move them in circles around your face.

3. Rinse with cool (but not icy) water to tighten the pores. Water that is too hot or too cold can cause broken capillaries.

glamorous then, but you won't be a pretty sight in the morning. Besides, your pores will clog.

Makeup Removers

Although a rinse-off cleanser will cut through most face makeup, eye makeup can be tougher to remove and requires a product with lots of oil. If your lifestyle includes the occasional heavy-makeup night with multiple coats of mascara, keep a makeup remover around. The best and cheapest way to remove stubborn eye makeup is to buy a bottle of sweet almond oil at the health food store ($4 for four ounces), shake a few drops on a cotton ball, and dab away. If you need an oil-free product, Klorane,

BEST CLEANSERS:

	PRODUCT & BEST FEATURE	COST
DRY SKIN	**CETAPHIL** *Clean, simple, contains only a few ingredients, not loaded with chemicals; leaves skin feeling soft and super-clean; the best drugstore cleanser, period*	$
	CLARINS GENTLE FOAMING CLEANSER *Contains shea butter, which moisturizes the skin as it cleanses*	$$
	DR. HAUSCHKA CLEANSING CREAM *Smells like almonds, softens skin. Because it contains minimal preservatives, keep an eye on the expiration date*	$$
	ESTÉE LAUDER PERFECTLY CLEAN FOAMING LOTION CLEANSER *Removes stubborn makeup; gentle on aging skin*	$$$$
	KIEHL'S GENTLE FOAMING FACE CLEANSER *Gentle, thorough, makes the skin feel really soft*	$
	LANCÔME ABLUTIA HUILE MOUSSANTE *Foaming (but not too foamy) oil cleanser*	$$$
	LANCÔME GALATEE MILK CLEANSER *Milky and moisturizing*	$$$
	MOLTON BROWN TOTAL FACIAL CLEANSER *Gentle, natural, contains rose hips*	$$
	ORIGINS LIQUID CRYSTAL *Grapeseed oil has antioxidant properties, refreshing mint makes skin feel fresh and tingly*	$$
	SHU UEMURA CLEANSING BEAUTY OIL *An oil that smells like cornflowers, foams up, and removes makeup beautifully*	$$$
NORMAL SKIN	**ASTARA BOTANICAL CLEANSING GELÉE** *Soothing calendula, comfrey, and a tangy tangerine scent*	$
	BEAUTY WITHOUT CRUELTY HERBAL CREAM FACIAL CLEANSER *Fresh smelling, light, and creamy*	$
	BLOOM FACIAL CLEANSER *Quality aromatherapy with lavender and grapefruit essential oils*	$$
	CETAPHIL GENTLE SKIN CLEANSER *Best drugstore cleanser, period*	$
	FACE STOCKHOLM FOAMING FACE CLEANSER *Balances out the skin and leaves it not too dry, not too oily*	$$
	KARIN HERZOG SOFT CLEANSING MILK *Contains only seven ingredients, so it's purer, and it lasts forever*	$$$$
	LAURA MERCIER ONE-STEP CLEANSER *For combination skin; dries up oil while softening skin*	$$$$
	NEUTROGENA EXTRA GENTLE CLEANSER *Nondrying*	$
	PRESCRIPTIVES ALL CLEAN *A bit oily; especially good if your skin is on the dry side of normal*	$$

KEY: $ = UP TO $10; $$ = UP TO $20; $$$ = UP TO $30; $$$$ = UP TO $40; $$$$$ = UP TO $50

soft, soothing, and really simple

PRODUCT & BEST FEATURE	COST
OILY SKIN	
CETAPHIL OILY SKIN CLEANSER *Best drugstore brand for oily skin*	$
CLARINS PURIFYING CLEANSING GEL FOR OILY SKIN *Attacks the oil but doesn't dry the skin*	$$
CLINIQUE WASH-AWAY GEL CLEANSER *A reliable classic; a bit drying, but doesn't leave skin feeling unnaturally tight*	$$
GUERLAIN EVOLUTION PURIFYING FOAMING GEL *Gentle but effective for aging skin that's prone to scattered breakouts*	$$$
LA FORMULE PURIFYING SKIN WASH *Effective and inexpensive French skincare; made with essential oils*	$$
LANCÔME CLARIFIANCE OIL-FREE GEL CLEANSER *Well formulated, with a luxurious, silky feel*	$$$
SHISEIDO PURENESS CLEANSING GEL *Gentle, soft, and sweet smelling*	$$
YONKA GEL NETTOYANT *Slightly astringent; smells like grapefruit*	$$$
BLEMISHED SKIN	
BEAUTY WITHOUT CRUELTY 3% AHA FACIAL CLEANSER FOR NORMAL/OILY SKIN TYPES *Smooth, softening, health-food-store-stuff, with alpha-hydroxy acids*	$
M.D. FORMULATIONS FACIAL CLEANSER BASIC *Tough, dermatological product containing AHAs*	$$
NEUTROGENA PORE-REFINING CLEANSER *Soaks up oil without drying the skin*	$
OIL OF OLAY AGE-DEFYING SERIES DAILY RENEWAL CLEANSER *Good, cheap, effective—don't let the creamy texture scare you*	$
PETER THOMAS ROTH BETA HYDROXY ACID 2% ACNE WASH *BHAs gently unclog pores*	$$
SENSITIVE SKIN	
ALBA BOTANICA FACE CITRUS CREAM CLEANSER FOR DELICATE SKIN *I use this on my daughter; gentle enough for children*	$$
ANNEMARIE BÖRLIND SYSTEM ABSOLUTE CLEANSER *Upscale, creamy, health-food-store product*	$$$
AVEDA ALL-SENSITIVE CLEANSER *Simple enough for the most sensitive skin*	$$
AVON CLEAR SKIN FOAMING CLEANSER *Inexpensive and gentle*	$
CETAPHIL GENTLE SKIN CLEANSER *(See description of Cetaphil on facing page.)*	$
NINA RICCI ROSÉE GEL PURIFICANTE *Sensual, smells like roses*	$$$
OIL OF OLAY SENSITIVE SKIN WASH *Drugstore runner-up, after Cetaphil*	$

THE DOPE ON SOAP:
WHAT TO AVOID

While Europeans avoid using soap at all costs, many Americans don't feel clean unless their skin is taut and tingly. But that feeling usually means the skin has been stripped too dry. If you *are* hooked on that squeaky clean feeling of "drag," Elizabeth Arden's One Great Soap and Clinique's Facial Soap are good choices because they're relatively gentle. Aveenobar is a gentle and less expensive drugstore alternative. But avoid the following products, which are all too harsh for the delicate skin on the face.

Cleansing products with sodium cocoate and sodium tallowate, unless your skin is extremely oily. These are strong soaps/detergents that strip oil from the skin and don't put it back.

Products that promise you the world. The claim "Cleanser-exfoliant-makeup-remover all in one!" is just plain silly. If a product cleans your face, it will also remove your makeup (except stubborn eye makeup, for which you may need a special product). If it doesn't, then the product hasn't done its job. And you really don't want to combine an exfoliant with a cleanser because you don't want to exfoliate every day.

Cleansers with alpha- or beta-hydroxy acids. Unless you have blemished skin, there's no point in putting on an AHA or BHA cleanser since you wash it right off. If they are going to work, they need to stay on the face for a while, not just hit and run.

"Complexion" or "beauty" bars. Although they're practically soap-free and they do contain moisturizers, the ingredients that keep them in a "bar" shape also make them too harsh to use on your face. Besides, the moisturizers used in these products—synthetic coconut-oil derivatives—can clog pores.

a drugstore brand, makes an inexpensive oil-free makeup remover that comes in a pretty blue bottle and works really well.

Spread the makeup remover on a tissue or a cotton ball, apply it to the area, and tissue it off with an *extremely light* touch. Always use delicate, gliding movements when caring for your skin to avoid wear and tear. If you're too heavy-handed, the day-in and day-out pull on the skin will eventually cause your skin to lose tone.

◼ STEP 2

Exfoliate

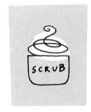

I like to think of healthy skin as a crush of well-fed little cells living in the fast lane, ever renewing and replenishing themselves. Approximately every three weeks, new cells push up from the lowest layer of the epidermis and move toward the surface, changing shape as they go. Healthy new skin cells make this trek to the surface every 28 to 45 days, and what happens to them throughout the course of their journey has a great effect on the skin's appearance. At the end of the cycle, at the surface, the flattened and dried-up cells are shed. Sometimes the old cells form a united front and stick around longer than they should. Exfoliation helps the natural process along by giving those cells a little extra push. Removing dead skin cells helps pave the way for plumper, healthier, smoother skin cells to surface, which can make a huge difference in your appearance.

Exfoliation is the one bit of skincare most of us tend to neglect, but I can't emphasize

ANATOMY OF THE SKIN

To understand what skin does, we need to take a quick look at what skin is. In this cross section of one square inch of skin there are millions of cells and hundreds of nerve endings, plus muscles, blood vessels, hair follicles, and sweat and oil glands.

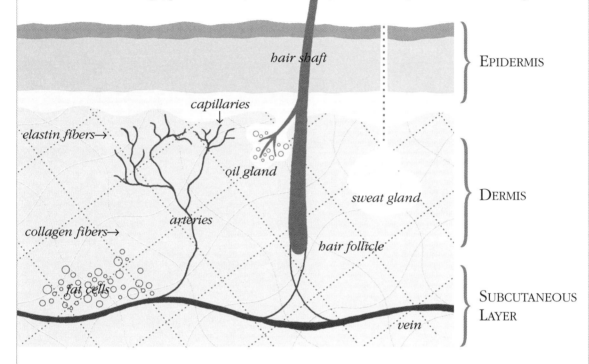

EPIDERMIS

The top layer (the stratum corneum) is actually 8 to 15 layers thick. Deep in the heart of the epidermis, farthest down in the basal layer, new skin cells are born from ingredients carried through the bloodstream.

DERMIS

The dermis provides the skin's support structure with two types of connective tissue: collagen, which gives skin its strength, and elastin, which gives the skin elasticity and snap. Oil travels up the hair follicle to the skin's surface, where it forms a protective coating.

SUBCUTANEOUS LAYER

The deepest layer is made of fat cells and strands of connective tissue. It functions as a kind of pillow, cushioning the internal organs, holding in body heat, and giving contour to the skin.

How To: rub your scrub

After you cleanse your face, take a bit of scrub into the palm of your hand. Wet it and lightly press the scrub into your skin. Then massage it gently around your face with the same easy pressure you use to shave your legs. The force of the abrasion should lie somewhere between that used to wash with 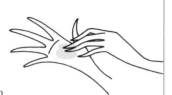 a washcloth and a loofah. (Never use a loofah on your face; it's much too abrasive.) To really get your circulation going, splash with cool, then warm water.

WARNING: Don't overscrub, because you need some of that surface stuff around to protect your skin.

---

enough how important it is, and what an amazing difference it will make on your skin. If you have oily or combination skin, use an exfoliant four or five times a week, after your cleanser. If your skin is dry or sensitive, once or twice a week will do. In warm weather, or in a warm climate, you need to exfoliate more often, because sweat acts like glue. (It clumps dead skin cells together and inhibits the skin's natural ability to shed like a snake.)

To exfoliate literally means to rub the top layer of the skin loose to make way for the fresher, younger generation of skin below. Exfoliation makes it easier for the skin to absorb moisture, removes surface debris, evens out the texture of the skin, and makes it look smoother, juicier, and less wrinkled. "If we've learned

anything from alpha-hydroxy acids," says Mark Potter, a cosmetic chemist and president of Atlantis Laboratories in Houston, Texas, "it's how much our skin benefits from exfoliation." (One of the reasons men of a certain age often have skin that looks so much better than women's of the same age is that men exfoliate daily when they shave.) Alpha-hydroxys (AHAs), beta-hydroxys, poly-hydroxys, Renova, Retin-A, glycolic peels, your humble oatmeal scrub, along with many of the dermatological procedures you will read about in chapter 4, all boil down to the same basic benefit: they help exfoliate the skin.

There are two types of exfoliants: physical scrubs and chemical exfoliants (such as alpha-hydroxys). Scrubs are composed of irregularly shaped bits of organic materials—ground walnuts, almond meal, apricot pits suspended in a cream base, or synthetic beads or granules. They're cheap, and they work well—provided you don't rub too hard (see box, above). Baking soda, powdered milk, or finely ground cornmeal or oatmeal, moistened with a bit of water, though not as elegant as the commercial

EPIDERMAL ILLUSIONS

When dead cells pile up on the surface of the stratum corneum around a wrinkle, they exaggerate the depth of the wrinkle. Exfoliate the dead cells, and you've razed what was a four-story building down to two stories. Exfoliation can also make the pores look smaller. Here's how: when the dry dead skin cells clump up like mini Mount Everests on your face, they cast shadows and make the pores look bigger. Get rid of the mountains, and you lose the shadows.

concoctions, work just as well. If you're heavy-handed and worry about nicking your skin, use a synthetic scrub. These contain abrasives that are perfectly round, with no rough edges.

Alpha-hydroxy acids (and beta- and poly-hydroxys) are chemical exfoliants that do the same job, except they depend on acid instead of a manual rub to loosen the hold between clumped-together skin cells. The best way to use these is in lotions and creams, not cleansers, because the acids need to stay on the skin for a while in order to work. They may tingle, or may even irritate the skin, at first—they are acid, after all—but this is the rare instance where an irritating product can actually help your skin. But, if your skin turns red or rashy after using one of these products, stop using it.

You should consider using AHAs only if you have what is euphemistically known in the beauty industry as "mature" skin—aka aging or sun-damaged skin (see chapter 4). AHAs can help correct, but cannot prevent, the appearance of aging on your skin, so there is no point in starting too early. Always use AHAs cautiously, since they can, literally, thin your skin. *Never* use both an AHA and a scrub—it's overkill. You can recognize the skin of an overzealous AHA user by its rubbery, "fake" look. If you do use an AHA, never leave the house without sun protection, as your skin will be especially sensitive to the sun and susceptible to sun spots.

A Word on Toners

For many women, toners are the logical next step in a skincare regimen, but I don't buy it. Literally. Whether they are called balancers, clarifying lotions, skin purifiers, or astringents

---

SWAB THE DECKS: TOP EXFOLIANT SCRUBS

Scrubs often contain a sweet-sounding list of ingredients like seaweed, sea lettuce, and other such treasures of the deep. Though rich in minerals, such nutrients drive up the price and are of questionable value in a scrub that stays on the face for less than 30 seconds. Avoid ingredients such as tea tree oil, eucalyptus, and mint in a scrub; in combination with scrubbing action, they can irritate the skin. These are some of the best scrubs: Kiehl's Milk, Honey and Almond Scrub, L'Oréal Plenitude Gentle Exfoliating Cream, Astara Daily Refining Scrub (for sensitive skin), Prescriptives Purifying Scrub, Clinique Face Buffing Cream. (See chapter 4 for alpha- and beta-hydroxy acid product recommendations.)

★ Best Products

(the strongest ones), toners are a pricey broth of water, color, preservatives, witch hazel, alcohol—and not much else. In fact, for most women, toners are a redundant product: toners are supposed to remove every last trace of oil, sweat, and makeup from your face—but so will a good cleanser. A toner *will* make your pores look smaller by swelling the tissue around the pore, but a moisturizer will do the same thing—and more. And those that contain alcohol do more harm than good. (The alcohol gives your skin that nice tingly feeling, but what is really happening is that as the alcohol dries, it dries the skin out, too.)

Granted, if you have very oily skin you

If you can't give up your toner habit, here are some gentle, alcohol-free toners: BeneFit Rosewater Tonic, Clarins Extra-Comfort Toning Lotion, FACE Stockholm Vegetable Toner for All Skin Types, Guerlain Odelys Soothing Toner, Iman Perfect Response Toner (especially for blemish-prone skin), Jurlique Herbal Extract Recovery Mist, Kiehl's Calendula Herbal Extract Toner Alcohol-Free, Lancôme Clarifiance Alcohol-Free Natural Astringent, Nivea Visage Alcohol-Free Moisturizing Facial Toner, Avon Moisturizing Alcohol-Free Toner, Reviva (good for oily skin), Shiseido Pureness Cleansing Water.

might benefit from using a toner, especially in the summer. (Use it only three times a week, however, to give the skin time to recover from the drying action.) But look for an alcohol-free toner with bacteria fighters like rose water, lavender citric acid (derived from lemon, a natural astringent), or even salicylic acid, for *really* oily skin. Use witch hazel sparingly because it contains alcohol. An alcohol-free toner will create the "shrunken-pores" effect you're after and cut through the oil just as well, without the bone-drying astringent properties.

Tip In warm weather, stash your gel, lotion, or cream in the fridge. The chill feels good on your skin and helps it look firmer, too. In cool weather, warm your moisturizer between your hands for a few seconds before you apply it to your face. It will absorb better.

■ **STEP 3**

Moisturize

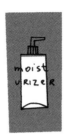

You must moisturize. This is a command, a rule, a law of beauty. No matter what type of skin you have, no matter what age you are, no matter what anyone says to the contrary, you must *moisturize.* And there is no good reason not to: it's easy, it feels good, and it is absolutely essential to your epidermal well-being. Besides, there are tons of good moisturizers out there to choose from (see chart on pages 36–37) in every price range.

When it comes to moisture, the skin is a democratic organ; it will respond to liquids and lotions, creams and gels. "I just moisturize with anything," says fashion designer Norma Kamali, "even olive oil, if nothing else is available." I wouldn't actually recommend using straight olive oil unless you're desperate, but it's true that your moisturizing options are almost limitless. And everyone needs it, even those with oily skin. (The only exception to this rule is someone suffering from a severe outbreak of acne—and even then, you'll need to moisturize when the acne clears up.)

Where moisturizers are concerned, the relevant question is not if, but how often and what kind of product to use: some of us benefit from a thick, oily cream several times a day, while others can get by on a couple of drops of light lotion or a dab of gel once a day. Listen to your skin; if it doesn't retain enough water, it will feel tight and dry. Pay attention and give it moisture.

THE RUB ON ALCOHOL

Women who know enough to avoid alcohol in their cosmetics often think they need to run from all alcohols, which is not the case. The simple alcohols—isopropyl, methanol, and ethanol—are the ones to avoid whenever possible. Ditto for the denatured alcohols (listed on the label as "alcohol denat" or "SD" followed by a number).

But the fatty alcohols are not really alcohols at all, but solid emollients, and they're actually beneficial because they moisturize rather than dry the skin. You'll find them in creams and moisturizers listed as cetyl, stearyl, caprylic, decyl, isocetyl, isostearyl, lauryl, myristyl, and oleyl, followed by the word "alcohol."

How Do Moisturizers Work?

Moisturizers keep the skin healthy and protect it from dryness in several ways. First, they attract moisture from the atmosphere and draw it into the skin cells, which keeps them plump and juicy. Second, they seal the moisture in with an occlusive coating—a kind of Saran Wrap effect. Third, they help fill in or remortar the gaps between the skin cells, which keeps the skin's barrier function holding strong and firm. *Humectants* that bind water to the skin, *barrier ingredients* that block water loss, and *emollients* that soften the skin and mimic its lipid structure make it possible for moisturizers to perform these functions.

One thing moisturizers will not do is prevent wrinkles—unless they contain sunscreen. Moisturizers can soften the *appearance* of wrinkles by plumping the skin tissue and swelling it with water, which is no small feat! But in order to actually prevent wrinkles you need to practice slavish daily devotion to a sun-protection product (see page 41). Your sun protection can come in the form of a moisturizer, tinted moisturizer, or foundation as long as it's rated SPF 15 and contains one of the following active ingredients: titanium dioxide, zinc oxide, or avobenzone (aka Parsol 1789). Dry skin is only slightly more prone to wrinkles than other skin types—unless it's been overexposed to the harmful rays of the sun.

WARNING: DON'T OVERMOISTURIZE. Overuse of a moisturizer is as bad as not using any—so don't slather it on. Too much moisturizer can lead to clogged pores and blackheads. It can also slow down your skin's turnover time: your dead skin cells will get "stuck," and they'll have a harder time sloughing off if your skin is oversaturated.

Types of Moisturizers

Moisturizers come in various types. *Balms* and *creams* are the thickest and greasiest; *oils* and *lotions* are lighter and more fluid; *gels* are clear or translucent, the lightest of all. Judging a moisturizer by its texture—and understanding what the texture tells you about its properties—will help you zero in on what you need. Here's a general rule of thumb: the thicker the texture, the more oil; the thinner the texture, the more water (unless the product itself is an oil).

Tip Always apply a thin coat of moisturizer before you enter a sauna. It helps prevent broken capillaries.

THE GOOD, THE BAD, AND THE OILY

The oil glands get a bad rap from the beauty industry; they're blamed for everything from acne to dry skin. To some extent, they deserve to take the heat, because more than anything else, the oil glands can make or break it for your skin.

Oil glands look kind of like Abstract Expressionist blotches clinging to the sides of the hair follicles. They secrete an oily substance called sebum, which is the skin's natural moisturizer. Sebum travels into the follicle, then flows out the pore onto the surface of the skin, where it forms a protective coating. (See page 29.) Because it seals in water, it keeps the skin moist and soft. But if the oil glands produce too *much* sebum and your skin is not properly cleansed and cared for, the sebum can clog pores and lead to blackheads, pimples, and acne—even in adults. If there's too *little* sebum, your skin will be prone to dry, flaky patches and fine lines. So it's a question of finding and maintaining the right balance.

If you have oily skin (especially if you're also prone to acne), you probably tend toward overzealous cleansing. But when you use soaps and harsh cleansers with alcohol (like Sea Breeze or Noxzema, which your adolescent skin could handle, but which are too harsh for you to use once you're old enough to drive), you strip so much oil from your skin that it can feel tight and dry. You can also develop a common skin condition called seborrheic dermatitis (flaking, red scales around the scalp and on the T-Zone) and begin to erroneously believe that you suddenly have dry skin. Since the skin looks and feels dry, chances are you'll overmoisturize. And if you use oily moisturizers with mineral oils, you'll only make the situation worse, because mineral oil doesn't absorb into the skin—it just sits on top of the skin, clogs it up, and causes more pimples. For solutions, see page 91.

Balms are thick, waxy moisturizers that contain mostly oil and no water. They look like ointments or salves, and they're terrific moisturizers for super-dry skin because they form a virtually impenetrable barrier against water loss. Regrettably, they can also be a slippery mess. Avoid petroleum-based balms like Vaseline (except on your lips). Instead, look for balms that are beeswax-based, because they are more absorbent. Balms are good bets for extremely sensitive or super-dry skin because they contain lots of oil and no water so they don't need preservatives, which may irritate sensitive skin.

Creams are thick because they are, essentially, a little water mixed into a vat of oil. Thick creams, night creams, and "maximum moisturizers" are mother's milk to European women, who are raised on the stuff. Because Americans tend to be averse to the hedonics of a heavy, gooey cream, the industry also offers lighter, less greasy, "low-fat" versions. Creams are good for dry or normal-to-dry skin.

Lotions are thinner, lighter, liquid formulations containing more water than oil. They are less greasy than creams—but also less moisturizing. Americans find these light formulations appealing: most moisturizers sold in the United States fall into this group. Most creams are also available in lotion form. Lotions are effective for dry, normal, or slightly oily skin.

Face oils have finally slid into the forefront of skincare. Because oils have a smaller molecular structure than lotions or creams, they are more easily absorbed and therefore moisturize better—except for mineral oils, of course. Certain plant and animal oils (see box, page 38) penetrate so well that they easily transcend the greasy, shiny stereotype that has given face oils an image problem. The finest oils penetrate the skin impeccably, plump it up, and leave it looking deliciously moist. Oils are good for dry skin or normal skin that doesn't break out.

Gels are mostly oil-free. They don't pack as much moisturizing power as creams, but because they are light and don't clog the pores, they're a sensible choice for oily skin.

Tip When you come home from work and your skin is almost as tired as you are, wash up and then slather on a face oil. Since you won't be going out again to face the world anyway, it doesn't matter if your face temporarily transforms into a reflector shield until the oil is absorbed. Once it does, your skin will feel like the proverbial baby's bottom.

Behind the Scene **Makeup Prep**

The hands of celebrated makeup artist Kevyn Aucoin have roamed freely over some of the world's most famous faces. Aucoin has created the seasonal makeup looks for Ralph Lauren, Todd Oldham, Richard Tyler, and Donna Karan, among others. Before he applies a dot of makeup to a woman's face, Aucoin always conditions the skin first with 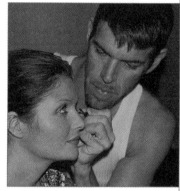 a moisturizer—and so should you. Dab some under the eyes and gently smooth it in all over the face, then blot the excess with a tissue. "Moisturizer plumps up the skin," says Aucoin, "and it's necessary, because nothing looks worse than a tight coat of foundation stretched on dry, taut skin."

Choosing the Right Moisturizer

You don't need a medicine cabinet full of moisturizers: sample several and pick the one that feels best, smells best, and, most important, delivers the best results for you. A good moisturizer will meet the following criteria: it should suit your skin type, be easy to use and readily absorbable, and not feel too greasy on the skin. It should *never burn or irritate*.

The best moisturizers are usually the simplest. Look for a product that is clear or white, without added FD&C dyes. Avoid products

BEST MOISTURIZERS:

PRODUCT & BEST FEATURE	COST
DRY SKIN	
CREME DE LA MER *If money is no object, it can't be better spent for two ounces of anything in a jar; also comes in a light lotion*	stratospheric
KIEHL'S ULTRA FACE MOISTURIZER *Thick as a shake; incredibly luxurious and occlusive*	$$
CLARINS FACE TREATMENT PLANT CREAM "BLUE ORCHID" FOR DEHYDRATED SKIN *Soaks right in for immediate gratification; contains cucumber to soften and orchid extracts to tone the skin*	$$$$
DR. HAUSCHKA MOISTURIZING DAY CREAM *Light, smells like an herb garden, carries an expiration date instead of synthetic preservatives*	$$
SHISEIDO BENEFIANCE DAYTIME PROTECTIVE CREAM *Oily, occlusive, heavily fragranced; not for everyone, but an excellent moisturizer*	$$$$
CLINIQUE DRAMATICALLY DIFFERENT LOTION *Looks like egg yolk and feels as rich; nongreasy and soaks right in to the skin*	$$
L'ORÉAL PLENITUDE HYDRA RENEWAL DAILY DRY SKIN CREAM *Good antioxidant for aging skin*	$
NIVEA CREAM *Super-greasy, for super-dry skin; contains mineral oil*	$
OIL OF OLAY *The classic pink lotion in the glass jar; it's light and plumps up papery thin skin*	$
NORMAL SKIN	
CHANEL PRECISION HYDRAMAX *Light antioxidant lotion; soaks right in to plump up the skin*	$$$$
ESTÉE LAUDER DAYWEAR SUPER ANTI-OXIDANT COMPLEX *Vitamins C and E, green tea, plus SPF 15; good for aging skin*	$$$$
CLARINS HYDRATION-PLUS MOISTURE LOTION *Lightweight but heavy-duty; contains botanicals that soften all skin types*	$$$$
ELENA SCHELL RUMANIAN VELVET OR ABORIGINAL OIL *Contains kalaya oil, which is used in Australia by aboriginal peoples as a cure-all and by cosmetic surgeons as an aid to healing; extremely absorbent, off the beaten track but worth it*	$$
FACE STOCKHOLM ORCHID OIL MOISTURIZER *Orchid extracts tighten up and tone the skin; for all skin types*	$$$

KEY: $ = UP TO $10; $$ = UP TO $20; $$$ = UP TO $30; $$$$ = UP TO $40; $$$$$ = UP TO $50

the scoop on lotions, potions, and creams

	PRODUCT & BEST FEATURE	COST
NORMAL SKIN	**SHU UEMURA DAILY EMULSION** *Terrific moisturizer to wear under makeup because it's extremely light and absorbs quickly*	$$
	L'ORÉAL PLENTITUDE ACTIVE DAILY MOISTURE LOTION *Good antioxidant for aging skin*	$
	DERMA-E *90 percent natural, good quality botanical ingredients*	$
	AVEDA TOURMALINE CHARGED HYDRATING CREAM *Contains grapeseed extract, a powerful antioxidant, along with other soothing flora*	$$$
OILY SKIN	**KARIN HERZOG VIT-A-KOMBI 1 CREAM** *An "oxygen" cream with hydrogen peroxide; kills bacteria, controls oil, and dries up pimples without drying the skin*	$$$$
	LORAC OIL-FREE MOISTURIZER *Soaks right in and plumps up skin; my personal favorite in the genre*	$$$$
	CREME DE LA MER OIL-ABSORBING LOTION *Mattes out the oil for hours, leaves your skin unbelievably silky*	stratospheric
	LANCÔME CLARIFIANCE OIL-FREE HYDRATING FLUIDE *Light and barely there*	$$
	SHISEIDO PURENESS MOISTURIZING GEL *Dries up oil but not your skin*	$$
	NEUTROGENA OIL-FREE MOISTURIZER SPF 15 *Nothing fancy, just an excellent basic moisturizer*	$
	BEAUTY WITHOUT CRUELTY OIL-FREE MOISTURE CREAM *Uncomplicated health-food-store goodie; simple, healthy ingredients*	$$
	CHANEL PRECISION HYDRAMAX OIL-FREE HYDRATING GEL *Smells lovely and soaks up excess oil fast*	$$$$
	L'ORÉAL PLENTITUDE REVITALIFT OIL-FREE LOTION *Good antioxidant for aging skin*	$$
SENSITIVE SKIN	**DECLEOR CORRECTIVE CARE WITH PLANT OILS FOR SENSITIVE SKIN** *Calms down skin that acts high strung*	$$$$
	BENEFIT VITA HYDRATING CREAM FOR SENSITIVE/DRY SKIN *The packaging is quirky, but the product doesn't play around*	$$
	PENNY ISLAND HYDRATING FACIAL MOISTURIZER *As gentle as they come; one of the few truly "natural" products on the market*	$
	SOTHYS IMMUNISCIENCE CREAM FOR SENSITIVE SKIN *Extremely soothing and beats redness, too*	$$$$

FAVORITE FACE OILS

Several summers ago, when my friends heard I was off to Paris, they begged me to bring back Huile Prodigieuse, France's latest skincare miracle. So I headed for the local *diététique* (the closest thing in France to a health food store), where the proprietor sold me her last precious bottles of the sweet almond and neroli oil. I've been hooked on the gentle glide of face oil ever since. Buy these oils in facial preparations, look for them as ingredients in creams, or use them on their own.

Rosa mosqueta (aka rose hip seed oil) is great for softening little lines around the eyes. My favorites are Aubrey Organics, Rosa Mosqueta Oil, and Natura Bisse Rosa Mosqueta Oil for Dry Skin.

Sweet almond oil is an extremely absorbent oil that's not only a terrific all-around moisturizer but calms the skin down fast after waxing or any other irritating event. At $4 a bottle, it's your best health-food-store buy. (Store it in the fridge.)

Evening primrose oil softens papery-dry skin and soothes eczema. I like a cheap balm called Common Sense Chamomile & Primrose Salve, from Rutland, Vermont, which grandmas, toddlers, and everyone in between can share.

Carrot oil moisturizes dry, aging skin and also dries acne; Dr. Hauschka's Facial Skin Oil is a good source.

Neroli oil moisturizes dry or sensitive skin; I like Aesop Fabulous Face Oil.

Kalaya oil is a by-product of the emu, a big Australian ground bird. Before you get grossed out, let me tell you there are few products that absorb as well, soothe scars as well, or make the skin smoother than this: Elena Schell Aboriginal Oil.

Lavender is the basic, all-around, magical oil that always takes me on an olfactory journey back to Provence. It also helps soothe irritations and dry up pimples. You can find it in health food store preparations, or try Clarins Face Treatment Oil "Santal."

containing TEA (triethanolamine), an ammonia derivative that is harsh on the skin. (If a product lists collagen, royal jelly, or aloe vera on its label but doesn't require refrigeration, don't waste your money on it, because the amount is minuscule.)

If you have oily skin, avoid mineral oils, mineral waxes, and other pore-clogging ingredients. Mineral oils can clog pores because they trap perspiration, sit on top of the skin, and don't get absorbed—the chemical composition of the molecule is just too big. Unfortunately, the vast majority of mass-market cosmetics manufacturers use petroleum and mineral oil in their moisturizers, because they are much cheaper than top-quality alternatives like beeswax, sweet almond oil, hyaluronic acid, collagen, vegetable squalene, or shea butter.

HOMEMADE MOISTURIZER

If your skin is extremely dry and super-sensitive, here's how to make your own moisturizer: mix 1 cup liquid oil, such as avocado or almond, with ½ cup beeswax. Place over low heat until the beeswax melts, remove from the heat, and whisk until cool. Add the contents of three capsules of Vitamin E and a few drops of pure essential oil for aroma (lavender, sandalwood, rose, whatever you fancy), pour into a sterile jar, and store in a dark, cool place.

(Mineral oil costs 50 cents per pound compared with glycerine at $2 a pound or collagen, which starts at $7 per pound.) They also have an eternal shelf life. Ingredients that are 100 percent derived from petroleum are mineral oil, carbomers, paraffin, microcrystalline wax, and petrolatum. (You can recognize petroleum-based ingredients on a label when you see the words "ethyl," "butyl," "methyl," "octyl," "propyl," "ene," "eth," and PVP.) So if you have oily skin, you may have to spend a bit more to get the right moisturizer.

Look for an *oil-free* moisturizer where humectants take the place of oil. Often, silicone is added to give the ingredients a pseudo-creamy, slippery feeling. (On the ingredients label, silicones end with "-cone": dimethicone, cyclomethicone, and so on.) Because silicones can be slightly drying, they're good for oily skin.

How to Use Moisturizer

The best time to apply moisturizer is right after you wash or shower, when the skin is already damp and the moisturizer can seal in

How To: maximize your moisturizer

1. Gently apply a dime-sized dab to your skin (too much is a waste of money).

2. Use an upward, circular motion to lightly massage the moisturizer into your face. Make sure not to pull or tug on the skin. If your skin is oily, don't massage too much: facial massage stimulates the oil glands to produce more sebum, which is the last thing oily skin needs.

3. When you apply cream under the eye, do it gently. (This is the most delicate skin on the face.) Use your fourth finger (the weakest) and pat the cream back and forth under the eye, starting at the outer corner and working inward. Do this twice a day, once in the morning before applying makeup and once at night after removing it. Don't put eye cream on your upper lids before bedtime or you'll wake up with puffy lids.

the moisture. Make sure you pat your face dry first (always pat, never rub), because if the skin is *too* wet, the cream will just slide right off your face. Most important, always apply moisturizer to a clean face with clean hands. For most people, one application in the morning and one at night should be enough, but use common sense. If your skin feels taut or dry during the day, moisturize it.

Most people don't need moisturizer on the nose. The nose has an extremely high concentration of oil glands that usually don't need any extra encouragement.

Don't forget about your neck. Stroke upward, so that you don't pull the skin down.

Fashion editors over 40 have managed to make turtlenecks look chic—even in summer—for this reason: the neck is one of the least-tended areas of the body, even by women who are scrupulous about using moisturizer and sun protection on their faces. No matter how vigilant you are about moisturizing your face, if you forget about your neck, the contrast will be painfully obvious.

Say no to night cream. You don't need a separate moisturizer for your neck, nor do you need a separate night cream. Admittedly, the thought of an overnight transformation can make night creams tempting. But most of us, most of the time, don't need another beauty product to help us tell day from night. At the end of the day, our skin doesn't really know the difference. "There is no physiological reason to use a heavier moisturizer at night," says dermatologist Dr. Ellen Gendler. In fact, unless your skin is dry, you don't need moisturizer at night at all. Give your skin a breather, and let your natural oils do their work overnight.

If your day cream has sunscreen in it, use a separate night cream. At bedtime, the sunscreen is not only unnecessary, it's apt to irritate the skin if used around the clock.

Spritzing

When your skin tells you it's thirsty, give it a drink. Keep an atomizer of water handy—especially during the summer, in a climate-controlled office, or on an airplane, where the air is exceptionally dry—and spray your face lightly throughout the day to hydrate your skin. Then blot it dry with a tissue.

A quick spritz on the go can help rinse, refresh, and rehydrate the face. The commercial versions are known as "exhilarators," "fresheners," "hydrators," "tonics," and "floral waters." But you don't need to buy a pricey commercial spray. You can make your own by mixing a few

THE TAPE TEST

At home, you can check the effectiveness of your moisturizer with a simple Scotch tape test. Two hours after you apply moisturizer, put a piece of tape on your lower cheek, near the jawbone, and lift it off. If the tape is coated with scaly shards of skin, it's time to find a new product. Even without the tape test, your skin should tell you—by the way it looks and feels—whether your product is working or not.

drops of essential oil with ½ cup of water, or pour rose water (or plain water) into a plastic spray bottle and leave it in the refrigerator overnight. If your skin is oily, spray your face with lemon water, and use a cotton ball to pat it lightly around your face.

Though the moisturizing effect of a spritzer is temporary, it feels good—and it smells good, too. As New York City dermatologist Dr. Diane Berson says, "Water evaporates quickly, unless you seal it in with a good moisturizer. But spraying and spritzing feel good. And if it feels good, do it." That pretty much sums up the very foundation upon which the beauty industry is built.

Eye Creams

I strongly recommend using a special eye cream. It's an expensive luxury, but one that I've come to consider a necessary splurge. The eye is surrounded by the shallowest tissue on the face. The skin under the eye has no subcutaneous (fatty) layer and not much support structure, which is why it wrinkles easily and isn't very resilient. (I'm still waiting for someone to market a magical eye cream specifically for contact lens wearers, who need it more than anyone because we're constantly pulling on our lower eyelids but must avoid gunking up our lenses with cream!)

It's not necessary for an eye cream to be thicker than a face cream—that's a matter of taste. The undereye area is a good place to directly apply a high-quality oil like kalaya, jojoba, rosa mosqueta, or evening primrose. Because oils spread smoothly and absorb easily, you won't have to disturb that delicate skin area by touching it too much. And when you wake

> **Tip** When makeup artists get to work on models straight off the red-eye, what do they use? There's always Visine, of course. But nothing takes the redness out of bloodshot eyes as well as a French product called Colyre Blue: it makes blue eyes seem bluer, and the whites of the eyes whiter. For puffiness around the eyes, keep an eye gel in the fridge, and apply it morning and night.

up, your undereye area will look notably smoother than it did the night before.

WARNING: If you use your regular moisturizer in the undereye area, make sure it doesn't contain coal-tar colors (listed as FD&C or D&C on the label). The FDA prohibits their application around the eyes because they can irritate the eyes and lead to blindness. And even if you're careful, eye creams do occasionally travel into the eyes.

▨ STEP 4

Use Sun Protection

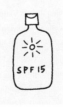

Although dry skin is more prone to wrinkles than oily skin, dry skin *does not cause* wrinkles and moisturizers *do not prevent* them. Ninety percent of your wrinkles are caused by the sun's ultraviolet (UV) light. It used to be that women concerned about their appearance took great pains to protect their skin from the sun—with parasols, gloves, and wide-brimmed hats. But ever since the 1920s, when a bronzed Coco Chanel returned from a Mediterranean vacation and made a tan the hottest fashion accessory

THE EYES HAVE IT:
the best creams and gels

I prefer undereye creams to gels, because gels can make the skin feel taut and dry. But if your eye area is puffy or your skin is blemish-prone, a gel may be a sensible choice for you. These are some of the gentlest and most effective eye products.

PRODUCT & BEST FEATURE	COST
ALMAY STRESS EYE GEL *Tightens and soothes; good for normal to oily skin*	$
AVON EYE BLOCK ENVIRONMENTAL PROTECTION CREAM *Contains SPF 15 for UVA/UVB protection*	$
BEAUTY WITHOUT CRUELTY GREEN TEA NOURISHING EYE GEL *This health-food-store fave feels cool on the skin and tightens a bit; good for normal to oily skin*	$
CHANEL FIRMING EYE CREAM *Really tones the undereye area and absorbs well*	$$$$$
CLARINS EYE CONTOUR BALM *This lush botanical balm is good for every woman*	$$$$
CLINIQUE DAILY EYE BENEFITS *Straightforward and nongreasy*	$$$
KARIN HERZOG EYE CREAM *The hydrogen peroxide and Vitamin A in this formula are extremely effective against wrinkles, dark circles, and blemishes*	$$$$$
KIEHL'S ORIGINAL FORMULA EYE CREAM *Light, emollient, balmlike texture that soaks right in; great for normal to dry skin*	$$
L'ORÉAL REVITALIFT EYE ANTI-WRINKLE AND FIRMING CREAM *Tightens and softens wrinkles*	$$
MARIANA CHICET BONE MARROW CREAM *Sounds icky—but it is easily absorbed by the skin; completely addictive*	$$$
NEUTROGENA HEALTHY SKIN EYE CREAM *AHAs soften wrinkles*	$$
NINA RICCI EYE CONTOUR CREAM *Surprise—a superb cream from a French couturier; very soft and gentle on the skin*	$$$
PHILOSOPHY EYE BELIEVE *A gentle, everyday moisturizer, good for 30-somethings*	$$
RENÉ GUINOT EYE-LIFTING CREAM *A rich, slightly greasy cream, good for dehydrated and/or aging skin*	$$$
SAMUEL PARR EYE CONTOUR CONCENTRATE *A light lotion, for those who don't need too much help*	$$
SHISEIDO BENEFIANCE REVITALIZING EYE CREAM *A good choice for dry skin . . . a bit greasy, but good for you*	$$$

KEY: $ = UP TO $10; $$ = UP TO $20; $$$ = UP TO $30; $$$$ = UP TO $40; $$$$$ = UP TO $50

NOTE: *For deep, dark circles, try an eye cream with Vitamin K, which doctors use before cosmetic surgery because it reduces bruising.*

of the season, it's been a real problem to reverse the popular perception that a tan is not only more attractive but healthy. Yet sun damage is the number one cause of premature aging in women. It's also the one cause of aging that you *can* control.

It is absolutely vital to wear sunscreen. Even in the dead of winter, you should never leave the house without sun protection. In fact, applying sunscreen is so important that I've made it a necessary fourth step in every morning skincare regimen. It should become as automatic as brushing your teeth.

Ultraviolet light, even at low-level exposures, erodes the skin's support structure. It breaks down collagen, causing wrinkles and sagging. It stimulates the skin to create abnormal elastin fibers, so the skin loses its bounce. Prolonged exposure to UV light damages the skin cells' ability to divide properly and inhibits the growth of healthy cells. It can lead to dark spots and turn your skin yellowish or sallow. Chronically exposed skin also develops a thick, leathery texture because the body speeds up cell growth to thicken the top layer in a feeble attempt to block the UV light.

Until recently, it was assumed that the UVB rays, which cause sunburn and suntan, were the only ones to worry about. But despite the fact that many of us were drenching ourselves in SPF sunblocks, skin cancer rates increased in recent years, which puzzled scientists. It is now believed that while SPF products protect our skin from damaging UVB rays, the UVA rays are the ones that cause the real problems.

UVA rays are responsible for photoaging and melanoma, the deadliest skin cancer (see page 100). UVA penetrates deep into the underlying support structure of the skin. It also

THE SKINNY ON SKINCARE

Japanese companies put a premium on skincare. They spend huge amounts of money on research, their standards are extremely high, and, as a result, their skincare lines (especially Shiseido, Awake, and Shu Uemura) are excellent, particularly for dry skin. The major French skincare lines tend to be heavily fragranced (except for Chanel Précision). Their creams are thick and they are also skewed toward consumers with dry skin. Smaller French companies like Clarins and Decléor emphasize plant-based skincare with essential oils, especially for the eye area, and Clarins tinted moisturizer is one of the best. Mass-market moisturizers almost always contain mineral oil, which clogs oily skin. (Good alternative: Kiehl's, which carries a "no mineral oil" tag.)

M.D. Formulations and Exuviance are rugged dermatologists' lines that bring heavy artillery (glycolic acid, salicylic acid) to fight the good fight against extremely oily skin prone to breakouts. Penny Island, a pioneer in developing soothing ingredients for sensitive skin, is one of the best health-food-store brands on the market and makes terrific moisturizers.

Have you ever noticed that the Nivea you bought in Europe feels richer than the one you bought in the United States? Well, you're not crazy: it *is*. When you buy skincare products in Europe, they're often significantly different from the ones you buy here, even though they share the same name. A mask that you purchased in Paris may be green, while the same label bought in Chicago is brown. Certain ingredients may pass muster abroad but don't here. And European products are aimed toward a market with different tastes and expectations.

If you don't use foundation with an SPF 15 rating, you need to apply an SPF moisturizer, a tinted moisturizer, or a standard sunscreen. Many moisturizers don't contain sun protection—in fact, lots of the good ones don't—and here's why: SPF moisturizers, for the most part, contain chemical sunblocks—PABA, the -cinnamates, the -salicylates—which absorb into the top layer of the skin and become oxidized by UV radiation, undergoing a chemical reaction that can sting or irritate the skin. Tinted moisturizers are a better bet, because they contain titanium dioxide, which is inert and nonreactive. My favorites are Aveda Moisture Plus Tint SPF 10, Lancôme Immanance SPF 15, Clarins Tinted Moisturizer SPF 6, Shiseido Vital Perfection Performance Protective Tinted Moisturizer SPF 10.

✦ Best Products

If you choose a standard sunscreen, you'll get the same protection from a drugstore brand as you would from an upscale product, but many cheaper brands will irritate or dry the skin. Suggestions: Clinique City Block or Special Defense Sunblock, Origins Let the Sun Shine, Estée Lauder Advanced Suncare Line, Clarins Crème Solaire Bronzage Sécurité, Elizabeth Arden Suncare Daily Face Protector, Peter Thomas Roth SPF 30, B. Kamins Sunbar. A good, inexpensive drugstore brand is Neutrogena Chemical-Free Sunblocker.

blasts apart collagen, destroys elastin, damages the immune system, and causes lines and wrinkles—all over the body. And although sun-protection products with SPF ratings protect us from UVB rays, they are totally useless when it comes to UVA radiation.

If you want protection from both UVB and UVA (and believe me, you do), your sunscreen must list one of three ingredients—titanium dioxide, zinc oxide, or Parsol 1789 (avobenzene)—as an "active ingredient." These are the *only* active ingredients that offer sufficient UVA protection, and sunscreens that list these as active ingredients are the *only* ones to buy. Titanium dioxide and zinc oxide are the only sunscreens considered by the FDA to offer "broad-" or "full-spectrum" protection, which means the product offers sufficient protection from both UVA and UVB rays.

Heard enough? Well, then, get smart. *Whenever you go outdoors,* use a moisturizer, foundation, or sunblock with titanium dioxide and a minimum SPF rating of 15. (SPF stands for "Sun Protection Factor," and the SPF number tells you how much protection the product will provide. If your skin normally turns pink after 8 minutes of exposure to the sun, SPF 8 means it will take 8 times as long, or 64 minutes, before that will happen. An SPF 15 gives you 120 minutes, and so on.)

Even if you're just hopping into the car to run an errand, dashing down the street to pick up your kids, or lounging in an outdoor café, you should wear sunscreen. Even on days when the sun *doesn't* shine, enough UV rays come through the clouds to do significant damage. UV light is ubiquitous, and it is persistent. It reflects off sand and snow. It penetrates at least three feet underwater. It is brazen, indiscriminate, and merciless; and it is your skin's single greatest adversary. If you're getting only incidental sun exposure (such as a stroll around town), you don't need a heavy-duty sunscreen as you would if you were spending a day at the beach. For ordinary exposure, an SPF 8, 10, or 15 moisturizer, a tinted moisturizer, or a foundation with titanium dioxide is enough for the face—and don't forget your neck! If possible, apply sunscreen at least 20 minutes before going outside to give the active ingredients a chance to be absorbed.

Sun damage is cumulative and irreversible, unless you submit to cosmetic dermatology or surgery (see chapter 4). But if you protect your skin from the sun now, you can avoid all that later. It's impossible to overstate the importance of this rule. **If you choose to follow only one beauty tip in this book, remember to protect your skin from the sun.** And don't ever feel that it's too late or that the damage is already done. Even if you've been lax in the past, if you start now, you can prevent further damage to your skin.

TO TOSS OR NOT TO TOSS?

- If a skincare product looks or smells funny, get rid of it.
- Keep makeup out of sunlight; keep sunscreens out of sun when at the beach.
- Creams and lotions in tubes last longer than products in widemouthed jars.
- Keep containers closed; air speeds up product degradation and bacteria sneak in.
- Never add water or saliva to a product that has dried out: you can introduce bacteria.
- If a product has separated, shake it. If the emulsion doesn't mix back together, toss it.
- Throw skincare products away after a year.
- When in doubt, throw it out.

What Not to Do to Your Face

Don't pick or extract blackheads or whiteheads yourself. If you do a bad job of it (and most amateurs do), you can spread the contents deep into the oil gland and surrounding tissue and cause an infection. And you can stretch the pore permanently. To have blackheads extracted properly is the main reason to go to a good facialist (see next chapter).

Don't use a tweezer on anything except eyebrows and splinters. Tweezers are a woman's worst enemy. If you pluck facial hair, it will grow out flattened or curled in the wrong direction, with a coarser texture. So restrain yourself. Wax, depilate, or find a good electrologist to remove hairs permanently.

Don't allow haircare products to stray onto the face because some of their ingredients can aggravate the skin.

There's a lot of information in this chapter, and the array of products may be dizzying, but my advice is not. If you just remember my basic four-step program—cleanse, exfoliate, moisturize, and protect yourself from the sun—you will know all you need to know. And if you supplement your at-home skincare regimen with regular visits to a facialist, you'll be doing all you can to make your skin as beautiful as it can be.

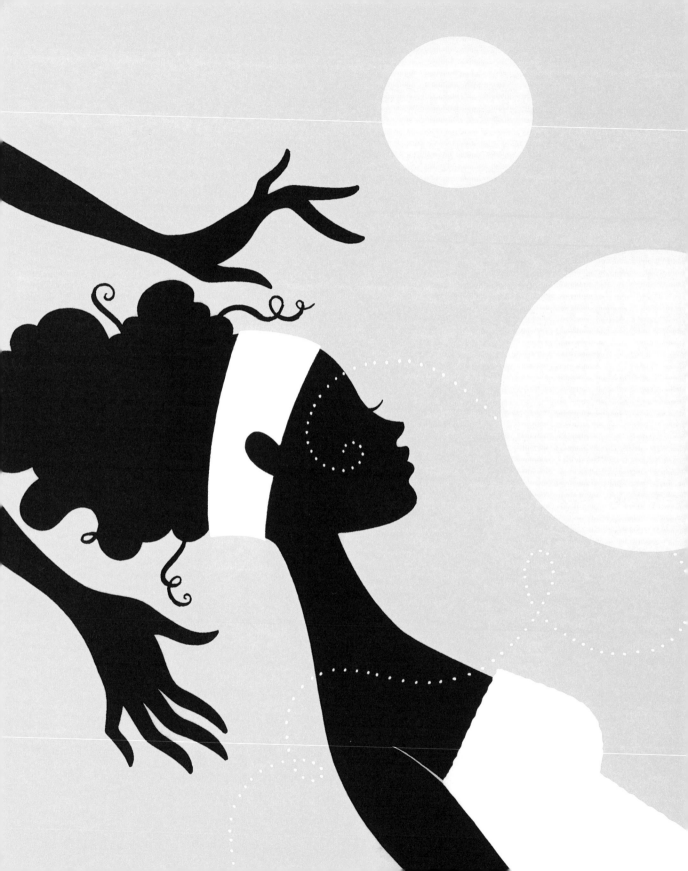

facials

She looked as new as a peeled egg.

—DOROTHY PARKER

In my search for great skin, I have offered up my face to Himalayan rejuvenation facials, Colombian tropical fruit masks, and the healing powers of Chinese herbs. In salons and spas from Manhattan to Marin County, I've been marinated in papaya enzymes, wrapped in sea algae, steamed in chamomile, and quite overdone. Off I go, each time, like some Saint Joan of the skincare set, to lead the charge against broken capillaries, adult acne, brown spots, enlarged pores, wrinkles, fine lines, scars, sagging, and sun-damaged skin. To seek out skin that is, like one of F. Scott Fitzgerald's heroines, "lit to a lovely flame, like the thrill flush of children after their cold baths in the evening . . . with color breaking close to the surface."

It's a mistake to think of facials as the exclusive province of Holly Golightlys or rich ladies who lunch. Good skin is the great leveler, after all. The average cost of a facial is $60, and it's worth every penny. A facialist will

deep-cleanse and rehydrate your skin, leaving it smoother, healthier, and more supple than when you arrived. But the main reason to have a salon facial is to have someone do things for you that you cannot do as well (massage) or should not even try (extracting blackheads) at home. Even if you can't afford to go regularly—say, every eight weeks—splurge at least once. You'll learn the basics of skincare, so that you'll be better able to take care of your skin properly at home forever after.

Years of facials account for the flawless skin Frenchwomen seem to own as their birthright. "In Europe, women are raised on facials," says Aida Thibiant, the grande dame of salons and founder of the Aida Thibiant European Day Spa in Beverly Hills. "They're a rite of passage, passed down from mother to daughter." And though facials are not yet exactly an American tradition, that doesn't mean we can't take a lesson from European women, who consider facials an important kind of preventive care, as

WHAT YOUR FACIALIST SHOULD KNOW ABOUT YOU

If it's your first time with a facialist, she'll ask you questions or have you fill out a questionnaire. If she gets right to work without a consultation, stop her and ask her what she plans to do. Here's what it's important for her to know:

- Your age
- Your normal skincare regimen
- Any allergies
- Any medications you are taking, including antibiotics or the birth control pill (this might account for blotchiness)
- Whether you use alpha-hydroxy acids, Retin-A, or Renova (if you do, your skin is hypersensitized and she should skip the exfoliation)
- If you have sensitive skin or your skin has had a reaction to essential oils
- Your history of acne and/or how often your skin breaks out

Beauty Day!

basic as teeth cleaning. And as with preventive dentistry, it pays to start early so you won't need to repair the damage caused by neglect later on.

A facialist is like a therapist for your skin. She's a professional who has had intensive training and knows how to diagnose common skin conditions and their causes. She's trained to analyze your skin, discuss potential problems and how to solve or avoid them, recommend an appropriate skincare regimen, and suggest the best products for your skin type and condition. Plus—and this is a big one—a good facialist can extract blackheads without scarring, help you clear up breakouts, and control acne (see page 87).

The best way to find a facialist is by word of mouth. Get recommendations from friends and colleagues who have good skin. Or splurge on a facial at the hotel spa while you're on vacation or a business trip. If you're pleased with the results, ask the spa manager to recommend a day spa or salon closer to home.

Another way is to start with products you like and find out which salons use those products in their treatments. Most companies have a toll-free number, and if you call, they'll direct you to a place in your area.

Here's what to look for once you find a facialist:

CURRENT LICENSE. By law, both the facialist and the establishment must be licensed, which means the facialist has been trained in an accredited school, completed 600 hours of classroom education with hands-on training, and passed a test.

EXPERIENCE. When you phone for an appointment, ask how long the facialist has been in the business and how long at that salon. Facialists develop their expertise by touching people. Practice helps!

CLEANLINESS. The salon should be neat and tidy; tools sanitized and sheets, headwraps, towels, and robes freshly laundered. The facialist should have short fingernails and hair that is pulled back and out of the way.

RELAXED ATMOSPHERE. The treatment room should be tranquil and inviting; the staff friendly; and you should feel comfortable. If you're not comfortable, you won't relax. And if you're not relaxed, you're losing out on one of the main benefits of having a facial.

What Every Facial Does

Most women have facials at a salon or a day spa. Each place stamps its own special imprimatur on what is, essentially, the same basic treatment: cleansing and massage, steam and extractions, masks and moisturizing. Beyond these basics, the success of a facial depends on the products the facialist uses, how skilled her touch is, and whether she has a well-trained eye for skin analysis. Here's the basic treatment you can expect wherever you go.

1. Skin analysis. A facialist will touch your skin and examine it under a magnifying glass to see whether you're predisposed toward broken capillaries, clogged pores, brown spots, and so on. Then she'll tell you your skin type, which will determine the kinds of masks she'll use. It will also help her set up a basic at-home regimen for you. A facialist is a trained diagnostician; she'll be able to tell, for example, that your skin discoloration is a result of the sun interacting with a topical or oral medication. She'll also recognize the signs of allergic

reactions, sensitivity, hives, eczema, or psoriasis, and refer you to a dermatologist if necessary.

2. Cleansing and massage. After securing your hair away from your face, the facialist will remove any makeup with a cleanser. Then, if your skin is normal or oily, she'll use a light scrub to exfoliate the top layer of dead skin cells. Dry skin can also benefit from a light exfoliation, which removes the top layer so that a moisturizing mask can penetrate more easily. (Stop her if the exfoliation feels uncomfortable.)

Massage stimulates the circulation and brings oxygen to the skin cells. (It's what gives you that postfacial glow.) Massage also releases tension and relaxes the facial muscles. If your skin is normal or dry, the facialist will apply a light moisturizer or oil (the moisturizer lessens wear and tear on the skin) and give you a facial massage, lasting anywhere from 5 to 15 minutes, depending on your skin type. The style may range from sweeping movements up and down the face and neck *(effleurage)* to acupressure (pressing specific points on the side of the face and sinuses to relieve tension).

If your skin is oily, the massage will be brief—sorry!—as the facialist won't want to overstimulate your oil glands. Instead, she might do a brief *tapotement*—a gentle tapping movement, like butterfly wings fluttering on the face—to get your blood moving.

3. Steam treatment. Many facialists use an L-shaped steamer that delivers a fine, warm mist to your face. Or they may have you hold your towel-swathed head over a bowl of boiled water infused with sweet-smelling herbs like lavender or chamomile.

Steam softens the skin, which makes it easier to extract blackheads. It also stimulates the circulation and activates sweat glands, which brings dirt and waste to the surface. Contrary to the common assumption, steam does not "open" pores. Pores don't open and shut like a window, but they do fill up and need to be unclogged. Your face should be steamed for about the same time it takes to steam vegetables—five to eight minutes. Too much exposure to steam can cause broken capillaries.

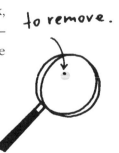

If your skin is fine-pored or sensitive and you don't have blackheads, the facialist may skip the steam treatment altogether. Instead, she might soften the skin with warm compresses so that it's more receptive to a moisturizing mask.

4. Extractions. A clogged pore is filled with

hardened sebum (oil), wax, and cholesterol—not dirt—which turn black when the sebum oxidizes through contact with the air. When pores fill with sebum, they stretch and appear larger

to remove.

and more dominant. If they remain clogged for a very long time, they can stretch permanently. When they're cleaned, they recoil and look smaller.

Using two fingers and a clean tissue or a special disposable tool, a facialist applies just the right amount of pressure to extract blackheads; if this is properly done, it causes little discomfort. A good facialist should be efficient and well organized in her approach to the extractions, but she should not try to clear up *everything* at once. If your pores have been clogged for a while, you might need to exfoliate at home and then return for another facial in six to eight weeks.

After the extractions, she will spot-treat the affected area with an antiseptic product, such as tea tree oil or witch hazel, to keep it free of bacteria.

5. Masks and moisturizers. Most facial-

ists start with a cleansing mask, followed by a moisturizing or rehydrating mask. If your skin is oily or aging, the first mask might be followed by a clay-based tightener.

If you experience tingling from a mask, tell the facialist as it may mean you are allergic or sensitive to an ingredient. (However, alpha-hydroxy

masks and mint- or camphor-based products are supposed to tingle.)

The richness of the moisturizer—lotion, cream, oil—will depend on your skin type. If your skin is dry, you might even get another massage at this point. Lucky you!

After the facial, your aesthetician will recommend a home regimen for you and most likely suggest that you use specific products available for sale at the salon. Remember, you are not obligated to buy any of them. At the end of a facial I was once handed a list of 10 products, including three cleansers—makeup remover, cleansing lotion, and wash-off gel. Although the facial was excellent, the hard sell really turned me off.

Sometimes skin gets worse before it gets better and breaks out after a facial. If your skin is oily and acne-prone and your pores have been clogged for a long time, it means the skin was overstimulated and lots of unpleasant stuff is coming to the surface. Liberating the pores at long last can initially stimulate the oil glands, too. They calm back down and regulate themselves in a day or so.

If you have clear skin and break out after a facial, it may mean that the products used were too rich or too oily for your skin. A good facialist will not make this mistake, so if this happens, don't give her your repeat business.

Pampering Plus

While some women prefer the grand, pampering extras of a facial in a full-fledged spa—plush terry-cloth robes, catered gourmet lunches, and bottomless Perrier—others prefer a cozy, boutiquey atmosphere or all-natural products and patchouli-scented candles. Unfortunately, the little gems without the big names are the hardest to find. But don't worry, I've done much of the legwork for you. Appendices C, D, and E include recommendations for good salons and spas around the United States. The one you choose will depend on your own personal tastes and needs. Given the pampering and stress-reducing component, a facial may seem like a luxury—and it is—but it's also good preventive maintenance. Even if you don't go regularly, at least go once or twice and apply what you learn to your at-home regimen.

The Natural

If you're the herbal-tea type, you may prefer a more "natural" approach. Because "natural" is so appealing these days, it's everywhere, but as we know, natural isn't always so natural. Some facialists make their own products to ensure the freshness and quality of the ingredients. Others use commercial products; two of the best lines in the truly natural category are Dr. Hauschka and Jurlique. Few others come close. On the mass-market level, Aveda is fairly "natural," too.

Aromatherapy. At Aveda salons around the country, aromatherapy facials are based on natural plant and flower essences, overlaid with a vaguely New Age "wellness" pastiche borrowed from Chinese and Indian philosophies. Aveda rates high on the politically-correct-o-meter, with barely a smidge of mineral oil or bioindustrial toxins to be found in their products.

Aromatherapy facials depend on essential oils, which penetrate the skin extremely well and, as a consequence, plump it up nicely. For European film stars, essential-oil facials are the Hollywood equivalent of a surgeon's scalpel. Proponents of aromatherapy claim that essential oils stimulate the circulation and help skin cells rejuvenate. Do they really? Who knows? But they do make skin look—and feel—great.

Behind the Scene — Red-Faced at Ringside

At a fashion show in New York City, Uma Thurman, seated in the front row surrounded by flashing cameras, asked the producers of *Entertainment Tonight* if she could beg off an on-camera interview. "I just got a facial," said Thurman, "and my face is red. Would you please not film me?"

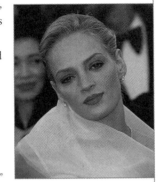

Thurman was lucky. The crew respected her wishes. But the actress should have known better than to have a facial right before a public appearance. So reader, beware: schedule a facial a day or two before a big event, or you may shine in a way you'd rather not.

Ayurvedic. Pratima Raichur, a doctor of naturopathy and owner of Tej, a day spa in Manhattan, believes that if you can't eat it, you shouldn't put it on your face. Raichur makes all of her own products and is a stickler for purity. She diagnoses you not by skin type but by body type (or "dosha"), then prescribes an individualized regimen based on the principles of ayurveda (a Hindi word that translates as "the science of long life") to balance the mind, body, and spirit through the preventive use of herbs, roots, flowers, minerals, and essential oils.

Tip. Forget about spending $50 per session for "facial toning," aka facial exercise. It's a waste of both time and money. There is a benefit to toning the facial muscles, which slacken as you age, but your face gets enough exercise in its normal range of movement. Besides, repetitive exercise can actually deepen existing lines in the skin.

The Euro

Ever wonder why so many of the best facialists come from Eastern Europe? The cosmetology schools there have curricula based on the study of medicine. Romanian facialists go to medical school, and in Bulgaria aestheticians study with dermatologists, pharmacists, and herbologists. When you're getting your face massaged, it's helpful to have it done by someone who understands the muscle groups and circulatory system.

The preponderance of facialists at the big salons like Georgette Klinger and Elizabeth Arden are Eastern European, so you can always count on getting a good treatment there and the ambience tends to be Old World. By now, of course, Arden's flagship Red Door and Klinger's eponymous salons have burgeoned into big beauty factories; Arden has 50 salons, worldwide, and Klinger is just opening its ninth. Because they are so large, they can be a bit impersonal—which may or may not be your cup of chamomile.

The Parisian. A couture facial at the jewel-box Institut de Beauté Yves Saint Laurent in Paris offers the ultimate in sensual pampering. Liberal dollops of heavily fragranced clotted cream were massaged into my face, neck, shoulders, and décolleté for a long, long time—at least 20 minutes. My face was cleansed with

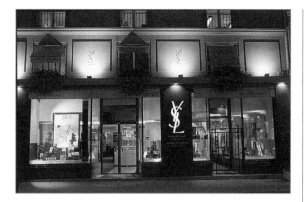

cream, steamed with cream—"to protect the delicate capillaries"—exfoliated, masked, and moisturized with cream. (There's no shortage of cream in France. It is the top-selling skincare product in the country.) If your face is dry and your pores imperceptible, this style's for you!

The Dermatological

If you're nervous about going for a salon facial and feel more comfortable under a doctor's care, you can now go for a facial in a doctor's office. Some special conditions, like whiteheads, plugged hair follicles, and cysts, are best

When AHAs broke into the market, around 1991, the FDA was not—and still is not—overly concerned about the safety of products from reputable companies. But in 1992, the FDA issued its first warnings on skin peelers after a salon product called Peelaway (made by Global Esthetics) was pulled from the market. It had more than lived up to its name and had seriously burned several women in the process. Unfortunately, this is not the only reported case of women suffering injuries at the hands of incompetent aestheticians. Never go to a facialist for a peel: glycolic, alpha-hydroxy, or otherwise.

treated by a dermatologist. Dermatologists use a needle or scalpel point to lance pimples or stubbornly clogged pores. They use comedone extractors, which apply equal circumferential pressure around the pore, to extract blackheads. After the dermatologist's initial treatment, a facialist, who has the same training as a spa or salon facialist, takes over. Not surprisingly, medical facials aren't as pampering as the ones in salons. The ambience is more clinical—no massage, no wafting aromatic plant essences, and no whale songs.

Glycolic. For many good reasons—ranging from consumer safety to professional self-interest—dermatologists are adamant about the importance of having facial peels performed in a doctor's office, and so am I. Glycolic acids are not new (dermatologists have been using them for years), but home and salon formulations are. They can be risky if used in too-high concentrations by practitioners who don't know what they're doing.

Although some salon facialists use over-the-counter products that have AHA concentrations of 3 to 7 percent, others use concentrations of 30 to 50 percent (doctors go from 30 to 70 percent, sometimes higher). This is why I advise against salon peels, because too high a concentration or an AHA that hasn't been buffered properly can result in burns.

The High-Tech

There are lots of elaborate gadgets and gizmos—like the electrically charged wand—that promise to penetrate and firm aging skin. Most of these treatments are incredibly expensive

THE AIR WE BREATHE

When Dr. Paul Herzog, a Nobel Prize–winning scientist and the inventor of the iron lung, trapped hydrogen peroxide (oxygen and water) in emulsion form, the resulting cream was used in hospital burn units, because it promotes cell metabolism and adds water into the cells. This product is now available commercially. Though pricey—$50 to $135 per jar—the line of Karin Herzog products (named after the inventor's wife) is the one most often used for oxygen facials. It works beautifully on oily and aging skin and also keeps ingrown hairs away.

(someone has to pay for that equipment, after all), though they will leave your skin bright and rosy. But so will a simpler-style facial—and chances are, it will be much more relaxing. Oxygen facials may be the most ethereal of the high-tech genre, but they do seem to help aging skin and acne.

Oxygen. Since free radicals are said to damage the skin by depleting oxygen from the cells, it's become popular to "restore" oxygen to the skin through oxygen-infused facials and products. At Bliss, a stylish New York day spa, the high-tech treatment is called ECHO2, an acronym for Exfoliation, Cleansing, Hydration, and Oxygenation. Founder Marcia Kilgore incorporates a light fruit acid peel, a massage with an antioxidant vitamin cream, and a "hydrating enzyme spray pack." She keeps an oxygen tank on hand for the coup de grâce: a 10-minute "finishing spray" of liquid oxygen infused with Vitamin A, glucose, and Vitamin E. Kilgore claims the oxygen adheres to the collagen and elastin molecules at a cellular level and

strengthens them, improving the elasticity of the skin. Oxygen is also great for acne, Kilgore says, "because when you shoot oxygen into the skin, you kill the acne-causing bacteria and cause the sebaceous glands to slow down."

Many dermatologists scoff at the notion of oxygen treatments: "We've got oxygen on our face all day," says one. I've tried oxygen facials. They may sound silly, but the result is out of this world. Unfortunately, so is the price!

Face Savers

1. If you're diligent about following a simple skincare regimen—washing daily with a cleanser, exfoliating regularly, moisturizing assiduously, using a sunscreen religiously—your skin will look good.

2. If you go for a salon facial on a regular basis—every eight weeks is ideal—it will make the difference between good and great skin.

3. Even if you can't go regularly, try to have a facial at least twice a year: at the end of summer and the end of winter. When the seasons change, your skin changes, too. A facial is like a spring cleaning: it will exfoliate your skin and remove any buildup of sluggish winter cells. As a general rule, in winter dry skin gets drier and oily skin gets oilier. In the summer, because you sweat more, your pores have a tendency to clog and your skin breaks out more. A facial can help clear it up.

4. Follow up your salon facials with occasional masks or facials at home. There's nothing a facialist can do for you that will make up for what you won't do for yourself at home.

At-Home Facials

At-home treatments can work wonders for both your skin and your psyche, they cost next to nothing, and they don't require an appointment. Some procedures are best left to professionals, but a relaxing mask applied in the comfort of your own home can make you feel fresher and cleaner, like a new and improved version of yourself, in just a few minutes. Apply a mask when your skin is showing signs of stress, when you're dehydrated after an airplane flight or a long day in a dry, climate-controlled office, or when you just need a pause from your frenetic life.

What Is That Green Goo?

Masks create an illusion—they make your skin *look* tauter, softer, smoother, healthier—but they also perform four important physiological functions. Depending on their ingredients, masks cleanse, tighten, exfoliate, or moisturize the skin. They can also make pores appear smaller and, by sweeping up the surface debris, they make your skin better able to absorb moisture. If you have dark skin, an exfoliating mask can also even out the ashiness in your skin tone. Choose a mask that suits your skin type and pleases your senses.

Tip **D**on't forget that your skin doesn't stop at your jaw. When you have time, apply the facial mask to your neck and décolleté, too. And always apply moisturizer and sun protection to the neck as well.

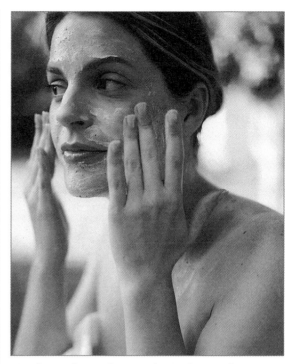

Gently pat the mask around your face and remember to give your T-Zone a little extra attention.

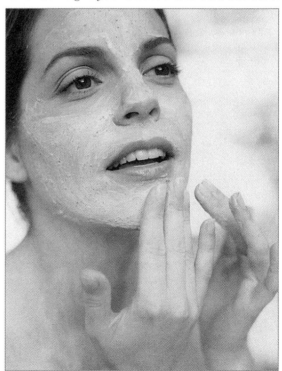

BEHIND THE MASK:

TYPE	INGREDIENTS	HOW IT WORKS
Cleansing and Tightening	Mineral-rich muds or clays like ▪ kaolin ▪ bentonite ▪ fuller's earth ▪ silicates; may also contain algae, seaweed, essential oils	Draws and absorbs excess oil from the skin; tightens the skin and makes pores look smaller
Exfoliating	Scrubbing particles AHAs enzymes (papaya or pineapple extracts) plant gums balsam	Peels or sloughs off dead surface skin cells, surface oil, and debris; loosens clogged pores
Moisturizing	Emollients ▪ essential oils ▪ calendula ▪ chamomile ▪ aloe vera ▪ ginseng ▪ dong quoi ▪ evening primrose oil ▪ sweet almond oil ▪ glycerine	Softens lines and wrinkles; smoothes flaking skin; soothes irritated skin
Blemish-Busting	Antibacterials sulfur salicylic acid benzoyl peroxide sulfates tea tree oil clay, AHAs	Dries excess surface oil; kills acne-causing bacteria
For Your Eyes Only	Anti-inflammatories ▪ algae ▪ amino acids ▪ cucumber extracts ▪ glycerine	Reduces puffiness; lightens dark circles; softens lines and wrinkles

the scoop on goop

FOR WHAT SKIN TYPE	GOOD CHOICES
All except very dry	AESOP PRIMROSE FACE MASQUE, AHAVA ADVANCED MUD MASK, AUBREY ORGANICS GREEN TEA AND GREEN CLAY REJUVENATING MASK, AVEDA DEEP CLEANSING HERBAL CLAY MASQUE, PRINCESS MARCELLA BORGHESE FANGO, MOLTON BROWN PURIFYING MARINE MASK, H2O SEA MINERAL MUD MASK, ORIGINS CLEAR IMPROVEMENT, REVLON 5-MINUTE MASK, CHANEL GENTLE CLEANSING MASK
Aging, normal, oily	ELIZABETH ARDEN MILLENNIUM HYDRA-EXFOLIATING MASK, CLARINS GENTLE EXFOLIATING REFINER, CLARINS GENTLE FACIAL PEEL, DECLÉOR PHYTOPEEL FACE PEEL, EDUCATED BEAUTY 10-MINUTE CRANBERRY PEEL, KISS MY FACE SCRUB MASQUE, LANCÔME MASQUE CONTROLÉ PEEL-OFF
All	**Gels:** AVEDA INTENSIVE HYDRATING GEL MASK, DECLÉOR T-ZONE REFINING GEL, CHRISTIAN DIOR INSTANT RADIANCE PURIFYING MASK, MILL VALLEY 99% ALOE GEL, PETER THOMAS ROTH CUCUMBER GEL MASK **Creams:** AUBREY ORGANICS ROSA MOSQUETA HERBAL MASK, BENEFIT MINT FIRMING MASK, DECLÉOR HYDRAVITAL MOISTURIZING MASK, GUERLAIN ISSIMA AQUAMASQUE, KIEHL'S IMPERIALE REPAIRATEUR MOISTURIZING MASQUE, ORIGINS DRINK UP, SAMUEL PARR MASQUE REVITALISANT, YVES ROCHER CHAMOMILE SOOTHING MASK, SHU UEMURA UTOWA MOISTURE MASK
Very oily, acne-prone skin	CLARINS ABSORBENT MASK, NEUTROGENA ACNE MASK, ORIGINS OUT OF TROUBLE, PENNY ISLAND PAPAYA AND HONEY FACIAL MASK, TISSERAND TEA TREE AND KALUKA GEL, VIT-A-PLUS HYDR-A-FIRMING MASK, ESTÉE LAUDER SO CLEAN DEEP PORE MASK
All	CARITA EYE CONTOUR, CLARINS EYE MASK, RENÉ GUINOT INSTANT EYE MASK, SHU UEMURA UTOWA FACE PADS

Sunday Night Special

Whether you fly solo or host a "beauty night" for your friends, a facial is good therapy for body and soul.

On a relaxing Sunday night, give yourself an extra-special treatment and put your best face forward for the week. Or gather some friends together for a "Girls' Night In." Order up your favorite food, lay on a good soundtrack, and let the gossip begin as you give each other manicures, pedicures, facials, and masks.

The Essentials

1. Wet your face and put some cleanser on a clean, wet cotton washcloth. The washcloth can be a little rough, but make sure it is absolutely clean. Cleanse your face by moving the cloth around gently in outward circular motions, which will also stimulate circulation.

Take another clean washcloth and wet it with warm water.

Gently blot your face—don't pull, don't rub—with the compress, all over, for two to three minutes to remove the cleanser. Then splash your face with warm water.

2. Put 1 to 2 tablespoons of loose herbs in a medium bowl. (Or use prepackaged facial steaming herbs, such as Essentiel Elements.) For dry or sensitive skin, look for an herbal blend

STEAMING STRESS AWAY

Steaming your face with herbs is not only relaxing, it's therapeutic," says Laura Peck Fenemma, CEO and founder of Essentiel Elements, a San Francisco–based aromatherapy skincare line. "By 'sweating' the skin, you're releasing toxins, softening the skin, and making it more receptive to a moisturizing mask." Peck's weekly regimen, a relaxing herbal steam followed by a mask, is a legacy of her previous career as a fast-track financial analyst on Wall Street. "I came to realize that it wasn't just my skin I was taking care of," she says, "but my overall health."

that contains lavender, chamomile, or rose. For normal skin, go for lavender, lemon balm, or rose. If you have oily skin, rosemary and sage are good choices. Comfrey works well on blemished skin. Pour boiling water on top of the herbs. Let cool for 30 seconds or so. Sitting about 18 inches away from the bowl, drape a towel over your head and the bowl to keep the steam in. Close your eyes, and breathe deeply. (If the steam feels too hot, it *is* too hot. Wait a few seconds longer before steaming.) Steam for only five to eight minutes, maximum, to soften your skin, loosen the dirt, and make your face more receptive to moisturizers. Then pat your face with a clean, warm, wet washcloth.

3. Choose an exfoliating mask from the chart on pages 56–57 or use one of the home recipes in this chapter. Lightly pat the mask on, avoiding the eye area, and gently rub in concentric circles around your face. Leave on for five minutes, then rinse with warm water.

4. Depending on your skin's needs, you can put on a commercial cleansing, tightening, or moisturizing mask. Choose one from the preceding chart or one that's homemade (pages 60–61). If you choose a commercial product, apply the mask a bit more heavily on the T-Zone, an area that needs special attention.

Lie down in a semidarkened room or in the bathtub, and put on some relaxing music. Shut your eyes and empty your mind, breathing as slowly as you can. Stay that way for 10 to 15 minutes. Rinse your face with warm water and pat dry with a clean washcloth.

5. Moisturize with your usual daily moisturizer, making sure to gently pat lotion or cream around the eye area using your fourth finger. (Remember, it's the weakest finger and exerts the least pressure on your skin.)

FIVE-MINUTE PICK-ME-UP

Never underestimate what you and a mask can accomplish with a few minutes together. Talk about instant gratification! A quick mask can improve the look and feel of your skin almost immediately. Here's a simple, satisfying, quickie facial:

1. Wash your face with warm water and a cleanser.

2. Apply a mask. Leave it on for five minutes, while you lie comfortably on the floor or bed with your eyes closed.

3. Rinse with lukewarm water.

4. Moisturize. You'll be much revived and ready to face the world again.

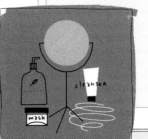

Make Your Own Mask

A friend once asked me why anyone would bother to make her own mask, with so many great products available on the market. Here's why: it's cheap, simple, and fun, and if you like to cook, you'll probably enjoy playing mad scientist in your kitchen, too.

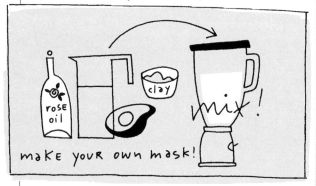

To make your own mask, all you need is some clay (available at health food stores) and some stuff from your pantry. Use green clay for dry, sensitive, aging, or sun-damaged skin. Use white kaolin or fuller's earth for normal or oily skin. To make a clay mask, mix two parts water to one part clay. Add more water—in driblets—if it's too dry. Also add honey, herbs, and so on. Then add your favorite essential oil, such as lavender, rose, or geranium. For a richer mask, substitute whole milk for water in any of the following recipes. Milk is soothing, and it contains Vitamin A and protein.

Before you apply any mask, always wash your face with warm water and a cleanser.

SWAMP THING

Sometimes you need a good dose of ugly to feel truly pretty. If you're willing to look like

EGG ON YOUR FACE

Egg white has been used throughout history to give a "tight" feeling to the skin and make pores look smaller. In fact, it does both. This principle is the basis of many of the "lift-creams," "tighteners," and "lift-less face-lifts" now on the market.

the Creature from the Depths for 15 minutes, you'll find that avocado is a very effective moisturizer and high in Vitamin E.

> 4 tablespoons clay
> 2 teaspoons avocado oil or ½ avocado, mashed
> 2 teaspoons water
> 4 drops lavender oil or rose oil (optional)

1. Mix the ingredients thoroughly.
2. Pat the mask on your face, avoiding the eye area.
3. Leave on for 15 minutes. Rinse off with warm water. Apply moisturizer.

THE QUEEN BEE

The buzz on this one? If that taut, tingly feeling makes you hum, this is the mask for you.

> 4 tablespoons clay
> 2 teaspoons honey
> 2 teaspoons water or milk
> 4 drops neroli oil or
>   wheat germ oil (optional)

1. Mix the ingredients.
2. Apply to face.
3. Leave on for about 15 minutes. Rinse off with warm water. Apply moisturizer.

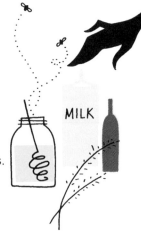

FACE FOOD

In his studies on "fruit hedonics"—the way fruit odors alter mood and behavior—Dr. Alan R. Hirsch, director of the Smell and Taste Treatment and Research Foundation in Chicago, had success treating migraine patients, insomniacs, and anxiety sufferers with inhalants of green apple, banana, or vanilla. Hirsch theorizes that something in these foods either changes the neurotransmitters in the brain, evokes pleasant memories, or increases alpha waves to produce a more relaxed state—which is not really news to women who've slathered, steamed, and soaked themselves in food-based, vitamin-rich beauty treatments for centuries.

"Food's friendly," explains Philip B., a celebrity hairstylist, author of *Blended Beauty,* and creator of an upscale hair- and skincare line. "Food represents mother. Nobody fears food. When you put carrot puree on your face, your skin feels better." If you use a homemade mask of fresh fruits or vegetables, you get the full potency of the raw food—no preservatives, no fragrances, no surprises. So the next time the baby doesn't finish her mashed bananas, slather them on your face for a few minutes. The potassium is good for your skin, and the laughter is good for you and the baby.

OATS AND GROATS (EXFOLIATING MASK)

This mask is as wholesome as breakfast on the farm. You can make other homemade exfoliants with a simple paste of baking soda, sugar, or salt and water.

> *½ cup dry cornmeal*
> *½ cup dry oatmeal*

1. Put the cornmeal and oatmeal in a blender and "pulverize."
2. Shake out a palmful and mix with warm water to make a paste.
3. Gently press the mask onto the face.
4. Leave on for 5 minutes.
5. Rinse off with warm water. Apply moisturizer.

LEMON AID

Lemon possesses astringent and exfoliant properties, making it a natural choice for oily skin.

> *4 tablespoons clay*
> *2 teaspoons lemon pulp*
> *2 teaspoons honey*
> *2 teaspoons water*
> *2 drops eucalyptus oil* or *jojoba oil*
> (optional)

1. Mix the ingredients thoroughly.
2. Apply to face.
3. Leave on for 15 minutes.
4. Rinse off with warm water. Apply moisturizer.

If you're in a hurry, you can mix equal parts lemon juice and water. Pat on your face, leave on until dry, then wash off with cool water.

Skin Tighteners and the Antigravity Facial

As we age, it's not just our skin that succumbs to the pull of gravity. The muscle underneath can lose its snap as well. A facial or a topical tightening cream obviously won't resuscitate flabby muscle tone, but it can temporarily tighten the look of the face or eye area. "Sleeping with a bra on is something someone told me in the seventies when I wouldn't consider a bra—day or night," says Norma Kamali. "But I decided to try it several years later," she continues, "and I think there is something to

fighting gravity." You might think of the tightening treatments in this section as the cosmetic equivalent of sleeping with a bra on your face!

If your skin is "aging" or sun-damaged, follow the directions for a home facial below, using one of the tightening products on this page. Tighteners are expensive and their transformative effects as fleeting as Cinderella's night at the ball, so you'll probably want to save them for a gala evening or an important meeting.

Cinderella's Mask

The effects of this tightening treatment should last you through a special day or evening. Then—alas!—the magic will wear off.

1. Splash your face with warm water and apply cleanser.

2. With the cleanser on, give yourself a brief massage to stimulate circulation. Starting at your nose, use your fingers to lightly pinch and knead your skin, as if you were squeezing a baby's cheeks, moving out to the sides of your face and down to your jawline. Knead along your jawline and out toward your ears. Then, starting at your collarbone, lightly push your skin upward toward your chin in smooth, flowing movements.

TIGHTENERS IN A JAR

For the most part, "tightening" products are glorified moisturizers. The primary tightening agent is often hyaluronic acid, a powerful humectant. It swells the skin by adding moisture and binding it in, making it look plumper, more toned, and less noticeably wrinkled. You can use a tightener as you would use a moisturizer, but they are expensive. Mariana Chicet, a Los Angeles facialist, makes one of the best skin-tightening moisturizers on the market, called Mariana Chicet Revitalizing Lotion Concentrate. Other good choices are Chanel Lift Serum Extreme, Guardian Sublift A.R.T., Sisley Botanical Tensor, Yves Saint Laurent Instantée/Instant Firming Gel, Elizabeth Arden Firm Lift Intensive Lotion for Face and Throat, and Estée Lauder Re-Nutriv Intensive Lifting Creme.

★Best Products

3. Remove the cleanser with warm water, and pat your face with a damp, warm washcloth.

4. Apply a tightening mask (pages 56–57) with clean fingers; use outward, circular motions. Leave on, lie down, and relax for 10 to 15 minutes.

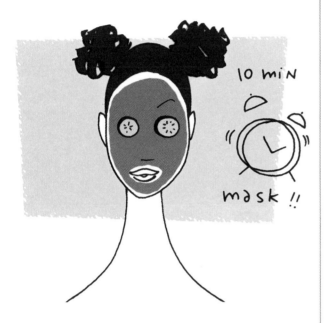

5. Remove the mask with warm water and a washcloth, and apply one of the products from "Tighteners in a Jar" (opposite page).

Try this favorite of fashion models and stylists: dab Preparation H on the puffy spots under the eyes. The shark liver oil in the product reduces water retention in the undereye area just as it shrinks hemorrhoidal tissues. Witch hazel and Listerine are other fashion favorites, but they'll dry out your skin in a big way. A caution for all of these products: Avoid direct contact with your eyes.

Trade Secret

LE PLUS ÇA CHANGE...

Some things change . . . and some things don't. Here is a quick look at beauty treatments in the past and now. Notice any parallels?

THEN: "Vapozone." A machine spewed ozone onto the face, an airy elixir that was said to help you "reclaim your youthful complexion."

NOW: ECHO2. A machine spews oxygen to "strengthen collagen and elastin at the cellular level."

THEN: "Tissulaire Injections." An electrically powered needle was attached to an instrument filled with "animal embryo serum" and injected into wrinkles to plump them up and rebuild tissue.

NOW: Collagen injections, botox injections.

THEN: "Supernemectron." An implement carried electric current into the tissues, which was said to "melt" the hardened sebum clogging pores and make it easier to unclog them.

NOW: Alpha-hydroxy acids. Chemicals "melt" the bonds between the skin's cells, exfoliate the upper layer, and unclog pores.

THEN: "Galvanopuncture" was a modified electroshock treatment for the face. The facialist put an instrument against the face that passed an electric current into the facial tissues. The electricity was thought to "plump" wrinkles and supposedly caused sagging facial muscles to snap to attention.

NOW: "Electric Face Lift." Claims to reduce wrinkles and lines by applying low-frequency electrical current to relax facial muscles. A "holo-electron neon iron" is an ice-cold glass wand that carries a crackling electric current and resembles the light saber used by the Jedi in *Star Wars*.

rona's skin remedies

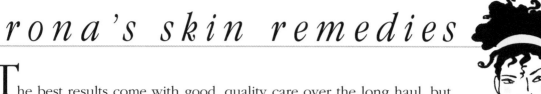

The best results come with good, quality care over the long haul, but everyone needs a quick fix once in a while. For the following pesky skin problems, try one of the homemade solutions or, if you're not the do-it-yourself-type, buy a recommended product.

PROBLEM	HOMEMADE SOLUTIONS	COMMERCIAL PRODUCTS
CHAPPED LIPS	■ Dab a bit of Vaseline on your lips and rub gently with an old toothbrush. No, it doesn't hurt! ■ Crack open a Vitamin E gel capsule and rub the gel on your lips. ■ Rub olive oil or sesame oil on your lips.	BURT'S BEES LIP BALM, HUDSALVA LIP BALM, MODE DE VIE SHEA BUTTER STICK, KIEHL'S LIP BALM #1, MUSTELA MUSTI HYDRATING STICK. Avoid products with camphor, which dries the lips. Look for products with shea butter instead.
DEHYDRATED SKIN	■ Mix 2 drops of lavender oil with baking soda and water until it becomes a paste. Put on face and leave on for 5 minutes. Rinse. Moisturize. This light, exfoliating mask makes skin more receptive to moisture.	CLARINS HUILE FACE OIL. Also try sweet almond oil from the health food store.
DULL, TIRED-LOOKING SKIN	■ Wrap grated cucumber in cheesecloth, lie down, and apply to face for 5 minutes. Rinse with cool water. ■ Refrigerate aloe vera gel for at least 1 hour. Pat it on your face, and lie down for 10 minutes. Rinse. ■ Lie on your back and hang your head over the side of the bed for 5 to 10 minutes. It will feed oxygen to your face, and improve your color and tone.	CABOT VITAMIN E GEL, JASON WITCH VERA HERBAL GEL, ROBERTS CUCUMBER STRESS GEL
FLAKY SKIN	■ Rub half of an apple on skin to help even out the texture. ■ Place a sprinkling of sugar in your palm and dampen with water. Gently massage on the flaky areas. Rinse.	ELIZABETH ARDEN EIGHT-HOUR CREAM, BENEFIT PEEL AND POLISH, ERNO LASZLO BETA COMPLEX, OIL OF OLAY AGE-DEFYING LOTION WITH SALICYLIC ACID

PROBLEM	HOMEMADE SOLUTIONS	COMMERCIAL PRODUCTS
INFLAMED, IRRITATED, OR SENSITIVE SKIN	■ Make a pot of chamomile tea. Pour into an ice-cube tray and freeze. Pop out a cube, wrap it in a thin cloth, and rub gently on face. ■ Soak a clean cloth in a small dish of milk, squeeze, and apply the compress to the affected area for 10 minutes. Rinse off with warm water.	AVEDA ALL SENSITIVE line, ANNEMARIE BÖRLIND ZZ SENSITIVE line, CHAMOCARE LIGHT THERAPY, COMMON SENSE CHAMOMILE & PRIMROSE SALVE, PENNY ISLAND OAT AMINO COMPLEX, DECLÉOR BALM FOR SENSITIVE SKIN, SOTHYS IMMUNOSCIENCE
OILY PATCHES	■ Keep a small spray bottle of rose water in the refrigerator. Give yourself a wake-up spritz in the morning, after you wash your face, or saturate a tissue and dab it on at night after washing.	CRABTREE & EVELYN ROSE-TINTED POWDER LEAVES, JURLIQUE LAVENDER SILK DUST, PRESCRIPTIVES SKIN BALANCER TOWELETTES, M·A·C OIL MATTE GEL (makeup artists' secret)
PIMPLES	■ Make a paste with water and coarse-grained sea salt, and apply it to the blemish twice a day until healed. Do not rub. ■ Dab a bit of toothpaste on your pimple(s) before bed. Repeat as necessary. ■ Dot a bit of clay mask on your pimple(s) and leave on overnight. In the morning, rinse off. Repeat as necessary. ■ Soak a piece of bread in milk. Place it on the pimple and lie down. Leave it there for up to 30 minutes. Rinse.	CLARINS ACNE CONTROL SKINCARE SYSTEM, CLINIQUE ACNE SPOT HEALING GEL, IMAN BLEMISH GEL, ORIGINS SPOT REMOVER, SAMUEL PARR AROMATHERAPY BLEMISH PEN
RED, BLOTCHY SPOTS	■ Put a few drops of Visine on red, blotchy spots. Because it constricts blood vessels, it will do for your skin what it does for your eyes. ■ Dab a yellow-based cream or pencil concealer on red areas after you apply foundation. Blend well with fingers.	AVEENO LOTION, DECLÉOR HARMONIE JOUR ANTI-REDNESS CREAM, LAURA MERCIER SECRET CAMOUFLAGE, PRESCRIPTIVES MAGIC RED NEUTRALIZER
UNDEREYE PUFFINESS	■ Apply damp, ice-cold tea bags (with caffeine, a diuretic) or hold a bag of frozen peas to the eyes for a few minutes to reduce swelling. ■ Wrap grated potato in two little cheesecloth sacks, lie down, and place the sacks under the eyes. Leave on for 10 minutes and rinse. ■ Place sliced cucumbers on your eyes; cover with a damp, cool cloth; and lie down for 10 minutes. ■ Place a satin eye pillow filled with buckwheat or lavender over your eyes as you lie back and relax.	BENEFIT EYE LIFT, CHAMOCARE UNDEREYE THERAPY, NIVEA SOOTHING EYE GEL, ORIGINS NO PUFFERY, POND'S CUCUMBER EYE TREATMENTS, SHU UEMURA MOISTURE EYE ZONE MASK

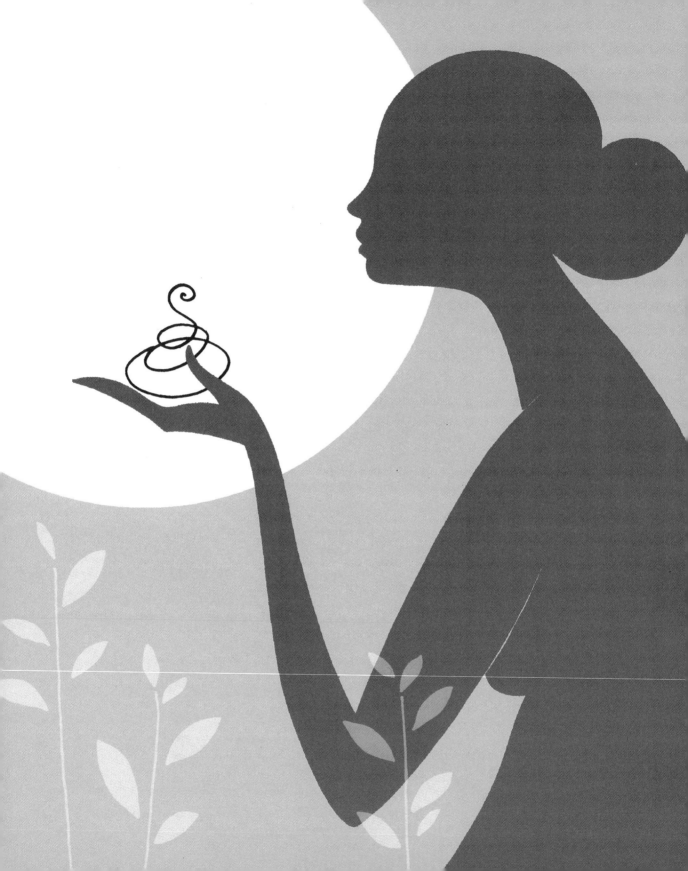

CHAPTER FOUR

aging

Beauty isn't about looking young, but about looking good.

—CLINIQUE

In 1900, what a woman could expect from turning 50 was to be dead. Now, according to the National Institute on Aging, 50 is the gateway to another 30 or 40 more productive years. Middle age is starting later, lasting longer—and looking better than ever before. "Maybe it's denial," writes Melinda Beck in *Newsweek,* "But whatever it is, it's working . . . through exercise, diet and dye, the StairMaster set has actually succeeded in pushing back the boundaries of 'middle age.' Boomers look, act, and feel younger at 50 than previous generations did."

Yet despite their long life expectancy, baby boomers are possibly the most age-phobic generation in history. The same demographic that vowed to "Never trust anyone over 30" apparently can't bear to look a day over 29, and they're whitening, tightening, peeling, and plumping their aging skin at warp speed. During the 1990s, sales of "age-repair" elixirs leaped from $325 million to $3.6 billion, and

cosmetic dermatology and surgical procedures have tripled in the last decade.

"If I have to diet, I'm gonna diet," says baby boomer Sharon Stone. "If I have to work out, I'm gonna work out. If I have to sleep upside down like a bat so I don't look like a basset hound, that's what I'm gonna do." And why *shouldn't* your face fit your youthful body or brain?

No reason. But what's disturbing is our growing dependency on invasive and sometimes risky procedures, and the ease with which we have come to depend on them at an earlier and earlier age, when there are so many other healthier options. Before you rush to the more extreme step of cosmetic surgery, I suggest that you try alternative (and gentler) approaches—good skincare, self-care, exercise, and a healthy diet. Perhaps the best way to start is by facing facts and shifting your attitude, rather than shifting your face or body parts.

As we age, our skin has different needs—

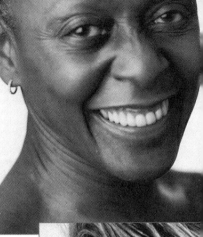

it's thirstier, finer, and doesn't snap back as quickly as it used to. So, first change your skincare regimen, give older skin extra nourishment and pampering on a daily basis, and turn to prescription drugs, cosmetic dermatology, and especially surgery, as a last resort. Even something as seemingly benign as a chemical peel is still an invasive procedure. The fact is, collagen injections, fat transfers—even face-lifts—will improve your appearance temporarily, but they won't prevent aging. In fact, they'll get you started on a course that's hard to stop. Surgery only leads to more surgery.

If you do opt for more aggressive treatments, make sure that you do them safely and well. Become fully informed about what you're getting into, and don't cut corners or look for bargains. Most important, choose your practitioner with care. This chapter will provide you with the information you need to make smart decisions. (The treatments are arranged in order of least to most invasive. Surgery is covered in appendix A.)

In the 1980s, in a refreshing moment of candor, Clinique took the high road when it rolled out a successful advertising campaign built around the slogan "Beauty isn't about looking young, but about looking good." If we could only take that message to heart, maybe we would soften our laugh lines and crow's-feet with gentle and pleasurable means, but not try to erase them altogether. Perhaps we could

Women who age beautifully and naturally (clockwise from top): Bethann Hardison, Diane Keaton, Lauren Hutton, Judith Jamison, Vanessa Redgrave, Dayle Haddon, Susan Sarandon, Candice Bergen.

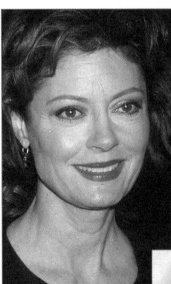

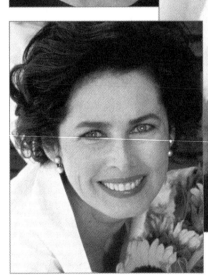

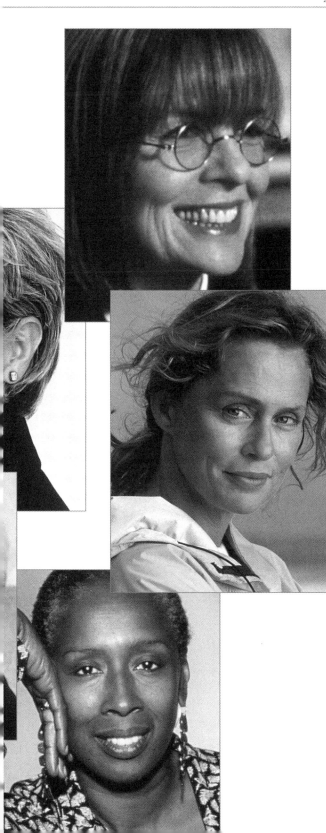

WHY DOES SKIN AGE?

There are many causes of aging skin. Some are avoidable, others are not. Here are the main culprits.

INTRINSIC

- Heredity
- Metabolic wear and tear
- Diminishing hormone production and oil secretion

EXTRINSIC

- Sun, pollution, and other environmental damage
- Free radicals
- Smoking, alcohol, poor diet
- Stress
- Use of harsh products that weaken the skin's natural barrier function over time.

even learn to accept them for what they are—expressions of a life deeply lived. "There are some people who prefer to look as if they haven't experienced life," says Diane Keaton. "My question is 'Why?'"

Granted, everyone wants to look good. But isn't there a deeper, more lasting beauty to aspire to—one that doesn't depend on cheating the clock? What about those extraordinary older women who choose to age naturally and gracefully: the crinkly elegance of Judith Jamison, Vanessa Redgrave, Susan Sarandon, Candice Bergen, and Lauren Hutton? None of these women looks young, but most of us still consider them beautiful.

After all, aging is not a disease. It happens to everyone lucky enough to live that long. So let's face facts and look at what, exactly, *is* happening to your face as it ages, and what you can do—not to look young but to look good.

Caring for Older Skin the Smart Way

Somewhere around age 40—give or take a few years—you'll begin to notice a few creases that won't go away or a hint of softness around the jaw. When you do, you've reached a point where you have to literally face up to the passage of time whenever you look in the mirror. And if you're not psychologically prepared for that moment, it can come as a shock. If your impulse is to run to a surgeon, wait a minute. Slow down. Whatever you do, don't panic. Despite all the antiaging hype, there truly are products that can reduce lines and wrinkles, smooth your skin's texture, and eliminate dullness and discoloration.

A HAIRY SITUATION

When you hit your 40s, chances are that as your head sprouts a few gray hairs, your chin will sprout a few errant ones as well. If you freak out about facial hair and pluck, you will damage the follicles, poke craters in tender facial tissue around the jawline and chin area—and generally wreak havoc on your face. So cease and desist!

Consider one of these options instead: wax (see page 97); depilate (drugstore depilatories like Mim Natural Hair Remover or Surgi-Cream work well); bleach; or find a good electrologist to remove facial hair permanently (see page 99). If you've already done damage to your chin, use a BHA on the area daily, and you should see an improvement within a week or two. Really.

But first, remember this simple fact: *the main reason that many antiaging treatments work is because they require you to care for your face daily.* When you moisturize your skin (which alpha-hydroxy acids do), you keep skin cells from drying out. When you use sun protection (a requirement when using Renova or Retin-A), you stave off wrinkles, blotchiness, and sagging. If you'd done these things all along, you wouldn't need an antiaging arsenal now. But enough about hindsight. Begin where you are. Even if you've never taken proper care of your face, now's the best time to start and take advantage of all the recent advances in skincare technology.

Adjust Your Regimen

As we age, skin cell turnover slows down, which is one reason our skin tends to look duller and dingier as we get older. When dead skin cells pile up on the surface, they can clog pores and exaggerate the appearance of wrinkles. As the blood flows more sluggishly and not enough oxygen reaches the skin, it loses color. White women's skin may take on a yellow tinge, and the skin of African Americans may look ashy. Sun damage now appears as dark spots and discoloration, and aging skin is also more vulnerable to dryness and broken capillaries. In addition, the cumulative effects of free radicals (unstable molecules that deplete the cells of oxygen) damage skin cells and cause the breakdown of collagen, which causes the skin to lose firmness.

Because the skin's needs change as you get older, you'll need to do a few things differently. In every case, stick with your gentle cleanser and be especially vigilant about sunscreen. That never changes. Now is the time to trade in your scrub (Step 2 in your daily regimen) for an alpha-hydroxy acid. This is the major change you will make in your daily regimen. AHAs speed up exfoliation without the risk of broken capillaries and make it easier for the skin to absorb moisture. Start by using an AHA three or four nights a week instead of a scrub after your nightly cleanser and see how well your skin tolerates the acid.

AHAs are now the number one skincare ingredient in the world. But they're not gentle, and they're not for everyone. It doesn't make sense to start using them before your skin needs them, because they are corrective, not preventive. Unless your skin is leathery or sun-damaged, AHAs are overkill for most women under 40. If you do use them, make sure your other products are especially gentle.

As you approach menopause and your skin gets thinner and drier, you may also need to change to a slightly heavier moisturizer (from lotion to cream) or incorporate a face oil into your regimen. High-quality face oils are not greasy; they penetrate well, plump up the skin (see page 38), and make it look juicy. Apply the oil or cream to your face in the morning, after you rinse, and leave enough time for your skin to absorb the oil before you apply makeup. There are also lots of appealing antioxidant creams that function as excellent moisturizers for all skin types and may help protect the skin.

Most people don't realize that AHAs are moisturizers as well as exfoliants.

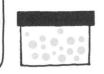

Red Alert

A HAs may sting for about a week, until your skin gets used to the acid. (This is the rare instance when an irritating product actually helps your skin.) However, there's a fine line between helping the skin cells' turnover process and causing irritation that can damage the skin. If your skin turns red or rashy after using one of these products, stop using it. If your skin is irritated or uncomfortable for longer than a week, it means either that the product isn't buffered well enough or that AHAs aren't for you. In that case, try a beta-hydroxy acid (BHA), which is less irritating, or a poly-hydroxy acid (PHA) designed for sensitive skin. Because AHAs make your skin more sensitive to the sun, it's essential to use sunscreen.

If you use an AHA, you may not need another moisturizer: most AHAs are set in a moisturizer base, and the acids themselves increase water retention and plump up the skin. And here's something else you may not realize: many moisturizers now contain AHAs, so if you *don't* want them, make sure to avoid products with these ingredients on the label—citric, tartaric, malic, lactic, or glycolic acid.

Rethink Your Makeup

Women in their 40s, 50s, and 60s often try to hide too much with makeup. When it comes to aging skin, less is more. The trick is to pay attention to the texture of the makeup you wear, and have it work *with* the texture of your skin.

"Some women need more coverage but not more color as they age," says makeup artist Sue Devitt. "Your skin loses some of its radiance, so you need to put on a luminous foundation, one that brings your skin to life and gives it a glow." Liquid foundation is much better than cream, says Devitt, because "it's not stiff, and it moves with your face." A sheer foundation can strike the perfect balance between an expressive, mutable face and some coverage. But avoid castor oil in foundation, because it tends to seep into little lines more readily than other ingredients do.

Tinted moisturizer is a good choice because it provides light coverage and adds moisture to older, drier skin. "The texture of makeup is important," says makeup artist Laura Mercier, "because it affects its performance." If your skin is good but marred by a brown spot, says Mercier, "camouflage it with concealer rather than covering the entire skin with makeup."

Powder eye shadow is also generally better than cream, which can seep into creases around the lids. Avoid dark, opaque colors, which will add years to your look. Light shades advance, while dark shades recede. Avoid matte lipstick, which also tends to set or harden the face. Cream is a better choice. And now is a good time to develop a close relationship with mascara, which can really bring out your eyes, especially if your lashes seem to have faded away. Wipe the wand first with a tissue so you won't apply too much, and use only on the top lashes.

Renova and Retin-A

AHAs, BHAs, PHAs, Retin-A, Renova, and even your humble oatmeal scrub all work on the same basic principle: they exfoliate your skin. If your skin is just beginning to show the signs of aging, AHAs will probably be enough treatment. If your skin is severely wrinkled and sun-damaged, consult your dermatologist and try the antiwrinkle prescription drug Renova. I prefer Renova to Retin-A because it's gentler on the skin. As Dr. Sara Colby, a San Diego dermatologist, explains, "Renova is the same as Retin-A, with the same active ingredient. The only difference is that it's in a moisturizing, emollient base so it's less irritating to older, dryer skin."

The active ingredient in both Renova and Retin-A is a Vitamin A derivative called tretinoin. Unlike AHAs, the tretinoin in Renova and Retin-A provokes actual chemical changes in the cells, which is why they're more irritating than AHAs. Tretinoin works on all layers of the skin, from the epidermis, where pigment changes occur (and where brown spots are born), to the dermis, where wrinkles begin. It is believed to correct the abnormal growth and differentiation of sun-damaged skin cells. But because it works on a deeper level, it takes longer to see a result.

As long as you follow the rules to the letter, Renova can make your face look smoother. But

Tip Though they don't often tell you the exact amount, over-the-counter AHAs generally contain concentrations of 3 to 7 percent acid—which is enough to exfoliate the skin. Some companies, such as M.D. Formulations, Exuviance, and Neostrata, offer higher concentrations—up to 20 percent— and in those cases you'll know exactly what percentage you're getting because they'll tout it. But I don't recommend high-level concentrations unless you're under a dermatologist's supervision—they're too irritating, and no one knows what the long-term effect on your skin will be.

WHO DOES WHAT BEST?

	MASS MARKET	PRESTIGE
AHAs	AVON, CHAMOCARE	ESTÉE LAUDER, ANNEMARIE BÖRLIND
BHAs	OIL OF OLAY	B. KAMINS, CLINIQUE
PHAs	L'ORÉAL	LANCÔME
Retinols	RoC, NIVEA	LANCÔME, ELIZABETH ARDEN
Antioxidants	NEUTROGENA	ESTÉE LAUDER

remember, the biggest benefit from Renova may be that your prescription forces you to use sun protection and moisturizer every day. (In a clinical study performed by Renova, 78 percent of the subjects showed improvement. But the placebo group, who were using Renova minus the active ingredient, showed a 43 percent improvement. My conclusion? The moisturizer alone improved the skin by 43 percent.) "It's not just the Renova, it's because you're staying out of the sun *and* using the moisture cream which is in Renova—regularly," says Dr. Ellen Gendler, a Manhattan dermatologist.

Although they are effective, I'm not a big fan of either Renova or Retin-A, and here's why: your skin will usually get worse before it gets better. The side effects include redness, dryness, itching, peeling, or a slight burning sensation, and they can last for a few weeks. Your skin will become extremely sensitive to the sun, and you'll have to wait up to six months for the full benefit. Plus, the

effects evaporate as soon as you stop using the product.

In any case, you need only one exfoliating product, not an entire battalion. If you use an acid, once a day is enough. Don't think that if a little is good, a lot is better. Piling it on only wastes money and can give your skin a fake, rubberized look. You won't have as many wrinkles, but if you use too much acid too

There's only one authentic Retin-A and one authentic Renova, and they're available by prescription only. Other products (Retinol-A, Rettin-A, and so on) may attempt **buyer beware** to mislead you into thinking you're getting the real thing, but you're not. (If you want Saint Laurent, would you buy Saint Laurie?) Cheaper versions are available outside the United States without a prescription, but there's no guarantee on quality control.

Beauty Buzz

Every Woman's Guide to the Antiaging Arsenal

Over the last 10 years, scientists have made enormous advances in the study of aging and its effects on the skin. There are now 1,700 different antiwrinkle creams on the market, and all promise to release "the real you," that baby-smooth self trapped beneath crusty layers of dried-up skin. Here's your state-of-the-art guide to the antiaging arsenal.

AHAS

These acid extracts exfoliate the top layer of skin. There are five types, all derived from natural or synthetic sources: citric (from citrus fruits), tartaric (from grapes), malic (from apples), lactic (from milk), and glycolic (from sugarcane). AHAs make the skin smoother, brighter, and softer. While they can help remove blemishes and discoloration, they can also irritate the skin, so use with discretion. Some AHAs claim to stimulate collagen production, but the scientific backup—though encouraging—is still inconclusive.

BHAS

These have the same effect as alpha-hydroxys but come from different sources (salicylic acid, wintergreen, benzoic acid, buteric acid) and may be less irritating. They'll also help keep your skin clear if you have acne. BHAs work especially well for oily skin with large pores, blemishes, and blackheads, because they can get inside the oil gland to exfoliate built-up skin cells that block the opening of the gland.

PHAS

Similar to AHAs, they moisturize better and don't sting as much.

AHA's...
Enzymes
PHA's
Renova
BHA's
Retin-A...

Unfortunately, the results aren't as good, because they don't penetrate as well. In other words, you don't get as much bang for your buck, but if your skin can't tolerate the burn from AHAs or BHAs, PHAs may work for you.

ANTIOXIDANTS

These ingredients, found in vitamins and other sources, moisturize dry, flaky skin and help repair, and possibly prevent, cell damage caused by free radicals—molecules that damage normal cells by depleting them of oxygen. (UV light, cigarette smoke, alcohol, and carbon monoxide all stimulate the production of free radicals.) The cumulative effects of free radicals are damage to skin cells and the breakdown of collagen.

The best way to get antioxidants is through your diet. The most potent are Vitamins A, C, and E and beta-carotene, but there is a long list of others also used in moisturizers. Vitamins in skincare products are listed on the ingredients label by their chemical names (see pages 16–17). They don't nourish the skin in the same way multiple vitamins provide nutrients to the body; if they did, you could just rub your vitamin pill on your cheek and be done with it. However appealing it may sound to drench your skin in vitamin creams, the jury is still out on whether or not they live up to their claims of actually exfoliating the skin, stimulating collagen production, and preventing wrinkles. Though promising, when it comes to the effects of topical antioxidants on the skin, the science is still hard to prove.

The most common antioxidants used topically in cosmetics are Vitamins C, E, and A. Ginkgo biloba and green tea, known as polyphenols, are the strongest known natural antioxidants. Beta glucans, derived from oats and shiitake mushrooms, are said to stimulate the immune system. Whether or not this is true, they do make the skin especially soft and smooth. Other antioxidants include grapeseed extract, green algae (flavonoids), lycopene (beta-carotene), ginseng, rosemary, juniper, horse chestnut, gluconolactone (the source of PHAs), licorice, lipoic acid, and alpha linoleic acid.

Hydroquinone and kojic acid. These skin lighteners bleach out brown spots. Hydroquinone, the more effective of the two, blocks the formation of melanin, which is egged on by sun exposure and hormones. It takes four months to work.

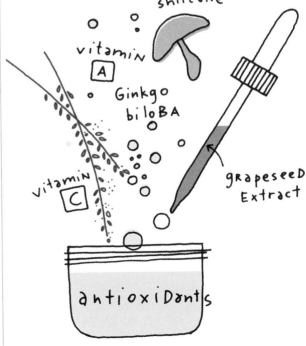

shiitake

vitamin A

Ginkgo biloBA

vitamin C

grapeseeD Extract

antioxiDants

VITAMINS

Vitamin A. Retin-A and Renova are prescription drugs that diminish wrinkles with a Vitamin A derivative called tretinoin. It improves the skin's texture and color and reduces fine lines and wrinkles, especially for deeply sun-damaged skin. (Retin-A also treats acne.) "Retinoids" are nonprescription "wanna-bes" that contain a less harsh—and less effective—Vitamin A derivative called retinol. Retinol exfoliates the skin and makes it smoother, but if your skin is really damaged, retinol is no substitute for its pharmaceutical distant cousins.

Vitamin C. Research shows that Vitamin C (L-ascorbic acid) is a powerful antioxidant that also offers some protection from UV radiation. Some products with Vitamin C claim to stimulate collagen production, but the jury is still out on this one as well. Unfortunately, Vitamin C in cosmetics is extremely unstable. It decomposes quickly (and turns orange) with exposure to heat and light. So as soon as you open your pricey jar, it begins to break down, and within a couple of days or weeks chances are it's worthless.

CERAMIDES

These synthetic lipids (fats) supposedly cleave to the skin's own lipids and help the skin retain moisture. When the lipids that hold skin cells together get poked full of holes through wear and tear, water evaporates, which causes dryness. Ceramides help remortar the wall.

CO-Q10

Coenzyme-Q10 An enzyme found in human cells, a version of Co-Q10 is taken internally to help prevent heart disease. Now used as an antioxidant, skin-smoothing, antiwrinkle ingredient in topical cosmetics, it's said to stimulate growth of new cells and produce firmer, smoother skin—but the scientific studies to back its efficacy aren't in yet.

COLLAGEN

Collagen in beauty products is either synthetic or taken from cows. Its ability to attract water to the skin makes it a superb moisturizing ingredient. Applied to the surface of the skin, however, it cannot rejuvenate our own collagen, which is mainly responsible for the skin's firmness.

ENZYMES

Derived from papaya, pineapple, or papain (a papaya derivative), these exfoliants can help even out your skin's color and tone and slow the breakdown of elastin. They're less irritating than AHAs, but, like Vitamin C, they're unstable. Chances are they've lost their effectiveness before you even open the jar.

HORMONES

The newest hormone creams contain wild yam extract (a plant source of progesterone), soy (a plant source of estrogen), and melatonin, an antioxidant hormone that naturally triggers the sleep cycle. But there's really no good reason to use hormones on your face. The dryness that accompanies lower levels of estrogen is best dealt with by using a good moisturizer.

MINERAL MAKEUP

When your face is especially raw or sensitive after a laser procedure or a peel and you want some coverage, most makeup is a no-go because it will irritate your skin. But not this stuff. It seems that the appeal—and efficacy—of mineral makeup lies largely in what it's not: mineral makeup contains no potentially irritating talcs, fragrances, preservatives, alcohol, FD&C dyes, or aluminum. The foundation is so pared down— it's literally ground-up rocks—that its purity makes it good for sensitive, acne-prone skin or skin recovering from laser surgery, cosmetic surgery, or other dermatological procedures.

Here are the top brands: Bare Escentuals, Bare Escentuals boutiques nationwide; Colorescience, Nordstrom, www.colorescience.com; La Bella Donna, Bergdorf Goodman; Youngblood, www.ybskin.com.

Cosmetic Dermatology

Cosmetic dermatology is now so popular that many dermatologists depend on quickie "lunchtime peels," injections, and implants for up to 90 percent of their business. Once relegated to the Siberia of medicine, dermatology has recently emerged as a glamor profession, along with plastic surgery. And as the demand for antiaging treatments has exploded—and as doctors' incomes have become severely restricted by the rules of managed care—many dermatologists have transformed themselves into beauty gurus. Their practices now include spa services and lucrative product lines, as well as the state-of-the-art medical stuff: peels, botox injections, and laser procedures.

Not all dermatologists are equally resourceful, of course. Many have not yet invested in expensive lasers, preferring to use the tried-and-true, older methods of treatment like dermabrasion and phenol peels, despite their drawbacks. The reason a doctor may recommend one procedure over another often has more to do with the doctor's confidence level in performing that particular procedure than with its actual effectiveness. For example, a doctor who is vastly experienced in dermabrasion may recommend it over a new laser treatment that he hasn't practiced very often. "Old therapies aren't necessarily bad therapies," writes Joan Kron in *Lift,* an excellent book on cosmetic surgery. "They're still around because they've stood the test of time, and doctors using them know what to expect."

assiduously—even the low percentages you'll find in cosmetic products—you can end up with what is, essentially, scar tissue. Your face won't have the flexibility, bounce, or glow of normal skin. Although some dermatologists suggest doubling up—an AHA in the morning along with Renova or Retin-A at night—always check with your doctor before using anything on your face when you are using prescription treatments. They are drugs, after all.

Nonetheless, laser procedures are clearly the wave of the future. They will probably take over eventually, but until then, the procedure you choose is only as good as the doctor who performs it.

Facial Peels

Some dermatologists make a peel sound as easy as a haircut, even though what they're doing is burning off layers of your skin with acid. Chemical peels treat fine lines and wrinkles; leathery, sun-damaged skin; acne and acne scars; blotchiness, brown spots, freckles, and irregular pigmentation. They can't correct sagging skin, deep wrinkles, scarring, or broken blood vessels. (Those require dermabrasion, laser treatment, or surgery.)

Even the most superficial chemical peel is best performed by a dermatologist, dermatologic surgeon, or plastic surgeon in a doctor's office or as an outpatient procedure in a clinic or surgery center. Here's the typical procedure for a dermatologist's peel:

After cleaning your face to remove residual surface oils and cosmetics, the doctor will apply a glycolic acid solution to your face with a swab. You'll sit for a few minutes with glistening acid on your face—it stings—while it penetrates. Next, a neutralizer (sodium bicarbonate —remember baking soda?) is applied to neutralize the acid, followed by a postpeel moisturizer. Before you leave, the doctor will advise a follow-up regimen that includes use of an AHA moisturizer and sun protection.

After the peel, you'll look like you have a light sunburn for anywhere from a few hours to three or four days, until your skin calms down.

The tender new skin below is smoother and initially more fragile and sensitive to the sun. The general rule with peels is: the more pain, the more gain. "The higher the level of acid," according to Dr. Mark Rubin, a Beverly Hills dermatologist, "the greater the delivery to the skin, and the greater the rejuvenating effects. However, the higher the potential for irritation." Deeper peels (up to 70 percent AHA) leave the skin redder and more irritated for a longer period of time, because they work at a deeper level.

Superficial peels (aka "mini peels" or "lunchtime peels") are less painful because the solution is less concentrated (about 30 percent concentration of glycolic or lactic acid). These heal more quickly, but the results are more

---

HOW TO FIND A GOOD DERMATOLOGIST

Remember, no matter how technologically advanced they are, tools are only as good as the talents of those who wield them. So choose your practitioner with care. For cosmetic dermatology—those procedures performed on the surface of the skin— seek out a qualified dermatologist or dermatologic surgeon. The American Society for Dermatologic Surgery will provide referrals to dermatologists or dermatologic surgeons around the country (800-441-2737; www.asds-net.org); so will the American Academy of Dermatology (888-462-3376; www.aad.org). Or ask your primary care doctor for a recommendation. When you have a shortlist of names, schedule a few consultations and shop around. If you're combining a surgical procedure with cosmetic dermatology, you will need to go to a plastic surgeon or cosmetic surgeon (see appendix A).

ABOUT FACE: THE ANATOMY OF AGING

Below the surface, the skin's support structure—the bonds between the connective tissues—loosen, and the elastin loses its "snap." Collagen production slows down naturally, the skin becomes thinner, and the face starts to droop. As we age, our body also loses calcium, and our bones, including the skull, shrink, but the surrounding skin doesn't, causing the problem Polonius complained of in *Hamlet* when he lamented, "My skin hangs about me like an old lady's gown." Here is what happens.

▪ Eyes. The upper lids loosen, the lower lids get puffy, and lines form alongside and underneath the eyes.

▪ Nasolabial folds. Lines etch in from the outside of the nose down to the corners of the mouth.

▪ Jawline and jowls loosen.

▪ Frown lines form between the eyebrows.

▪ Horizontal lines creep across the forehead.

▪ Dark, discolored spots develop and broken capillaries appear.

▪ Vertical lines groove the upper lip.

superficial. They can get rid of light wrinkles, rough skin, and blotchy spots. Unlike deeper peels like TCA or phenol (see page 80), they don't permanently lighten the skin, which means that they're a good bet for dark skin types, too. According to Dr. Thomas Romo, director of Facial Plastic and Reconstructive Surgery at the New York Eye and Ear Infirmary, a superficial AHA or glycolic acid peel "does what a Buf-Puf does—but with chemicals."

I recommend the Refinity peel, because it's the only physician-dispensed line, to date, that contains a built-in moisturizer. Also, this is the only one I've seen that's truly a "lunchtime peel." In other words, it takes only 20 to 30 minutes, and there is no lingering redness or irritation, even though it's a strong solution. Because Refinity contains an anti-irritant, your skin can tolerate a 70 percent peel right away, with better results.

TCA peels. This deeper peel is usually done with a 30 to 40 percent trichloroacetic acid solution in the doctor's office without anesthetic. It is used to treat hypopigmentation (whiteouts) and hyperpigmentation (dark spots), deep wrinkles, mild scarring, and blotchiness. Because it smooths the skin, a TCA peel (or a laser treatment) is sometimes performed in conjunction with a face-lift. Doctors also use TCA to remove age spots or precancerous spots or to lighten dark spots under the eyes. Because it lightens the skin, it's not advisable for women with dark skin.

DOWNSIDE: Because a TCA peel reaches the dermis, there is potential for permanent scarring, hyperpigmentation, hypopigmentation, and infection. Ask your doctor about these possible risks. And expect redness, swelling, and the need to stick close to home for a while. The healing time is seven days to two weeks.

Phenol peels. When doctors first started using peels, the deep phenol peel was the one and only. Phenolic acid is a coal-tar derivative also known as carbolic acid. It was used to burn off everything from freckles to severely sun-damaged skin. Because of its potential for permanent scarring and pigment changes, hardly anyone uses this treatment anymore, though it can be useful to smooth (and, to some extent, tighten) the surface of the skin.

DOWNSIDE: Deep peels are even less predictable than dermabrasion because acid penetrates the skin at variable rates that can't be manually controlled the way dermabrasion can be. Healing time is 10 to 20 days, and after the peel, your skin will be red and raw for a few weeks.

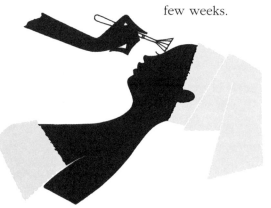

Collagen Injections

The most common way to plump up wrinkles, grooves, shallow scars, and hollows on the face is by using collagen and fat injections, known as SAM (Superficial Augmentation Material). The collagen comes from cows and is injected into wrinkles around the lips, the lips themselves, crow's-feet, shallow forehead wrinkles, and nasolabial folds. Collagen injections fill in a wrinkle and literally smooth it out. When injected into the lips, collagen makes them more pillowy. The procedure takes 20 to 30 minutes. The results are immediate. Occasional swelling and puffiness last a couple of days.

Not everyone can tolerate a foreign substance injected into the body, and for some people, these injections can compromise the body's ability to tolerate its own collagen. (If you have lupus or another autoimmune disease, discuss this risk with your doctor.) A dermatologist should always test your skin for allergic reactions—at least twice—before beginning treatment. He'll inject a bit of collagen into your arm, wait 48 hours, check for redness or swelling, wait a month, and look again. Some will test you a third time, after another month, to make absolutely sure that you're not allergic.

Instead of cow collagen, some doctors use a synthetic filler called Fibrel, a powder that is mixed with the patient's blood and then injected into the wrinkle. It is less likely to cause sensitivity, but, like collagen, the effect lasts only a few months, until it dissolves in the body.

If you really love yourself, another choice is to have your very own collagen cloned and injected. The doctor sends a bit of your skin off to a lab that cultures it, keeps it in liquid nitrogen, and "farms" it forever. *You* may be getting older, but your collagen's not.

DOWNSIDE: Some people suddenly develop an allergic reaction even after successfully tolerating collagen injections for several treatments. In these cases, bumps develop at the injection site. They can last up to three months, and they're no fun. Plus, collagen injections get expensive, because they need to be repeated every three to six months.

POKER FACE

In the Victorian era, a woman was advised to keep her face free of wrinkles at all costs—even if that meant keeping her face devoid of expression. In *Personal Beauty,* two 19th-century doctors, D. G. Brinton and G. H. Napheys, advised women to "Avoid frowning and grimaces which contract the muscles of the face, do not sit by a bright light, which forces you to squint and half close the eyes, and maintain as much command as possible over the facial muscles. . . . Undoubtedly, half the lines which seem the face of maturity are not those of years, but of passion, of chagrin, or of habitual contortion of the muscles. They can therefore be prevented, and when they are just beginning to show themselves, they can be diminished by a strong exertion of self-command."

If you think inhibition of our natural expressiveness is buried in the past, think again. Nowadays, we have botox injections, which temporarily paralyze the muscle that allows you to move the skin on your forehead, and we have technology that allows us to cut the procerus muscle and obliterate frowning permanently.

Lipo-Injection or Fat Transfer

Fat injections are the ultimate in recycling. And because the fat is your own, this technique avoids the allergic reactions that may result from introducing collagen into your body. The injections are often performed in conjunction with liposuction; the doctor practically has to do liposuction anyway to remove the fat for a fat transfer. Patients come back every four to six weeks until they're happy with the way they look.

If the transplanted fat becomes supplied with blood vessels, or vascularized, the transfer is permanent. Dr. Patricia Wexler, a Manhattan dermatologist, says that since only a small percent of blood vessels per injection will vascularize, she gives repeated treatments in small doses, in the hope of making the effect as permanent as possible. She extracts, processes, and stores fat in the deep freeze.

DOWNSIDE: The procedure has to be repeated every three months. Some swelling will occur the first day. The site may be bandaged for a day or two to help stabilize the fat.

Botox, or Botulinum Toxin

If you're a squinter or a scowler, you may have developed vertical furrows between your brows or horizontal creases across your brow. In the past, these would have been smoothed with silicone injections or a brow lift. The most modern option available—botox injections—could easily have sprung from the pages of a Stephen King novel.

In large enough doses, botox can cause botulism and can kill you by paralyzing your diaphragm muscles. It's long been used by pediatric ophthalmologists, however, to straighten out crossed eyes and calm muscular twitches and tics in children. In this case, the doctor injects minute quantities of botulinum toxin, or botox, into the offending scowl. The injection paralyzes the procerus muscle so that you are physically unable to squint, scowl, or grimace and, as a consequence, you no longer *can* wrinkle between the eyes. The results are noticeable

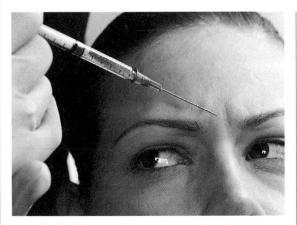

A little jab'll do ya. Botox injections have become a means to the end of scowl lines.

in three to five days and last for up to nine months. Whatever wrinkles you already had fade over time, because you are no longer reinforcing them through repetitive motion.

Doctors have expanded the botox repertoire to include erasing lines around the eyes and mouth, smoothing saggy neck skin, and eliminating laugh—or sneer—lines at the corners of the mouth. Botox injections are replacing collagen in popularity because they last up to nine months. And at about $500 a treatment, they end up being more cost-effective.

DOWNSIDE: Though you'd need at least 1,000 times the dosage used to cause botulism, if you end up in the hands of an inexperienced practitioner and too much botox is injected—an extremely rare occurrence—you can temporarily lose the use of other muscles in the area and develop droopy eyelids, a lopsided expression, or temporary vision impairment.

Dermabrasion

Dermabrasion is a technique used to remove deep acne and chicken-pox scars, rosacea, broken blood vessels, sun-damaged skin, tattoos, precancerous lesions, and other facial lacerations. It first became popular in the 1950s, when the main tool, a wire rotary brush, was introduced to scrape off layers of skin, and it hasn't changed much since.

Today, since peels and laser treatments offer a neater, cleaner, less painful alternative with a shorter healing time, dermabrasion would be considered a last choice.

DOWNSIDE: This is a bloody procedure, and the aftereffects can be uncomfortable; the skin swells, and you won't be presentable for a couple of weeks. You must wear sunscreen for a long time, or your skin can become pigmented.

Laser Resurfacing

"Lasers are at the cutting edge of skincare technology," says Dr. Ariana Scheibner, a Beverly Hills M.D. who devotes 90 percent of her practice to "perfecting complexions." Using a local anesthetic and a quick, concentrated beam of light, the doctor burns off the top layers of wrinkled skin, especially the furrows at the corners of the mouth, chin wrinkles, and smile lines.

Lasers are now used to do most things that doctors once did with deep peels or dermabrasion. Doctors are also using lasers instead of surgery, especially for cosmetic treatment of puffy lower eyelids. Because the laser cauterizes the cut, there is less bleeding and the surgeon can work faster, which means reduced swelling and bruising. According to the American Society for Dermatologic Surgery, the laser may offer advantages over traditional surgery because it's relatively bloodless, the risk of infection is small, it's precisely controlled to limit the injury, and

WEIRD SCIENCE

Several years ago, in France, the epitome of *richesse* was the "gold thread treatment," in which solid gold thread (an inert, nonreactive substance) was implanted beneath a wrinkle to smooth it out. More recently, scientists have developed cosmetic uses for materials that are more bourgeois—maybe that's why they call it "wash-and-wear" dermatology. For example, Gore-Tex, the material you wear on your back when it's raining, is now used to bulk up lips and nasolabial folds. Gore-Tex is popular because it's extremely biocompatible (strips of Gore-Tex have traditionally been used for hernia repair) and readily available.

Even though the lips are one of the most sensitive, blood-engorged areas of the body, the doctors I interviewed claim that Gore-Tex implants do not affect sensation in the lips. Doctors also say that you can't feel it afterward unless it's not implanted deeply enough, in which case you not only feel it but the area becomes inflamed. Sometimes the Gore-Tex shifts a bit, but doctors agree that if you don't like it, it's easy enough to take out. Or you can choose Soft-Form, a permanent injectable implant that is replacing Gore-Tex in popularity because it is more pliant. Like Gore-Tex, Soft-Form shores up grooves in the face. It, too, can shift a bit, and tiny Dr. Frankenstein–style stitch marks may be apparent at the site of implantation.

Alloderm, a freeze-dried patch of cadaverous dermis—that's right, skin from a corpse—is something Mary Shelley would have had a field day with. As with many breakthroughs in cosmetic dermatology, Alloderm was originally developed to aid burn victims. Your body doesn't reject this "second skin" because it's sterilized. Over time, your body "snatches" the dead tissue: your own tissue grows into it and incorporates it as its own.

Are these miracle treatments or signs of a macabre new world? Stay tuned.

there is less scarring than with scalpel surgery.

Lasers are used to remove vascular lesions, scars, brown spots, fine lines and wrinkles, tattoos, blood vessels, port-wine stains (like Mikhail Gorbachev's), and freckles. They can also repair sun damage, erase acne scars, and remove precancerous lesions. Lasers can be used to resurface dark-skinned and African American complexions without lightening the skin the way some peels do. And they can zap broken capillaries and help eradicate stretch marks.

DOWNSIDE: You can expect to feel a mild burning and swelling for 4 to 24 hours after a laser treatment. You will also look as if you have a terrible sunburn for a week or two. Doctors use Vitamin K cream to reduce the redness. To avoid problems after treatments, follow-up visits are essential.

Lasers can burn and scar the skin, and no one really knows the long-term effects. They may also leave your face looking shiny, and there's no way to predict in advance whether this will happen to you. Laser treatments take a long time to heal. Sometimes it's two months before all the irritation or redness fades and skin color returns to normal.

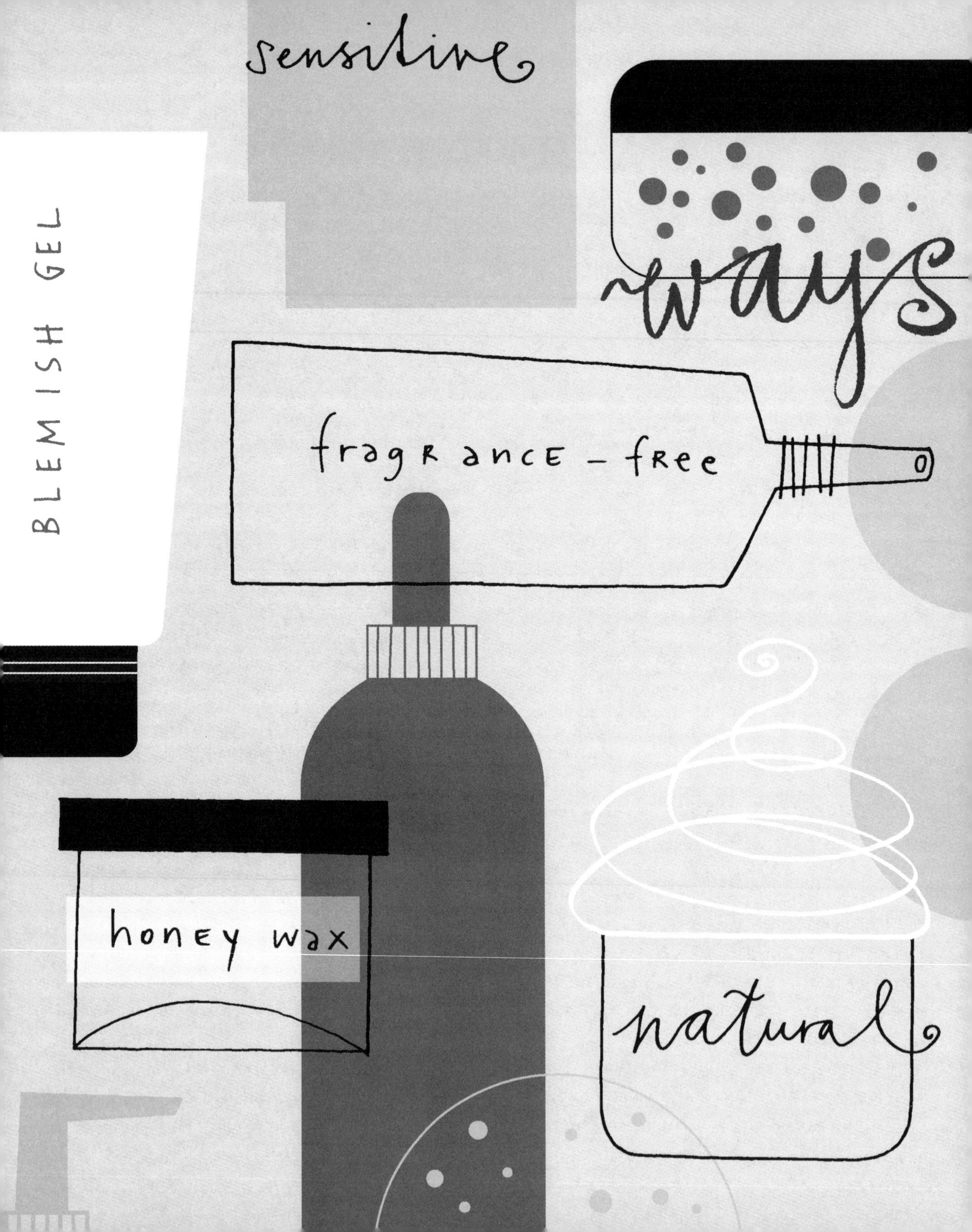

sensitive

ways

fragrance - free

honey wax

natural

of the flesh

If it's not one thing, it's another.

—GILDA RADNER

Most of us learn to live with, if not love, the little quirks that uniquely punctuate our all-too-human flesh. An insouciant mole or dimple on the cheek can easily add to our charm. But what about the more irritating recurrent conditions like red bumps, flaky patches, and adult acne? Do we have to learn to tolerate those, too? Or can we simply banish them forever?

There are close to 1,000 diseases and conditions that affect the skin. The skin is a vast and complex organ; every single cell sheds and replaces itself about every three weeks in layers that are fossil-thick on the soles of the feet and paper-thin on the eyelids. So it's not surprising that in this delicate dance of cellular rejuvenation, missteps can occur. This chapter will deal with the most common skin problems and tell you what you can do about them.

Adult Acne

If you thought you'd seen your last pimple at 15 and your face is breaking out again at 35, join the club. You weren't alone then, and you aren't now either. Adult acne is a big problem for one in five women between the ages of 25 and 40. And with an average of 900 oil glands per square centimeter on the face, upper neck, and chest, it's no surprise that more than 20 million Americans suffer from some form of acne.

Acne usually begins with blackheads. Contrary to popular opinion, blackheads are not dirt. They are the result of oil and dead cells that get trapped in a pore, block the duct, and mix with bacteria. The secretion turns black through exposure to the air. Women with overactive oil glands and large pores are most prone to blackheads and pimples. Red pimples (papules) develop when blackheads become inflamed, and they spread when touched with dirty fingers. If the pimple becomes infected, a whitehead or pustule can develop. This is the type of blemish that can burst and may eventually scar. The biggest, baddest blemish of all is a cyst—the red, swollen result of a deeper infection. If you develop cysts, you should definitely see a dermatologist; don't try to take care of these by yourself.

Many women develop acne for the first time in their 30s or 40s, after an unblemished adolescence. Adult acne usually appears on the face, neck, back, and shoulders. It is caused by proliferation of bacteria (so keep your hands and face clean!), oversecretion of the oil glands (minimize stress!), and hyperkeratinization, or dead cells clogging the surface pores of the face (exfoliate!). Many sufferers find that the condition worsens in the summer, when they sweat more. Anything that irritates your skin can lead to breakouts.

Causes of Adult Acne

Stress. When you're stressed out, the pituitary gland increases your hormone production, which stimulates the adrenal glands. The adrenals, in turn, secrete androgen, and too much androgen can enlarge the oil glands and stimulate excess sebum production, which can clog the pores and cause acne.

Bad Cosmetics Choices. Cosmetic acne is just what it sounds like—acne caused by oily, pore-clogging ingredients in your makeup and skincare products. It is so prevalent that it eventually spawned the growth of oil-free cleansers,

moisturizers, and foundation. Breakouts on your cheeks may also be caused by sensitivity to D&C red dyes in your blush.

Cosmetic acne looks like a raft of tiny pimples and shows up most often—but not only—on oily skin. If your skin is oily, avoid cosmetics, creams, and cleansers containing heavy oils like lanolin or mineral oil, which can clog the pores (see page 91). Stick to water-based foundation and loose powder rather than pressed. And avoid cream blushes and alcohol-based products, which can overdry and irritate the skin, upset its natural pH, and cause the oil glands to overcompensate and produce excess oil.

Hormones. Acne is common in adolescence, when raging hormones stimulate the sebaceous glands and they become more active. But hormonal imbalances can also trigger acne well after a woman passes through puberty. You may be among the 70 percent of grown women who experience breakouts two to seven days before menstruation because your sebaceous glands go crazy and your skin becomes oilier. Here's the standard scenario: for up to a week after your period, your skin can behave erratically—while it regains the proper balance. For the next two weeks, your skin behaves more or less well, until your estrogen levels rise again. If you're in your 40s, sudden breakouts in the lower cheeks and chin could be the result of the fluctuations in estrogen levels that lead to perimenopause.

Birth Control Pills and Other Medications. Sometimes the Pill can help clear up acne, while other times it can cause acne as well as hyperpigmentation. Some women break out after going on a pill high in androgen or discontinuing a pill high in estrogen. Tell your doctor if you're having a problem—switching to another type could help.

Common cold remedies that contain bromides and iodides can also trigger outbreaks of acne. So can barbiturates and high doses of Vitamin B$_{12}$. Lithium and steroids, especially cortisone, can also make you break out.

Treatments for Acne

You don't need to ban cheese or chocolate from your diet; it won't help. (Although for some women, acne can be aggravated by the iodides in the seaweed wrapped around sushi makki or the potassium iodide found in vitamin tablets.) But you should do something—and fast. Before you go to the dermatologist, first try a facial. A good facialist can treat acne nonmedically, which, in the long run, is the best way.

Acne Facials

After suffering from breakouts on one side of my face every month for years, I asked a colleague with beautiful skin for her recommendation. As it turned out, my colleague had been taking tetracycline to control her acne, under a dermatologist's care, from the age of 15 until her mid-20s. She finally got fed up and went to the Elena Schell Skincare Clinic in Manhattan, and Schell's natural products and treatments cleared up her face in three months. Fifteen years later, she still has beautiful skin. So I decided to give it a try—and I've been an ardent

BACK OFF!

If you have acne on your back or shoulders, go for a "back facial." Follow up the treatment at home by washing with a salicylic acid soap like SalAc or Sastid, which exfoliates the skin, or a beta-hydroxy acid body wash. (Salicylic acid is related to aspirin, so if you're allergic to aspirin, do a patch test first. If you have an allergic reaction, try Neutrogena, Aveeno, Basis, or Purpose soap instead.)

proponent of facials to control acne ever since. Every woman with acne whom I've ever sent for a facial has seen a vast improvement in her skin. The regimen for women with acne—sulfur, zinc, and camphor masks; conscientious exfoliation; blackhead extractions; and at-home follow-up care—works, if you become one of the faithful and stick with it.

"I am against medication for acne, because acne is not a disease," says Schell. "It's a condition of the skin. It can be controlled, but it cannot be cured, because no medication exists to slow down and control the seborrheic secretion (oil glands) except Accutane, and that has too many side effects."

But you don't need heavy artillery to treat acne or the chronic breakouts caused by oily skin. Why start with drugs if there's

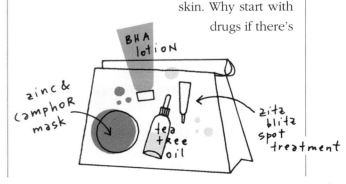

ZITS BLITZ

If you want to keep your skin free of bacteria, dead cells, and product residue, mix 1 tablespoon of apple cider vinegar or white vinegar into a cup of warm water, then pat on the face with a soft, clean cloth or cotton balls, says Tammy Ha, a cosmetic chemist formerly with Neutrogena. Applied once a week, it will keep pimples at bay, says Ha, "because the bacteria that cause pimples are not acid-tolerant, and they *die, die, die.*" Not even the strong will survive.

another way? Take my word for it: go for three facials at six-week intervals, and then judge the results. (See appendix C, page 361, for facialists around the United States.)

Doctors' Orders

The time to consult a dermatologist is when you have severe acne—if your entire face is broken out, or if you have chronic whiteheads or cysts. Dermatologists treat acne in a variety of ways. Most often they'll prescribe an oral antibiotic like tetracycline, which kills off bacteria and keeps your skin's oil secretions from going haywire. But because the oral antibiotic treatment of acne is a long-term commitment, there is cause for concern. Long-term use of antibiotics can make bacteria resistant to the treatment and possibly lower your immunity to other diseases. Plus, as with most medications, there are side effects that may include nausea, sun sensitivity, and vaginal infections. The effectiveness of some birth control pills is also diminished by tetracycline—so if tetracycline is prescribed, let your doctor know if you're on the Pill.

Retin-A (tretinoin), a topically applied, Vitamin A–based prescription drug, is another popular treatment for acne. Although it's now more frequently prescribed as a wrinkle peeler, Retin-A was first marketed as an acne medication some 30 years ago. Retin-A treats acne by peeling away the unwanted skin, unplugging the oil glands, and stimulating the growth of healthy skin. Side effects include redness, peeling, extreme dryness, and sun sensitivity. I'll never forget when a colleague at *ELLE* magazine slathered Retin-A all over her face, went out shopping on a sunny day, and was unable to come to work for three days afterward because she looked like a burn victim. If you use Retin-A, make sure to wear an SPF 15 sunscreen with active ingredients that include titanium dioxide, zinc oxide, or Parsol 1789.

Other newer topical prescription medications are also Vitamin A derivatives. Two of the most popular, tazarotene (aka Tazorac) and adapolene (aka Differin) loosen clogged pores and prevent new pimples. Sometimes these are prescribed in conjunction with oral antibiotics.

The drug of last resort is a powerful oral medication called Accutane. A synthetic Vitamin A derivative (retinoid), Accutane may be prescribed for serious and recurrent acne, the type that leads to deep cysts, pitting, and scars. Accutane inhibits oil production, which is how it dries acne. Although it works, its potential for harm far outweighs its ability to do good. Unfortunately, excessive dryness and chapping are among the least of its side effects, which can include headaches, hair loss, joint pain, elevated cholesterol and triglyceride levels, and liver problems related to excessive levels of

Vitamin A. But the biggest problem is the drug's potential to cause birth defects: therefore, doctors monitor its use very carefully among women of childbearing age.

At-Home Care

Adult acne can be traumatic, especially if you've never had acne before. Stick to this simple, daily regimen, designed to keep your skin dirt-free and oil-free—without overdrying it—and it won't be long before you'll see a definite improvement! Once the breakouts clear up, you can avoid future problems by maintaining your routine.

1. Wash at least twice a day with an oil-free, beta-hydroxy or gel cleanser. Even though "oil-free" products contain trace amounts of oil, they're minuscule, and these products are by far the best for you if your skin breaks out. If your breakout is more severe, beta-hydroxy cleansers will add a little extra "oomph" to your cleansing (see page 27).

2. Exfoliate four or five nights a week with a beta-hydroxy lotion or cream or a gentle scrub. (If you use a scrub, choose one with the soft consistency of baking soda or potato flour. No rough stuff!)

3. Apply a mask once a week. The masks (and spot treatments) in this chapter are especially good for keeping acne at bay. For those of you not inclined toward making your own masks, see pages 56–57 for recommended commercially available products.

4. Use an oil-free moisturizer. What's the use in clearing up pimples if you overdry your skin and develop flaking and dermatitis in the process?

5. Use a sunblock. Avoid products with pore-clogging ingredients (see page 91).

AUSSIE TEA TREE TREATMENT

Tea tree oil is an elixir to the gods of the bush in rural Australia. Aboriginal people use it for practically everything related to skin, but because it's antiseptic, analgesic, and anti-inflammatory, it will send your pimples packing.

> *1 drop tea tree oil (available at health food stores and some pharmacies)*
> *½ cup milk or water*

1. Mix the tea tree oil into the milk or water.
2. Swab on your face with cotton.
3. Rinse off after 5 to 10 minutes.

You can also use a Q-tip to swab this mixture directly on blemishes.

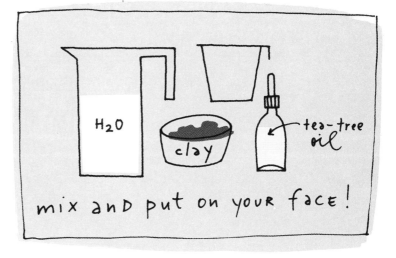

mix and put on your face!

CURDS AND CLAY

Yogurt kills bacteria and helps soften skin.

> 4 tablespoons clay
> 2 teaspoons plain yogurt
> 4 teaspoons water
> 2 drops tea tree or geranium oil
>   (or you can boil fresh thyme in water
>   and replace the water above with
>   4 teaspoons thyme water)

1. Mix the ingredients to form a paste.
2. Apply to your face with clean fingers.
3. Leave on for 15 minutes.
4. Rinse off with warm water.

BLACKHEADS BE GONE

And you thought parsley was only good for garnish . . .

> A bunch of parsley

1. Run the parsley through a blender.
2. Prepare steam according to directions on pages 58–59.
3. Apply the blended parsley to your clogged areas (T-Zone, anyone?).
4. Steam your face with the parsley mixture on it for 5 minutes.
5. Follow with an exfoliating mask or *gently* exfoliate your face with a scrub. And no matter how great the temptation—*do not pick!*

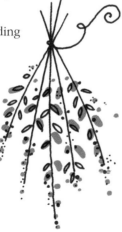

The "Clearasil" Panacea

At-home products are not going to clear up a massive breakout, but there are on-the-spot treatments that work quickly and effectively on a small area of blemished skin. More important is a consistent, healthy skincare regimen, which will keep the problem under control in the first place.

Beta-Hydroxy Acids. These contain salicylic acid, which exfoliates the skin and helps keep it unclogged. Try these products—Oil of Olay Age-Defying Lotion, Clinique Turnaround Cream—or wash with a BHA cleanser at night. If your skin is really oily, use the cleanser in the morning, too. For a quick fix, try Pond's Clear Solutions Overnight Blemish Reducers (medicated adhesive strips) or Bioré Blemish Bomb. Both deliver salicylic acid to the skin in an encapsulated form that makes it more effective.

Camphor, Sulfur, Mint Lotions. Many facialists create their own brew of acne lotions and gels, and many are excellent. Calamine, camphor, eucalyptus, mint, and sulfur are favorite ingredients because they dry up pimples. (Unfortunately, most sulfur lotions smell bad.) Clinique and Shiseido (Pureness) are the companies to turn to if you have oily, blemished skin.

FREE AND CLEAR:
HOW TO LIBERATE YOUR PORES

The ingredients in the left-hand column are comedogenic, which means that they clog pores and can cause blackheads, pimples, or cosmetics-related acne. You may be wondering why these substances are used in cosmetics at all if they clog the skin. The answer? They're cheap!

Most people don't realize that even lipsticks, eye creams, and hair pomades can spread to the surrounding skin and cause breakouts. Be sure to check the ingredients lists on your cleansers, moisturizers, makeup, and sunscreens, and avoid these potentially pore-clogging ingredients if your skin is prone to breakouts. Instead, look for the good alternative ingredients in the right-hand column.

PROBLEM INGREDIENT	FOUND IN	GOOD ALTERNATIVES
COCOA BUTTER, ISOPROPYL MYRISTATE	Sunscreen, moisturizer, massage cream, lipstick, blush, body lotion	Plant oils (except coconut), kalaya oil, vegetable glycerine, propylene glycol, polyethylene glycol, butylene glycol (these are partially petroleum-based but formulated not to clog oily skin)
-CINNAMATES, -SALICYLATES, OCTYL PALMITATE, PABA	Sunscreen	Titanium dioxide, zinc oxide, Parsol 1789
SHEA BUTTER	Moisturizer, soap, shampoo	Plant oils (except coconut), kalaya oil, vegetable glycerine, propylene glycol, polyethylene glycol, butylene glycol
COCONUT OIL, LANOLIN	Moisturizer, soap, shampoo, hair conditioner, pomade, massage cream, body lotion, blush, eye cream, foundation, cold cream, lipstick	
MINERAL OIL	Most inexpensive drugstore cleansers, moisturizers, and makeup; cold cream; eye cream; hair conditioner; sunscreen; makeup remover	
PETROLATUM	Moisturizer, cold cream, balm, wax depilatories, eye shadow, blush, cream foundation, lipstick, baby-care products	Beeswax, jojoba wax, carnauba wax, candelilla wax
PARAFFIN	Cold cream, wax depilatories, eyebrow pencil, lip balm, cleanser	Beeswax, jojoba wax, carnauba wax, candelilla wax
D&C RED DYES, FD&C RED DYES	Blush, lipstick, powder	Carmine, annatto, cochineal powder, caramel, grapeskin extract, iron oxide

There is actually a medical condition called *acne excoriae des jeunes filles,* a self-mutilating, obsessive-compulsive disorder that largely affects young women who can't stop picking their faces, to the point where they disfigure themselves. If your picking is extreme, consult a doctor.

Benzoyl Peroxide. This bacteria-killing medication is available in prescription and non-prescription forms, if your acne is bad. But overuse can overdry and peel the skin, so use it for only a week at a time. Wash with a benzoyl peroxide cleanser, or look for a 2 to 5 percent concentration of medication; anything higher is too strong.

Hydrogen Peroxide. An antibacterial ingredient that keeps your skin antiseptically clean, but it's too harsh on its own. Try Karin Herzog's Vit-A-Kombi 2 cream.

Azelaic Acid. An antibacterial cream prescribed by doctors to unclog pores.

Plant Oils. Tea tree oil is a highly effective, antiseptic, analgesic, anti-inflammatory oil derived from the Australian tea tree plant. Unfortunately, some versions smell so medicinal you may not care how well they work. Look for versions that blend tea tree oil with other oils. (It's still no olfactory picnic.) Try Desert Essence Organically Grown Tea Tree and Lavender oil or balm or Tea Tree Solutions tea tree ointment.

The Samuel Parr Aromatherapy Blemish Pen is a blend of oils, including clove, that you can pop in your purse and dab on a pimple throughout the day (it's invisible).

The Top Five Acne Don'ts

1. Never, never pick or extract blackheads or whiteheads yourself. "You can spread the contents deep into the oil gland and surrounding tissue and cause a cystic infection," says dermatologist Dr. Patricia Wexler. And you can stretch and disfigure the pore—permanently.

When you squeeze a pimple, you push the sebum down through the pore, and the pore can rupture. When it ruptures, the sebum enters the oil gland and possibly the surrounding tissue, which can cause irritation and scarring. If

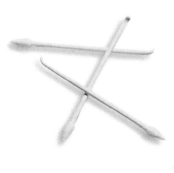

the only way to restrain yourself from squeezing is to wash your face with the lights out or stay away from mirrors, do it! But whatever you do, don't pick.

That said, let's get real. If you are going to squeeze a blackhead anyway, at least do it right. Wash your face and hands, and use two Q-tips (or two tissues, one in each hand) to gently ease the contents out of your skin. Do not use your bare fingers! Follow with an antiseptic dab from your Samuel Parr Aromatherapy Blemish Pen or tea tree oil, and *don't touch,* or you'll introduce bacteria and create an infection—in other words, a pimple.

2. Don't use astringents with harsh alcohols (see page 33) and soaps that overdry and strip the skin. They can make the acne worse because the oil glands will overcompensate and secrete even *more* oil. There's also a good chance that you'll develop dermatitis and skin that feels taut and dry—and get caught up in a cycle of overmoisturizing.

3. If you have developed mysterious bumps on your forehead, especially around your hairline, check the haircare products you use. Alcohol, emollients, and the fragrances in some gels and sprays can aggravate the skin. Either discontinue use of the product or put a thick terrycloth headband around your forehead whenever you apply it.

4. Don't go for a facial more often than every six weeks. (Although an at-home mask every week or two is fine.) This is a case when too much of a good thing—extractions, massage, exfoliation—can inflame or irritate the skin.

5. Don't rest your chin on your hands, and keep your hands off your face. Didn't your mother tell you that?

Acne Impersonator

A pimple is a pimple is a pimple, right? Wrong. There is a certain skin condition that looks and feels like acne but isn't. Once you understand and unmask the true culprit, you'll be able to treat it, get rid of it, and get on with your life.

Tip To avoid the red swath of pimples on the cheeks that characterizes rosacea, avoid the same foods that can trigger migraines: alcohol, red wine, chocolate, and spicy foods.

You think you've got pimples and red, rashy skin, but you may actually have rosacea, an inflammation of the oil glands. Rosacea generally starts with pimples around the nose that sweep across the cheeks and forehead. Large swaths of skin become red and flushed. Blood vessels and spider veins enlarge and look like broken capillaries on the face. Women with rosacea are often mistakenly judged to have a drinking problem, since the nose swells and turns red. (W. C. Fields suffered from a severe case of rosacea, or what he called his "gin blossoms.") But rosacea is not caused by drinking: it's a genetic condition, made worse by alcohol and caffeinated beverages, which dilate the blood vessels and cause a flush, and by extremes of temperature.

If you have these symptoms, go to a dermatologist for treatment. If left untreated and you've got a bad case, it can cause the nose to swell permanently—no kidding. In the meantime, the best cosmetic to camouflage redness is Secret Camouflage by Laura Mercier. A product called B. Kamins Revitalizing Booster Concentrate can take the red out of rosacea and also helps soothe lasered and radiated skin.

Sensitive and Allergic Skin

Although only 5 percent of the American population is born with truly sensitive or "atopic" skin, 40 percent of American women have suffered—or think they have—from the condition known euphemistically in the beauty industry as "weakened skin." Those of us with weakened skin are prone to eruptions of red,

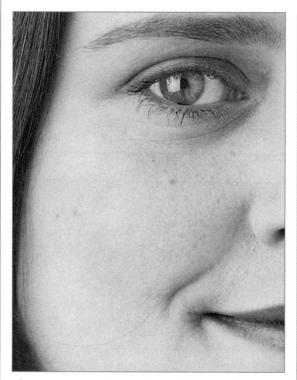

If you are among the very few who have truly sensitive skin, here's your Rx: Avoid fragrance and color in all products and baby your skin.

flaky, scaly, extremely dry, itchy patches known as dermatitis. Dermatitis can be caused by many things, but the most common triggers are an allergy or physical contact with something that irritates the skin. Contact dermatitis, the most common type, is often triggered by a sensitivity to irritating or drying cosmetic ingredients, harsh detergents, and contact with certain metals. (Earlobe dermatitis can be a reaction to nickel in pierced earrings; if you're prone, stick with stainless steel.) It can flare up immediately, but it is usually the result of repeated exposure over a period of months or years. If you're allergic, you will react immediately when exposed to any amount of a substance, no matter how small.

According to Dr. Richard Noodleman, a San Diego dermatological specialist in chemical sensitivity, "Many people are sensitive. But few are truly allergic." How can you tell? "Most people who are allergic swell up, turn bright red, and have a much more severe reaction," says Noodleman. "People who are easily irritated can help themselves by using gentle products and avoiding heavily perfumed or brightly colored products." But as far as I'm concerned, *all* skin responds best to gentle treatment—whether it's super-sensitive or as tough as hide.

If you have dry skin, you are most at risk of sensitivity reactions, but anyone can develop sensitivity to a specific ingredient in a product. Fragrances, colorings, talcs, alcohol, FD&C dyes, aluminum, and synthetic preservatives are the most common irritants. And although it may be tempting to ban preservatives from the beauty menu, they're necessary in any beauty product that contains water, since water is a breeding ground for bacteria, and without preservatives, you'll contaminate a product each time you dip in your finger.

Check the labels of your beauty products. The most common preservatives are ethyl-paraben, propylparaben, diazolidinyl urea, disodium EDTA, potassium sorbate, and sodium

I f you have sensitive skin or are allergy-prone, do a patch test before you try any new product. Apply a small amount to your neck or upper arm and wait for 24 hours to see whether you develop a rash. If you do, either consult a doctor who can help isolate the source for you or systematically eliminate the ingredients listed above in order to see where the problem lies.

benzoate—and these are also frequent causes of irritation (others are phenoxyethanol and imidazolidinyl urea). Look at your cosmetics labels, and you'll see that most of the products you use probably contain at least one of these. (Other ingredients to watch out for include nickel, PABA, lanolin, quaternium compounds, DMDM hydantoin, essential oils, formaldehyde, amines, and dyes.)

If you are highly allergic or super-sensitive, look for natural alternatives to synthetic preservatives: Vitamin E (tocopherol), citrus seed extract, grapefruit seed extract, Vitamin C (ascorbic acid), Vitamin A (retinyl palmitate), wheat germ oil. Or try a balm or oil instead of a lotion or cream, because these water-free products do not contain preservatives.

Eczema

If you have sensitive skin, you may be more prone to eczema. Eczema is a type of dermatitis that appears as red, flaky, scaly patches of dry skin. There are many different types of eczema, which is why it's so difficult to treat. One of the most common forms, asteotic eczema, can actually be caused by excessive dryness. In extreme cases, eczema blisters and scales, and in all cases it itches. It can be mistaken for seriously dry skin, but it's not as easy to get rid of. Sometimes eczema flares up as an allergic reaction, and, in fact, childhood eczema, which can appear all over the body, is common among asthmatic, allergy-prone children.

In adults, patches of eczema are common around the eyebrows, the hairline, and in front of the ears. Heavily perfumed soaps, shampoos, and moisturizers can aggravate the

OLDIE BUT GOODIE

Few products have had a shelf life like Elizabeth Arden Eight-Hour Cream, a soothing skin balm that's been on the market since 1930. Because it soothes chapped skin—lips, cheeks, cuticles, feet, elbows, and almost anywhere else you can imagine—and protects against windburn, abrasions, and razor burn, its users range from makeup artists shooting a fashion spread on the slopes at Saint-Moritz to mountain climbers shooting a charging moose on the icy tundra. If your grandmother didn't use it, your mother probably did, as did Sir Edmund Hillary when he climbed Mount Everest in 1953.

Eight-Hour Cream looks like orange Vaseline, and, unfortunately, it doesn't smell too great, but it really works. (A friend reports that it soothed her skin after radiation treatments.) The formulation includes petrolatum—an occlusive used in cold creams, moisturizers, and baby creams to prevent the evaporation of moisture from the skin and protect against irritation. Salicylic acid, another active ingredient in the cream, is an antiseptic and antimicrobial, and has been used by dermatologists for over 100 years to exfoliate the skin. Although I don't generally recommend the use of petrolatum-based moisturizers, this one also helps fight bacteria, and the salicylic acid exfoliates rough, scaly patches, which is why it is sometimes helpful in the treatment of eczema.

condition. So can clothing made of synthetic fabrics that don't allow air to pass freely. Eczema thrives on humidity, though sometimes moisturizers can help soothe the flaking and eliminate the red patches. But they can also make it worse, especially if you apply a

OTHER UNWANTED SKIN CONDITIONS

COLD SORES, aka fever blisters. These blisters at the sides of your mouth fill with fluid, ooze, and crust over. In other words, they're no fun. Because they're caused by the herpes simplex virus, they come and go, but they never go for good. They're highly contagious, *so don't touch them.*
They can be stimulated by the sun (along with hormones, stress, and a compromised immune system), so an opaque lipstick or a lip sunblock with SPF 15 helps prevent them.

The minute you feel a cold sore coming on, try Zilactin, an over-the-counter medication that can head it off at the pass. Or try this FOLK REMEDY: split a fresh clove of garlic in half, and apply it to the sore. Leave it there for a few minutes, and before long, the budding sore will actually start to go away. If one is already in full bloom, mix ¼ teaspoon water with 2 teaspoons of goldenseal powder from the health food store. Apply it and leave on for about 45 minutes. The sore will go away quickly.

PSORIASIS. These thick, red, scaly patches are most common on scalp, elbows, hands, and knees, but they can appear anywhere. Psorasis is a chronic, genetic condition caused when the skin sheds cells too quickly and they pile up like cars in a train wreck. For mild cases, retinoid creams may help. For more severe cases, doctors generally recommend UV light therapy, cortisone creams, coal-tar shampoos, antihistamines for the itching, PUVA (a medication called psoralen in conjunction with UV light therapy), Accutane, Dovonex, or other prescription medication. Consult your dermatologist.

VITILIGO. These fading patches of skin happen to people of all races but are, of course, more devastatingly obvious if you have dark skin. Vitiligo attacks the melanocytes, which give the skin its pigment. Consult your dermatologist.

WARTS. There are four main types of these growths caused by a virus: plantar warts (on the soles of the feet), hand warts, genital warts, and flat warts (which can appear anywhere, but in children they're most often on the face; in adult women, they're on the legs). They're contagious—and capricious. Sometimes they'll disappear on their own, sometimes they lie dormant until they make an encore appearance. Dermatologists burn them off with lasers or freeze them off with a nitrogen solution. At-home treatments include over-the-counter liquid salicylic acid solutions, but be very careful with these: they can fade the pigment in your skin, and they're photosensitive, which means they can leave permanent white spots. Consult a dermatologist for treatment as soon as you see warts because they can spread.

FOLK REMEDY: A friend had flat warts on her forehead, and she treated them slowly and deliberately with liquid salicylic acid, under a dermatologist's guidance, for eight months. They never went away. She had a trip to Hawaii planned and was concerned about photosensitivity caused by sun and salt water. According to a folk tale she heard, warts disappear when they are covered, so she decided to give it a try and wore a stylish little bandanna tied around her head for five days, 24 hours a day. When she took the bandanna off, the warts had disappeared completely. Two years later, she's still free and clear. Go figure!

moisturizer with sensitizing ingredients, because the skin is already inflamed and hypersensitive from the eczema. Use one of the gentle balms or moisturizers for "sensitive skin" listed in the chart on pages 36–37. For a quick fix, try Oil of Olay Age-Defying Lotion (it contains salicylic acid, which exfoliates the flaky patches and soothes the redness within a day). Other useful products include Clinique Turnaround Cream, Exorex Eczema Formula (strong stuff, but it works), and oat-based products like Penny Island Moisturizer and Estée Lauder Diminish (an antiaging product), both of which contain beta-glucans.

A quick oat bath in Aveeno can soothe the skin, but don't soak for too long. Wash your body with A-Derma O.A.T. or Penny Island Shower Gel. If the eczema occurs around your scalp, try Penny Island Oat Amino Complex Shampoo.

Evening primrose oil can also help. It contains gamma-linolenic acid (GLA), which is what eczema sufferers need. Try skincare products with evening primrose oil, or get GLA through your diet by eating salmon two or three times a week or by eating flaxseeds (or taking flax oil capsules), which you can buy at the health food store. In a blender or clean coffee grinder, grind enough for two tablespoons a day and sprinkle on foods like cereal or potatoes. Both salmon and flaxseeds provide omega-3 fatty acids.

FOLK REMEDY: A serving of watercress every day is said to keep eczema at bay, along with a daily drink of parsley, spinach, celery, and wheat grass. It may not be the tastiest juice you've ever tried but, like chicken soup, it can't hurt.

Hair, There, Everywhere

Aside from the promise of laser hair removal—which is still unfulfilled—there hasn't been much of a change in the depilation arena since I was a teenager. At that precise developmental moment in my life, I watched a friend's European mother drag her to the salon to have her upper lip and legs waxed. Because she got a head start, by the time she hit 30, my friend was as hairless as a newborn babe. I, on the other hand, like so many typical American teens, suffered through years of razor burn and Jolen Creme Bleach.

Waxing

Waxing is my favorite method of hair removal for the upper lip, chin, and eyebrows. (It's also great for legs, bikini lines, and underarms—if you can bear it—because a couple of waxes will get you through an entire summer.) After waxing, the hair grows back finer, because, unlike shaving, waxing pulls the hair out below the surface of the skin. It also requires less maintenance, because regrowth takes from three to five weeks. Before you try it on your own, however, have it done at a salon at least once so that you know what it feels like and what to expect. It does hurt when the hair is pulled out, but you get used to it. If the cost or inconvenience is off-putting—depending on where you live, a lip wax can cost from $7 to $17—it's easy to do the upper lip yourself and give yourself little touch-ups whenever you need them. Salons use hot wax, but cold wax is better when you do it yourself at home.

Waxing your eyebrows lasts longer than

plucking, and you get a beautifully clean line. Don't ever wax your eyebrows yourself, though, because you'll make a mess of it. You can't get the same angle on your face as an aesthetician can. She has a magnifying mirror to help her ferret out and eradicate all the tiny hairs. Besides, the skin around the eyes is very thin, and you can really irritate it if you don't know what you're doing.

If you want to wax facial hair yourself, there are lots of concoctions available at the drugstore or beauty supply store. The best I've found are Elle and Moojan cold wax strips ($4.39 for 12 applications). They look like translucent Band-Aids, are completely natural with no chemical additives, and they're a total no-brainer to use. Warm them between your palms for a few seconds to loosen the wax, peel the strips apart, place one on your upper lip, and pat in the direction of the hair growth. Then hold your skin taut and quickly pull the strip across the lip in the opposite direction. You can repeat this a couple of times until you get most of the hair, but don't go too crazy or you can irritate the skin. After you've waxed, apply aloe gel, eye gel, or a face oil—but first check out the ingredients, and make

Tip **W**hen waxing, hold your upper lip taut by sticking your tongue out behind it. Afterward, apply a gentle gel like aloe to the lip. The skin usually remains red for 15 to 20 minutes.

sure *never* to apply any product with alpha- or beta-hydroxy acid to freshly waxed skin.

Sugaring is a less painful, gentler salon alternative to waxing. Instead of wax, the depilatory is a mixture of sugar and honey, which is less irritating because it's not hot. The treatment generally takes longer than waxing, and it's more expensive.

Depilatory Creams

Depilatory creams literally melt away the hair with substances like calcium or sodium thioglycolate, or sulfides in a pastelike form. These are the same ingredients used in permanents and hair straighteners, but they're much more concentrated in depilatories and they actually *remove* the hair.

The problem with these alkaline products is that they are so concentrated, they can burn the skin, especially if you make the mistake of leaving them on too long. (They should be on for at least five minutes but no longer than eight, depending on the coarseness of your hair.) Another downside is that depilatories, unlike waxing, remove hair only on the surface, not at the root, which means that the hair grows back within a few days. Most depilatories with sulfides also have a strong, unpleasant smell.

There are lots of depilatories available at drugstores, and they're cheap, but you do need to use them frequently, so it adds up! Make sure you use one made specifically for the face. Any respectable cosmetologist would recommend Surgi-Cream for the Face, one of the oldest depilatories

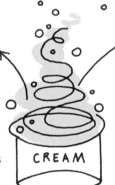

CREAM

around—and so would I. (Most cream depilatories, including Nair, haven't changed much in the past 40 years.) If you depilate the lip, make sure to remove the cream a minute or two *before* you're supposed to, in order not to burn your skin. *Never* use depilatories around the eyes or on broken skin, and never in conjunction with a facial peel, Retin-A, or Renova.

Bleaching

If you have dark hair but it isn't thick and coarse, try bleaching. The hair won't go away, but it will become less noticeable—unless you have dark skin or a tan, in which case it will be more noticeable. Most bleaches are still formulated with peroxide, which turns the hair yellowish blond. It works best on small areas of skin, such as the upper lip, but you can also use it on your arms. Follow the directions carefully, and don't leave it on too long—it, too, can burn the skin. One of the oldest—Jolen Creme Bleach—is still one of the cheapest and best.

Electrolysis

Electrolysis was invented in 1875, when Dr. Charles Michel, a St. Louis ophthalmologist, first used an electric needle to treat ingrown eyelashes. Since then, it has remained the only permanent method of hair removal, although laser technology is advancing at the speed of light. (It won't be long, I'm sure, before lasers become a safe and painless alternative. At the moment, laser hair removal is available, but it is not yet permanent. Stay tuned.)

Electrolysis uses an electric current to kill hair at its source—the cluster of capillaries called papillae that feed the hair at its root. A sterile needle is inserted into the hair follicle and given a jolt of electricity, which destroys the hair's ability to regenerate. In effect, the electricity that courses through the electrologist's needle cuts off the hair's food supply and destroys the root, thereby preventing new growth. Sometimes you need three or four treatments until a single hair is removed permanently, and sometimes it works on the first try.

So far, electrolysis is the only depilatory to cut the growth at its source. Some electrologists use disposable needles, while others sterilize and reuse their needles. In the latter case, they are required to follow strict guidelines developed by the Centers for Disease Control and Prevention (CDC). Any reputable electrologist will offer a free consultation, and that is the time to ask whether he or she uses disposable needles and, if not, what sterilization procedures are followed.

The number of treatments needed varies depending on things like the rate of your hair growth, the amount of hair, and the coarseness of its texture. Electrolysis can be expensive (about $30 for 15 minutes) and painful (which is why most sessions are limited to 15 minutes)

After a treatment, your skin may be red or slightly swollen for a few hours. Depending on your skin type, your electrologist will recommend a lotion for the irritation. Occasionally, a whitehead or small scab may form at the site, but it goes away after a short time. Since it's neither cheap nor painless, electrolysis is best confined to small areas. The most common are the chin, bridge of the nose, upper or lower lip, cheeks, eyebrows, and hairline.

Finding a good, qualified electrologist is essential. If your practitioner is not competent, the hair can grow back, because the needle doesn't always reach the root. In the wrong hands, electrolysis can also cause scarring or infection. (For this reason, never try to do it yourself with one of those electric "pens" advertised in the back of magazines.) Lucy Peters International is an excellent electrolysis center, with branches all over the country.

Ask your doctor for a recommendation, or call the American Electrology Association (AEA) (203-374-6667) or check out its Website (www.electrology.com) for a referral in your area. The AEA is a reputable trade association that has established national board certification for its members. To become certified, an electrologist must take an approved course of study, pass a test, and be retested regularly. (Make sure your electrologist has a CPE certificate on the wall, or call the International Guild of Professional Electrologists at 800-830-3247.) Note: if you're pregnant, consult your doctor before going for electrolysis, as there is always a slight risk of infection.

Danger Zone: Skin Cancer

Of all the problems covered in this chapter, none is as preventable—or as potentially dangerous—as damage to your skin from overexposure to the sun. The range of problems is vast—from the nuisance of the brown spots that begin to appear on the face, hands, and other exposed parts of the body as you get older, to full-blown melanoma, which can kill you.

Each year, there are approximately one million new cases of skin cancer in the United States. Before the 1950s and 1960s, malignant

BODY CHECK

Here are the American Cancer Society's "ABCDs" of melanoma detection. If you notice anything on your skin that resembles the photos below, consult a dermatologist immediately.

(A) ASYMMETRY
Normal moles are mostly round and symmetrical. Melanomas are asymmetrical and odd-shaped. One half is often markedly different from the other half.

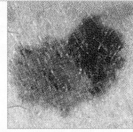

(B) BORDER
Normal moles are smooth around the edges. Melanomas often have jagged, irregular, or scalloped edges.

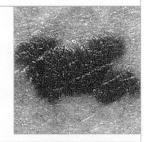

(C) COLOR
Normal moles are a single shade, most often brown. Melanomas can vary in color from one area to the next, or they can be black, blue, pink, or multicolored.

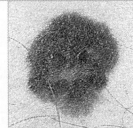

(D) DIAMETER
Most normal moles are less than a quarter of an inch in diameter. Melanomas spread outward and become larger.

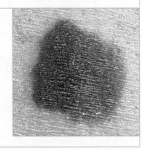

melanoma, the deadliest form of skin cancer, was extremely rare. But over the past 30 years, there's been a significant increase in cases. No one really knows why, though some attribute it to the depletion of the ozone layer, which is allowing more UV light to penetrate the atmosphere, along with the particularly harmful effects of unprotected—and increased—UVA exposure. Melanoma is known as a "white-collar" disease, because it most often afflicts those who spend the majority of their time indoors and then go off on vacations where they expose themselves to sudden and intense bursts of UV radiation. The two other types of skin cancer are associated with long-term exposure, and basal and squamous cell carcinoma are fairly easy to remove.

According to the *New England Journal of Medicine,* in the United States malignant melanoma is the leading cancer in white women between the ages of 25 and 29, and the second leading cancer in women 30 to 35. Fair-skinned blonds and redheads face a risk that's two to four times greater than everybody else's. African Americans and those with darker skin are less prone to melanoma because their skin naturally produces more melanin, and melanin not only creates color but also offers protection from UV exposure. Nonetheless, no matter what your skin tone, you can still tan or burn, and no one is immune to skin cancer.

Early detection of skin cancer can save your life. Because 70 percent of melanoma tumors develop from preexisting moles, it's important to examine your skin regularly. If you see a change in the way a freckle or mole looks, or if a mole starts to itch, see a dermatologist.

Other possible signs of skin cancer include sores that won't heal, or new growths that won't

★Best Products

For the best suncreens to use on your face, see page 44. For the best products for the entire body, try one of the following: Neutrogena Oil-Free Sunblock or Sensitive Skin Sunblock SPF 30, L'Oréal Ombrelle Sunscreen Lotion SPF 30, B. Kamins Sunbar SPF 30, Clinique Cityblock SPF 15, Origins Let the Sun Shine In SPF 21, DDF (Doctor's Dermatologic Formula) Organic Sunblock SPF 30, Peter Thomas Roth Clinical Skincare Oil-Free Sunblock SPF 30, Shiseido SunCare.

go away. For example, a reddish patch that won't go away, even after six months or more; a whitish area that looks like a scar; an open sore that won't heal, even after four weeks; a blemish with a wavy border and depressed center, which gets bigger rather than heals; a smooth, shiny bump that looks like a mole, in odd colors (black, purple, white) or normal ones (brown, red). Anytime you see a new or unusual growth that won't go away, see a dermatologist and get it checked out. And if you've had a melanoma in the past, you must go back to your dermatologist every six months to a year for a full-body check.

The only active ingredients that offer full-spectrum protection from the UVA rays that cause melanoma are titanium dioxide, zinc oxide, and Parsol 1789 (avobenzone). Make sure your sunscreen lists one of these three as an active ingredient and an SPF 15, and use it *every day,* not just at the beach. The other FDA-approved sunscreens—octyl methoxycinnamate, octyl salicylate, and oxybenzone—will protect your skin from UVB, *not* UVA, rays. And, because they chemically absorb UV energy rather than physically blocking or scattering it, they can irritate your skin.

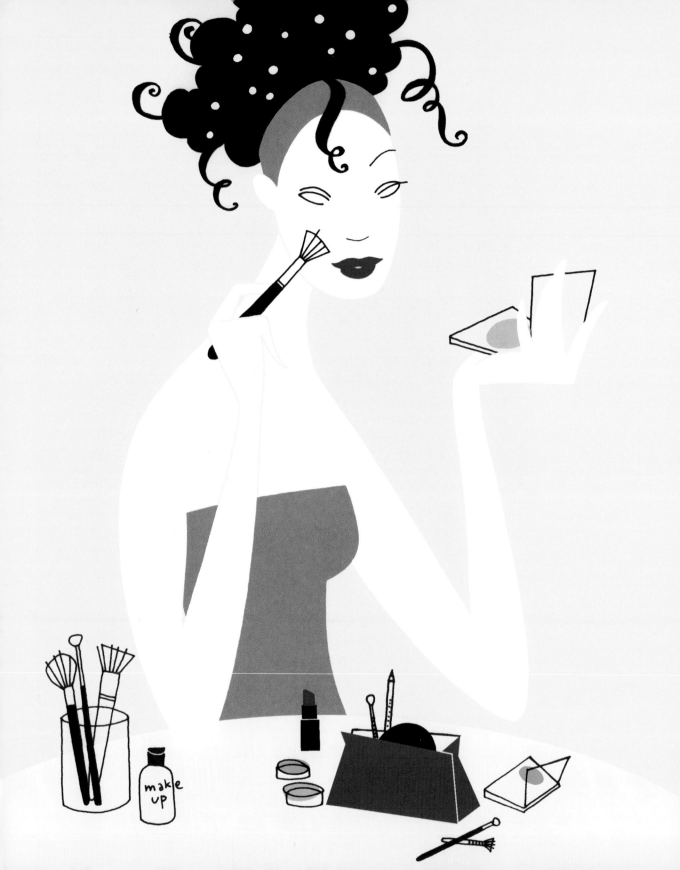

CHAPTER SIX

makeup

Lots of women buy just as many makeup things as I do . . . they just don't wear them all at the same time.

—DOLLY PARTON

Some women collect cashmere sweaters, Prada handbags, vintage pumps. I collect makeup. Others, less kind, might call it an obsession. But at least makeup is a small investment compared to cashmere or even a good pair of shoes.

For me, each chubby new pencil or glistening pot of gloss holds sweet promise. The fact that I almost always end up wearing some variation on the same three things—lipstick, concealer, and eye pencil—is not the point. As every woman knows, makeup is not a practical matter. Makeup is all about intangibles, the little tube or magic wand full of tantalizing possibilities. As one friend said recently, "It's only a lipstick, but it can change your life." Besides, makeup is fun.

Playing with pots of color and brushes, magic wands and tubes of paint, a woman can be as expressive as she was with her paintboxes as a child. It's almost as much fun to rifle

through a bulging makeup bag as it is to put the stuff on. And when you do put it on, makeup offers instant gratification: a stroke of blush, a tiny dab of silver shimmer, a rub of ruby lip gloss can make you look instantly better. In less than 10 seconds, any woman can become a prettier, more dramatic, or trendier version of herself.

Makeup can be understated, as in a Ralph Lauren advertisement, or overdone, like Dolly Parton's, but it always reveals much more than it can ever conceal. Makeup sends a message to the world. Like it or not, people will form opinions about you based on your lipstick color. What your makeup conveys, above all, is how you feel: chic, rebellious, pretty, flawed, or powerful.

Today most of us choose to err on the side of discretion and keep it simple—to eliminate the artifice and focus on the artistry of makeup application. Because ultimately, what every woman wants is for makeup to make her

Behind the Scene

Makeup Spectacles

The Japanese expression "Stop eating when you're 80 percent full" applies to makeup as well as food, says makeup artist Shu Uemura.

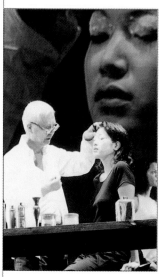

In his native Japan, Uemura stages "makeup spectacles." He packs a stadium with thousands of fans who come to watch makeup artists apply makeup to models who sit on elevated stools on small platforms, with their video images projected onto huge screens. It is, literally, like watching paint dry.

appear more naturally beautiful. In the 1980s, Revlon capitalized on that basic truth and launched "The Nakeds," the first makeup line devoted exclusively to neutral shades that emphasize whatever is uniquely yours. The Nakeds and the scores of imitators it inspired are still going strong.

"In every person's face, there is one place that seems to express them most accurately," says the heroine in Mona Simpson's novel *Anywhere But Here.* "With my grandmother," she continues, "you always looked at her mouth." I was lucky to learn from my grandmother, too. Grandma's signature burgundy lip stain taught me my most important lesson

about makeup: Take your most expressive feature—big eyes, bow lips, high cheekbones, strong brows, dainty chin—and play it up. Never diminish whatever it is that gives you your unique style of beauty and makes you look even more like yourself. But don't overdo it either.

Always start with a light touch. You can layer more on later. The last thing any woman wants is to have her makeup enter the room before she does. Fortunately, technology has made this a lot easier to avoid. Whether you shop at Kmart or Christian Dior, formulations are finer, pencils are softer, colors are sheerer than ever before. And if you do end up with something you don't like, you can layer it beneath another color, swap with a friend, or simply throw it away.

Here are some guidelines, tips, and tricks to make it less intimidating and more fun to play with color. "After all, what's the point of makeup," says Thierry, Yves Saint Laurent's international makeup director, "if it's not fun?"

Color

When it comes to makeup, color is where women mess up most of the time. I believe that we know, in a vague and general sense, what range of colors works best for us. But mastering the tiny nuance that makes a good look great or a polished look perfect—now, that's a challenge.

Let's start with the basics. When you set out to find the range of colors that will look best on you, first consider skin tone. Makeup looks best when it complements the undertone (the color below the skin's surface that shows through) in

THE FOUR COSMETICS C'S

■ **COMFORT.** It's amazing how often I hear questions like "If I wear powder, do I *need* foundation?" "If I wear lipstick, do I *need* something for balance on my eyes?" Never mind what you "need." Think about how much makeup feels comfortable and leave it at that. Makeup is a want, not a need. Some women don't feel fully dressed without foundation, others feel embalmed when they wear it. If you love lipstick but you're uncomfortable with eye makeup, go with the lips—or vice versa.

■ **COLOR.** Stick to the same color family. It's a major blunder to mix a warm lip shade (rust) with a cool blush (pink). The advice throughout this chapter will help you find the shades that work best for you.

■ **CONTOUR.** Blend, blend, blend. Use brushes, sponges, velours, puffs, and fingers to soften the lines of demarcation. Nothing looks worse than rigid lines of color that divide the face into a harsh grid.

■ **CONFIDENCE.** A little attitude goes a long way. Even if you don't feel secure about your ability to apply makeup, fake it until you learn. Get yourself a good mirror, and, whenever possible, apply your makeup in natural light. Remember, makeup application is not rocket science; it's supposed to be easy and fun. But a lot of women are held back by the fear of doing something wrong. No matter what the counterperson or you best friend says, if you don't think it looks good, it won't look good, because you won't have the confidence to pull it off. Go with your gut, but take a risk once in a while, too. Remember, you can always wash it off!

your skin. Yes, your hair and eye color also play a part, but that can be factored in later.

All skin can be broken down into two basic undertones: pinkish blue (cool) or yellow (warm). Conveniently, all makeup can, too. The cool category generally covers complexions on the extreme ends of the spectrum (very pale and very dark), while warm covers most women in between. In

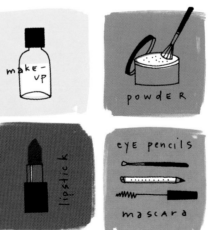

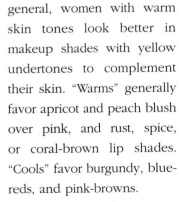

general, women with warm skin tones look better in makeup shades with yellow undertones to complement their skin. "Warms" generally favor apricot and peach blush over pink, and rust, spice, or coral-brown lip shades. "Cools" favor burgundy, blue-reds, and pink-browns.

If you don't know your color, here's a trick that really works (for all except dark skin tones). Look at one of your elbows and squeeze gently.

What Color Are You?

Although it may seem impossible, every skin tone (and makeup shade) on the planet breaks down into two basic categories: warm and cool.

warm

REACTION TO SUN

tans easily

COMPLEXION

not too pale, not too dark, almost all medium shades in between, including olive, Mediterranean, and honey tones

UNDERTONE

yellow

BEST CLOTHING COLORS

bright colors (e.g., reds, blues) or earth tones (rust, olive, khaki, brown)

BEST MAKEUP COLORS

cheeks: apricot, peach, bronze
lips: bronze, plums, spice, cherry reds, yellow-reds, brick-reds, apricot-browns, soft peach, soft beige, cocoa, toast, brown-peach, peachy-bronze

WORST COLORS

pinkish blue; dull, pale pinks

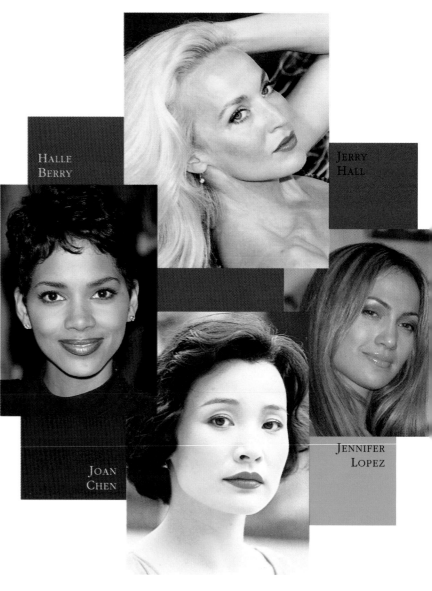

HALLE BERRY

JERRY HALL

JENNIFER LOPEZ

JOAN CHEN

Once you figure out whether you're warm or cool, it becomes much easier to zero in on the makeup that will look most fabulous on you. These celebrities were chosen not only because they're personal favorites, but also because their skin tones illustrate the warm/cool breakdown so perfectly that you can use them as a guide. Are you a pale brunette like Winona Ryder? Cool. A honey-toned blonde (sometimes!) like Jennifer Lopez? Warm (though, in her case, many would say hot!). If you're in doubt between the two choices, you're probably warm (unless you're really pale or dark). The guidelines below will help you.

cool

REACTION TO SUN
burns easily

COMPLEXION
extreme shades on either end of the skin tone spectrum: pale, rosy or ruddy, or dark ebony

UNDERTONE
pinkish-blue

BEST CLOTHING COLORS
deep jewel tones (burgundy, navy, deep indigo) or chalky pastels

BEST MAKEUP COLORS
cheeks: pink, rosy
lips: blue-reds, berry, soft rose, mauve, burgundy, maroon-brown, raisin, eggplant, pink-browns

WORST COLORS
yellow, orange

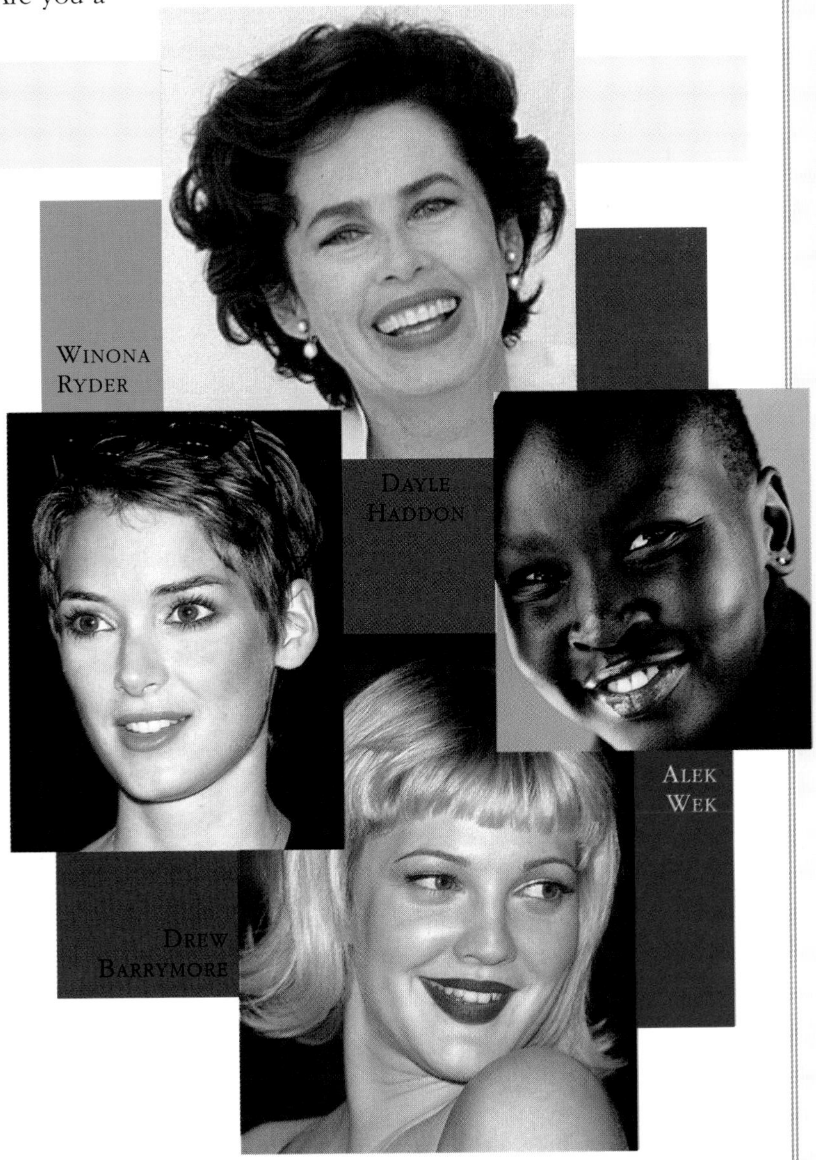

DAYLE HADDON

WINONA RYDER

ALEK WEK

DREW BARRYMORE

A concentrated yellow or pink undertone is always obvious in that area. Once you figure out whether your undertone is pink or yellow, you know what makeup family you're in. Most women know, instinctively, whether they are a "warm" or a "cool," or at least know which colors look best on them when they shop for clothes. Those colors look good because they pick up something flattering in their skin. It's the same with makeup.

Whether you're warm or cool, you don't ever need to eliminate a color that you like. *Any woman can wear any color she likes—red, pink, brown—as long as it's the right shade.* For example, anyone (even a redhead) can wear red lipstick, but if you have a cool skin tone you'll want a blue-red shade; if you're a "warm," your lipstick should be a yellow-red shade.

The Best Makeup Artists' Colors

A makeup artist's line is a great place to learn how to perfect your sense of color. Makeup artists have seen it all—every type of skin, every color, every illusion that women want to create—and that experience is reflected in the types of products they make and the way they're formulated. Their lines tend to be small and well edited, and the quality is high. Plus, their development time is quick, which means that the colors are up-to-the-moment: if a makeup artist senses a trend—or a need for a new color—she or he can bring it to the market quickly.

The makeup artists below have a distinct image, focus, and forte that is obvious through their product lines. Each one has a knack for simplifying color, and what each one does, he or she does extremely well.

■ BOBBI BROWN ESSENTIALS

FOUNDER: Bobbi Brown, magazine and runway makeup artist, coauthor of *Teenage Beauty*

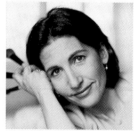

THE IMAGE: Neo-Natural

SPECIALTIES: Yellow powder; brown, brown-pink, and neutral lip shades; black and brown mascara; lip "stains" and "shimmers"; navy blue, bone, and pink eye shadows

QUOTE: *Strong women don't need strong makeup.*

IMAN

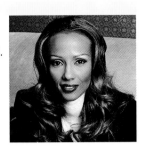

FOUNDER: Iman, the Somalian fashion model. (Unlike most models who "front" makeup lines, Iman, though not a makeup artist, is involved in the development of hers, every step of the way.)

THE IMAGE: Multi-Culti Cachet

SPECIALTIES: Lip pencils, oil-control foundation, deep-colored eye shadows and lipsticks (although originally created for women of color, her line has expanded—and the colors work beautifully even on pale skin), blemish gel

QUOTE: *I was lucky to have access to makeup artists who taught me how important it is to mix and blend.*

LAURA MERCIER CLASSIQUE

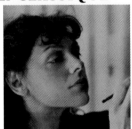

FOUNDER: Laura Mercier, magazine and runway makeup artist, creator of *The Flawless Face* video

THE IMAGE: French Chic with a twist

SPECIALTIES: Secret Camouflage, Secret Concealer, bronzing powder, sheer lip glacés, the subtlest, shimmery cream to powder eye shadows

QUOTE: *Makeup can not only make you more attractive, it can boost your attitude and celebrate your uniqueness as a woman.*

LORAC

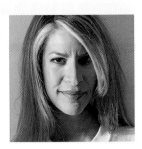

FOUNDER: Carol Shaw, Hollywood makeup artist

THE IMAGE: Understated Glamour

SPECIALTIES: Oil-free foundation, oil-free cleanser, oil-free moisturizer, cream concealer, purple-plum-pewter eye shadows and lip glosses, Vitamin E stick, lipsticks inspired by—and named after—Shaw's Hollywood clients. It's easy to order your lipstick if you match your coloring with the name of a star. For example, if you're a pale redhead, try "Geena," after Geena Davis. If your coloring is closer to Demi Moore's or Drew Barrymore's, try "Demi" or "Drew." It's a shrewd marketing gimmick, but it actually helps you choose well.

QUOTE: *I want women not only to look gorgeous but to have the products benefit the skin, too.*

M·A·C

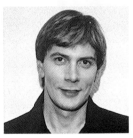

FOUNDER: Frank Toscan, former makeup artist and political activist; the company is now owned by Estée Lauder

THE IMAGE: All Races, All Sexes, All Ages

SPECIALTIES: Moisturizing matte lipsticks, Viva Glam, Vino; lip pencils (Everywoman's neutral: spice), shimmer face powder, Oil Matte

QUOTE: *It's not about how much or how little, but how it's done.*

◼ NARS

FOUNDER: François Nars, magazine and celebrity makeup artist

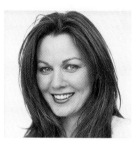

THE IMAGE: Euro-Hollywood

SPECIALTIES: Deep, rich, brightly colored lipsticks; khaki, mustard, "warm-toned" eye shadows; Multiple Sticks

QUOTE: *If you make the makeup look more transparent, you can get away with more color.*

◼ SHU UEMURA

FOUNDER: Shu Uemura, Japanese makeup artist and pioneer

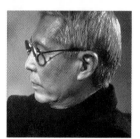

THE IMAGE: Zen simplicity and purity in a vast range of colors

SPECIALTIES: Lighter-than-air SPF mousse foundation, pale eye shadow, perfect lipstick shades, Cleansing Beauty Oil

QUOTE: *Makeup is your decoration, not a mask.*

◼ STILA

FOUNDER: Jenine Lobell, music video and editorial makeup artist

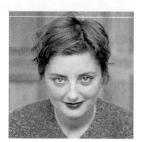

THE IMAGE: Intelligent Makeup for Real Women

SPECIALTIES: All-over shimmer, lip rouge, four-in-one Quad Lip Palettes (#1 or #2) in easy natural colors that are completely addictive

QUOTE: *Don't paint someone else's face onto your own. Don't fall victim to trends.*

◼ SUE DEVITT

FOUNDER: Sue Devitt, makeup artist

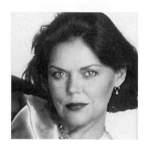

THE IMAGE: Smooth Sophistication

SPECIALTIES: Beautiful brushes, satiny foundation, good self-tanners, rich eye shadow colors

QUOTE: *My makeup has a lot of elasticity; the formulations move with your expressions. Women are so active these days, we need makeup that can move.*

◼ TRUCCO

FOUNDER: Geri Cusenza, former makeup artist and co-owner of Sebastian International (now owned by Wella)

THE IMAGE: Totally Trendoid

SPECIALTIES: Funky eye shadow color, lip stains and glosses

QUOTE: *We're retraining our eye to look in a different way—to enhance the face, not disguise it.*

Tools of the Trade

Good tools are essential. To a makeup artist, a good brush is what a good set of knives is to a chef: indispensable. And the biggest, baddest makeup hazard to afflict women—*the stripe*—is caused by a bad brush. Any woman who wears makeup should make a small investment in a few good, natural-bristle brushes. Good brushes (if well cared for) will literally last a lifetime. They'll also help your makeup go on more easily and look a lot better.

The best brushes are made of natural bristle, with wooden handles. (Plastic is too slippery.) The handle should sit well in your hand, so that you can get a good grip. Natural bristle—made from sable, goat, or squirrel—is best because the hairs have cuticles that "grab" the powder or blush and allow it to go on more evenly. (Don't worry, no animals are harmed in the process.) Synthetic brushes, though cheap, aren't supple enough for a smooth application. They usually cause streaks, and they're almost impossible to clean.

Soft bristles work best for a soft look. But if a brush is *too* soft, it won't be able to pick up and put down color. If it's too hard, it won't feel good and could irritate your skin. To find a good brush, try before you buy. If a brush sheds more than a few bristles when you run it along the back of your hand, the quality is bad. Gently pull on the bristles. If more than a few come away in your hand, don't buy it.

Value: Mass vs. Class

Max Factor was one of the first to mass-market cosmetics, and his name is still a household word today. In 1909, Factor, a Russian Jewish immigrant, opened a makeup studio in southern California that became a hub for stage and screen performers. He developed "flexible greasepaint," a natural-looking makeup for the screen in 1914, and eventually created "Pan-Cake" foundation, cinematic makeup adapted for everyday use. (Factor's nephew Dean continues the family tradition with Smashbox Cosmetics, a hip, young company that also draws on—and updates—the Factor family connections.)

As mass-market, brand-name cosmetics like Max Factor grew, companies that wanted a piece of the profit without the manufacturing headache turned to private-label manufacturers. They would cook

The Toolbox

A small investment in good tools will pay off big time.

There are zillions of brushes out there. But after years of peering over makeup artists' shoulders backstage at fashion shows and on photo shoots—and interviewing them about their craft—I've concluded that you really need only three or four good brushes and a few basic tools. Your fourth finger, the best tool a primate could have, will do the rest.

The Essentials

Blush brush. *Invest in a good medium-size brush with a rounded tip. To create a natural look, use the same brush for highlighting.*

Powder brush.
A large, soft brush will apply face powder or bronzing powder flawlessly. Use the same brush to remove the excess powder from your face so that you don't look like a Kabuki dancer.

Eye shadow brush.
A small brush with bristles angled on one side will help you get the line you want when you use powder eye shadow to line your eyes or shade your lids. It also fills in spotty brows.

Lip brush. *A lip brush is tapered on both sides to a rounded point. It not only gives you a perfect lip line and an even application but also prevents waste by scraping the last smidgens of color out of the tube. Look for one with a protective top.*

Triangular makeup sponges. *These spread foundation or concealer evenly and take it into all those nooks and crannies around the eyes and under the nose.*

Circular sponge or velour. *The sponge or velour applies pressed powder lightly and evenly. Because it picks up the oils on your face, you'll need to replace it when it looks shiny or caked.*

Tweezer. *A tweezer lasts forever, so buy a good one. The best is one with a pointed or slanted tip, like Tweezerman, because it is the most versatile and grabs hair easily.*

Pencil sharpener. *Keeps your eye and lip pencils ready to work.*

Eyelash curler. *Eyelash curlers may look like medieval torture instruments, but they do what they claim: they curl the lashes, which opens up the eyes and makes them look bigger—and you look wider awake. They're cheap and easy to find*

BEST BRUSHES

Not surprisingly, makeup artists' cosmetics lines carry the best brushes, because makeup artists know, firsthand, what works best. Shu Uemura, Bobbi Brown, Lorac, Stila, M·A·C, Make Up For Ever, Nars, Trish McEvoy, Vincent Longo, Sue Devitt, and Alcone are a few makeup artists' companies with great brushes. Chanel and Yves Saint Laurent make good ones, too, but they're more expensive. Prices generally range from $16 to $45 per brush.

in the drugstore. Make sure the curler has foam padding, which is gentlest on the lashes.

An old toothbrush. *Recycle your old toothbrush—it can have more lives than Shirley MacLaine. Use it to brush excess mascara from your lashes so that you don't get little raccoonlike "paw prints" under your eyes, or to "comb" unruly eyebrows into place.*

Baby wipes. *Keep a travel pack of baby wipes in your purse. They're especially handy on airplanes and cars. Use to remove smudges, take makeup off your hands, and clean your face for a spot touch-up when you're going out straight after work.*

Makeup bag. *Even if you travel light, with just a lipstick and compact, find yourself a petite makeup bag to carry them around in. That way you'll avoid fumbling for your lipstick at inopportune moments.*

CARE AND HANDLING

Makeup brushes as well as sponges, powder velours, and puffs should be washed and air-dried thoroughly on a regular basis, because they can harbor bacteria. A dirty brush can cause skin breakouts.

Soak your brushes in a mix of hot water and an antibacterial soap like Kiss My Face or Dr. Bronner's lavender soap for 10 or 15 minutes. Leave them out to air-dry. Between cleanings, use tissues to wipe off your brushes. If the bristles stray off in different directions after prolonged use, simply cut them back.

UNDER $10

Even top makeup artists still troll the drugstore bargain bins, where they find all kinds of great stuff—and so can you. If you're adventurous, start at Ricky's—a

funky, fashion-forward drugstore with branches in New York City, London, and Seattle. Mattesse makeup, the house brand, is modeled after the Chanel colors (stylish-to-the-minute) *and* it's cheap. It has a terrific shimmery silver eye shadow ($9) and taupe lip gloss. Also look for Burt's Beeswax ($3) for lip shine and conditioning.

At big chains like CVS and Rite Aid, look for Wet 'N Wild eye pencils—you can also stroke them on your lashes for definition. Also try Lehcaresor Papier Poudre, oil-blotting paper that pinch-hits for powder, and Lord & Berry Lipstique (smooth, creamy, and stays on your lips). Other beauty bounty: jane clear gel for brows and lashes and jane lip gloss, Reviva Vitamin E stick, Rite Aid makeup sponges, Dramatize Line and Shade Eye Pencil, Maybelline Expert Eyes Pencil, Prestige lip liner, Neutrogena cosmetics (sophisticated colors, polished textures), Duane Reade Lypstique pencils.

up standard-issue products for many different companies, repackage each with its own private label, and claim it as a unique and special formulation. Because the products were so similar, packaging was the only way to distinguish them. Department stores and mail-order catalogs used this method extensively, and many still do.

Today, mass-market cosmetics are the cheaper brands normally found in drugstores, outlet stores, and discount stores; they're commonly sold through infomercials, on the Internet,

or by the "Avon Lady." Prestige brands—such as those pioneered by Elizabeth Arden, Estée Lauder, and Helena Rubinstein—were originally sold only in upscale venues like department stores, salons, and boutiques. They still are, although they're now sold in discount outlets, too.

So what's the difference in brands—aside from the price? In some cases, it's quality, based on the amount of money a company spends to support its research and development. In others, it's the shade and sophistication of color—an area in which high-fashion houses like Chanel and Yves Saint Laurent obviously have an edge over Cover Girl and Coty. With some products—lipstick, for example—it's the nuance, above all, that separates the so-so from the sublime. Most women understand that there is good reason to break the bank on the season's latest Chanel lipstick.

When you come right down to it, some cosmetics (like foundation and powder) demand a splurge, some are well worth it (concealer, lipstick, blush), and some just aren't (mascara, pencils). To find out why, read on.

Foundation

ORDER OF APPLICATION

1. FOUNDATION
2. CONCEALER
3. EYE SHADOW
4. EYELINER
5. MASCARA
6. BLUSH
7. POWDER
8. LIPSTICK

No matter how much or how little makeup you wear, if you want to look your best, apply your makeup in the order shown at left. It blends better this way and is less likely to smudge. Of course, you can skip as many steps as you like.

WHO DOES WHAT BEST?

	MASS MARKET	PRESTIGE
Blush	L'Oréal, Bourjois	Bobbi Brown, Origins
Concealer	Cover Girl	Shiseido, Laura Mercier
Eyeliner	Revlon	Yves Saint Laurent
Eye Shadow	Jane	Shu Uemura
Face Powder	Max Factor	T. Leclerc, Chanel
Foundation	Neutrogena	Awake, Christian Dior
Lipstick	Revlon, Bourjois	Lancôme, Chanel
Mascara	Maybelline, Sephora	Estée Lauder
Pencils	Wet 'N Wild	M·A·C

If women are loyal to any cosmetic these days, it's foundation—probably because it takes so long to find the right one to begin with. Foundation (also called base or primer) is the number one consumer loyalty category in cosmetics. And as far as I'm concerned, it's the number one makeup product it makes sense to spend money on. Good foundation evens out your skin tone. It covers spots, freckles, blemishes, blotches, and whatever else you'd prefer the world not to see. Foundation gives the rest of your makeup something to adhere to. Most important, because it contains titanium dioxide (the ingredient in full-spectrum sunblock) it protects your skin from exposure to UV light. It also shields your skin from dirt, a special problem if you live in the city.

Good foundation won't streak, overdry, or change color as the day wears on. It feels as comfortable as a second skin. Bad foundation can look truly awful—especially when it sits like a mask on your face or turns a putrid shade of orange. And what about those lines of demarcation that separate your jawline from your neck like the Arctic timberline? When you consider that you wear foundation *all over your face, every day,* isn't it worth it to spend a little more? Besides, unlike mascara, foundation is good for up to two years after it's opened— which is another reason to justify the expense.

One of the biggest myths about foundation is that it's bad for your skin. This is simply not true. It's bad only if you make a bad match—if you put an oily foundation on oily skin, or if your skin is sensitive to certain ingredients in the particular product you are using. Good foundation doesn't contain pore-clogging ingredients like lanolin or mineral oil, or irritants like alcohol, which are contained in most drugstore versions and can cause contact dermatitis (flaking or redness) or cosmetic acne.

The natural look of healthy skin is what you're after. If you've got it, you're lucky. If not, foundation can really improve the look and feel of your skin. Most women reach for the spackle when they begin to see changes in their skin, like lackluster color or leathery texture. But often, they end up using too much. Less is definitely more when it comes to foundation. For example, a tinted moisturizer or sheer foundation may be just the trick to "warm" pale, dull, or ashy skin, add moisture, and make it look supple, especially if you're over 40. (Heavier foundation can seep into your lines and actually end up emphasizing what you're trying to conceal.) In general, if your skin is just a tiny bit oily, powder alone can do the trick.

Most foundation contains three main ingredients: titanium dioxide, pigment, and oil—as well as a lot of cosmetic chemicals, of course. If you want chemical-free foundation, try "Mineral Makeup," page 77. (In oil-free versions, water replaces most of the oil, although even oil-free foundations contain some silicone oils to give them "glide.") And for every foundation shade in the world, chemists use just four colors—white, black, red, yellow—most often derived from the mineral iron oxide.

What to Look For

There are three things to consider when you buy foundation: (1) the color that matches your skin perfectly, (2) the finish that feels comfortable, and (3) the coverage that's best for your skin type.

Liquid foundations give sheer to medium coverage; creams give the heaviest. Within these two basic categories, you can get a variety of different "finishes," which also tell you how much coverage you'll get. "Matte" has a flat, polished, heavier finish. "Satin" is semisheer, with a "dewy" finish. For a little sheen, look for "light diffusers" or "iridescents," which are sheer but contain tiny particles of silica-coated mica to reflect light. The one you choose will depend on the look you prefer and what feels most comfortable on your skin.

To find a foundation that blends naturally into your skin, go to the cosmetics counter without any makeup on your cheeks. (Testing foundation with a layer of makeup on is a waste of time.) Ask the salesperson to guide you to the right colors for your undertones. Foundation in a jar should look like skin color: pinkish beige, yellowish beige, brownish pink, and so on. Anything that's sold as a "corrective" and looks too weird in the jar—orange or green, for example—will look weird on your face, too.

Rub a tiny round of several shades of foundation into your lower cheek. (Don't test foundation on your hand—that's not where you'll wear it and your hand is darker than your face.)

Tip Forget about oil-free cream foundation or powder-based foundation; they're too drying.

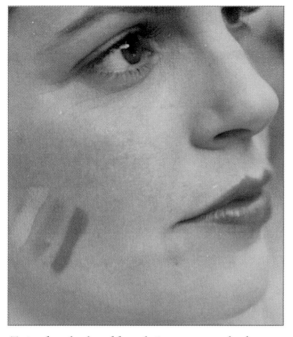

Test a few shades of foundation on your cheek, preferably in natural light. You'll know the right one when you see it blend seamlessly into your skin.

Give the foundation a couple of minutes to dry. Then tell the saleswoman you want to see it in natural light and head for the exit with a hand mirror. The best shade is the one that completely disappears. The best texture is the one that feels like it isn't there.

If you're pale and want more color in your face, do not buy a foundation a shade or two darker than your skin, because it will just look like you're wearing a mask. Color is what blush is for. And if you've gotten too much sun and want to lighten up, don't buy a foundation that's too pale. The color of your neck will be a dead giveaway.

Custom Blending. Most prestige-brand cosmetics companies offer about 12 shades of foundation in several different textures. Mass-market

Behind the Scene Model Skin

Ever wonder how the models like Kate Moss (below) get such dewy-looking skin? Some, obviously, are born with it, but most aren't. They benefit from their makeup artists' favorite sleight-of-hand trick: a thin coat of Vaseline on the face. How about your favorite film stars? Well, there will always be lens filters on Hollywood sets, but advances in makeup technology are helping to lessen the demand for them. Instead, makeup artists on set use spray-on makeup—applied through a pressurized wand—that literally "airbrushes" the face with a makeup mist. Sort of like photo retouching your face. Here is some light-reflecting makeup you can use to create the effect yourself: Magic by Prescriptives, Benefit High Beam, Clinique Zero Base.

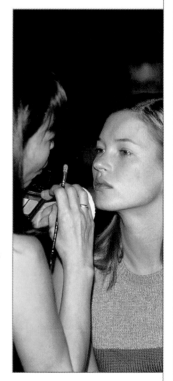

brands usually offer fewer. Considering the zillions of subtle shadings and skin tones in the world, it doesn't sound like much, does it?

Custom blending, the cosmetic equivalent of couture, may be the answer. Elizabeth Arden and Prescriptives (with over 100 shades) lead

FOUNDATION:

	TYPE	GOOD FOR	THE SCOOP
LIQUIDS	**OIL-BASED**	Dry or mature skin	Feel the greasiest, because they contain the most oil. Some of these turn orange because of an unfortunate interaction betweeen the oils and pigment.
	WATER-BASED	All skin types, expecially sensitive or combination skin	Give light coverage because the base is water, which is lighter than oil. Usually contain some silicone oil for glide.
	OIL-FREE	Oily skin; many actually soak up excess oil throughout the day and keep your face matte	The pigment is suspended in water instead of oil, although most contain some silicone oils for "glide." Some contain talc, which regulates excess oil on the face.
	TINTED MOISTURIZER	Normal or dry skin; especially good for mature skin because coverage is light; it doesn't seep into lines and wrinkles.	Provide the sheerest coverage, because they are, quite simply, lotion mixed with a bit of pigment. Use if you want light coverage or if you have wrinkles—they plump up the skin. Often contain sun protection.
CREAMS	**CREAM FOUNDATION OR CREAM POWDER (DUAL FOUNDATION**	Normal or combination; not good for older skin	Usually come in a compact or a stick. Oil-based, they look creamy and greasy in the pan but actually go on matte and powdery. Cream foundation is best applied with a sponge; cream powder can be applied with a brush as a powder or with a wet sponge as foundation. If you don't use too much, they can make your skin look flawless.

the best base for your face

FINISH	COVERAGE	BEST PRODUCTS
Matte	Medium to heavy. In many cases, a little can go a long way.	CHANEL TEINT NATURAL LIQUID MAKEUP, LORAC SATIN FINISH MAKEUP, LAURA MERCIER MOISTURIZING FOUNDATION, SHU UEMURA UV LIQUID FOUNDATION, CHRISTIAN DIOR TEINT DIOR LIFT SPF 15, L'ORÉAL VISIBLE LIFT LINE MINIMIZING MAKEUP
Sheer, satin	Light: they look natural and blend beautifully.	CHANTECAILLE REAL SKIN FOUNDATION, LANCÔME EAU DE TEINT PURE COMPLEXION WATERCOLOR, VINCENT LONGO WATER CANVAS, LORAC NEUTRALIZER, ORIGINS AS GOOD AS IT GETS, STILA LIQUID MAKEUP
Matte or satin	Medium.	AWAKE OIL-FREE FOUNDATION, BOBBI BROWN ESSENTIALS OIL-FREE FOUNDATION, CHANEL TEINT PUR MAT, CLINIQUE STAY TRUE MAKEUP OIL-FREE, IMAN SECOND TO NONE OIL-FREE MAKEUP, LORAC OIL-FREE MAKEUP, LAURA MERCIER OIL-FREE FOUNDATION, PRESCRIPTIVES EXACT COLOR MAKEUP OIL-FREE, NEUTROGENA HEALTHY SKIN SPF 20
Sheer	Light: especially good in warm weather, when you want the sheerest coverage.	BOBBI BROWN TINTED MOISTURIZER, CLARINS TINTED MOISTURIZER, AVEDA MOISTURE PLUS TINT SPF 10, SHISEIDO VITAL PERFECTION PERFORMANCE TINTED MOISTURIZER SPF 10, LAURA MERCIER TINTED MOISTURIZER SPF 15, MAX FACTOR INVISIBLE MAKE-UP SPF 6, M·A·C ENVIRONMENTAL PROTECTION TINTED MOISTURIZER, PRESCRIPTIVES TRANSPARENT FACECOLOR, SHU UEMURA ANTI-UV SPF 17 MAKEUP MOUSSE
Matte	Medium to heavy: creams can make you look heavily made up, so apply carefully.	ELIZABETH ARDEN SPONGE-ON CREAM MAKEUP, CHRISTIAN DIOR FOND DE TEINT COMPACT FOUNDATION (especially great for women of color), DERMABLEND COMPACT COVER CREME (for heavy coverage), YVES SAINT LAURENT POWDER CREAM VEIL, STILA ILLUMINATING POWDER FOUNDATION, SHU UEMURA NOBARA FOUNDATION, TRISH MCEVOY POWDER FOUNDATION DUO

How To: apply foundation

1. Shake the foundation bottle well. Dab some into your palm, and mix with a few drops of moisturizer (or apply moisturizer to your face first).

2. Dip in your fingers or a triangular sponge, and dot on your cheeks, your chin, your forehead, and your nose.

3. Smooth it over your face and gently blend in upward, outward motions, making sure not to forget the side of your nose, under your eyebrows, along the jawline, blending an inch below the jawline and chin.

4. Gently blot the face with a tissue when you're done, to soak up any excess oil. Your foundation should feel light and natural. In fact, if you can feel it at all, you've put on too much.

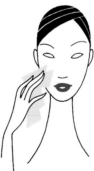

Tip If your water-based foundation dries out, add a few drops of alcohol-free toner and shake to get rid of clumps. A bit of toner will also make an oil-based foundation sheerer and less oily. (Note: oil-based foundations separate; shake each time before you use them.)

the small herd of companies that will individually "custom-blend" foundation for you. With custom-blended foundation, you'll have more choices, although in the end, you're still striping color on your face to see which melts into your skin—and you'll be paying a premium for it. Here's my suggestion for a thriftier alternative: if you find yourself in between shades at the cosmetics counter, try two—the one that's closest to your skin tone and the one that's next to it— and mix them together. Experiment by mixing a little of each in the palm of your hand, and see if you come closer to a match. If you do, buy both. They will last twice as long!

Concealer

If I could take only two cosmetics to a desert island, I'd choose lipstick and concealer. Concealer covers dark circles or tiny veins that show through the thin skin beneath the eyes and against the sides of the nose. Most people have natural shadows beneath their eyes, because of the way the eyes are set into the head. Add that to the fact that the skin is thinnest in the undereye area, and we're ready to talk concealer.

What concealer will *not* do is "treat" or "heal" dark circles. But because of its thickness, it will cover them—and keep them covered. Concealer can also be used to cover up an errant pimple, or redness at the sides of the lower part of the nose, but don't spot it on in too many different places or you'll draw attention to what you're trying to hide. Foundation or tinted moisturizer will sometimes do, but most of the time they're not occlusive enough. Plus, they tend to nestle into the little lines and stay there.

How To: use concealer

1. Put a small amount on your fourth fingertip and dot it on, moving from the outside corner of the eye inward, and back out again. The most important and easily overlooked place to put concealer is the inner corner of your top lid. Put a bit slightly below your dark circles to avoid the raccoon-like look.

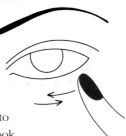

2. You can apply concealer over or under foundation, but no matter which way you choose, be sure to blend, blend, blend. If you prefer, use a triangular makeup sponge to blend in a gentle back-and-forth dotting motion. (Do not pull or rub: you'll stretch your delicate thin skin!)

3. After applying, smile into the mirror and check that it's evenly applied and hasn't crept into the little lines around your eyes. If that happens, blot gently with a tissue.

Concealers generally come in stick, liquid, or cream form. Like the porridge in "Goldilocks and the Three Bears," stick concealer can be too thick and the applicator may pull your skin; liquid concealer is too thin and runny; but cream is just right for almost everyone. Cream concealer is as low-tech as you can get. It usually comes in a little pot, and you apply it with your fourth finger or a triangular sponge, which helps get it into the corners around your eyes. Because it's smooth but creamy, it's easy to dot on and easy to keep on.

I'd also recommend a pen concealer. It's thicker than most liquids, and it's packaged in a thin, pen-shaped cylinder with a brush at one end. The concealer glides onto the brush and goes on very smoothly and gently. Then you can blend it in with your finger.

Choose concealer that's a shade lighter than your foundation. (If your circles are really dark, go two shades lighter.) You won't have as many choices with shades of concealer as you do with foundation, but make sure that if your foundation has a pink or yellow undertone, your concealer does, too. And beware of the following:

■ If your concealer is too dark, you'll get that raccoon look: your eyes will look smaller, and you'll create the illusion of pushing them deeper into your head.

■ If you choose a shade that's too light, your concealer will emphasize the area you wish to hide: a sort of reverse raccoon effect.

■ Dot and dab to apply, but never, ever pull.

■ If you use concealer to cover pimples, spider veins, beauty marks, acne, or acne scars, use only a little bit. If you use too much, by 4 P.M. those speckles of concealer will show through in a polka-dot design on your face.

Tip

THE FOURTH FINGER

Makeup artists swear by concealer brushes, but I believe that you'll get the best and most even coverage if you apply concealer with your fourth finger. The fourth finger exerts the least pressure, so it doesn't pull on delicate skin and its warmth blends better. Just be sure to pat *gently*. The fourth finger is also great for applying eye cream and eye shadow, as it gets into all the little nooks and crannies around your eyes.

Steer clear of oddball, "color-corrective," weird-looking colors. I've seen yellow, blue, green, white, pink, and peach versions. Avoid them all. You'll look like a science experiment.

Here are some good cream concealers: Laura Mercier Secret Concealer, Stila Eye Light, Shu Uemura Nobara, Shiseido Concealer, Prescriptives Virtual Skin Concealer, Revlon New Complexion Concealer, Estée Lauder Smoothing Skin Concealer. If you use a stick, Cover Girl Concealer and Neutrogena Under Cover Concealer Stick are good and inexpensive options. But apply it with your finger, not directly from the tube.

Blush

To any woman who squeezed her first tiny tube of Bonne Bell Cheek Gel around the age of 12 or 13, the magic of blush is obvious. Blush is fast-fix beauty: it warms up the skin, contours the cheek, highlights the cheekbones, exaggerates an attractive hollow, and, ideally, creates a bloom on your face that looks like it comes from within.

Blush comes in three basic shades: pink (for cool undertones), peach (for warm), or a soft shade of brown (for either warm or cool). Powder blush is the easiest to apply. It's also easiest to blot off with a tissue if you apply too much.

Cream Blush. As you get older, you lose color in your face, and blush can come in really handy. Since your skin is drier, too, powder blush may start to look cakey. If you notice this happening, try a cream blush, which will bring

How To: apply blush

Blush warms with the heat of the body to a more intense hue, which is one reason to apply it very sparingly.

1. First, throw away the brush that comes in the compact; it's too stiff and small to create a natural look. Use a good blush brush.
2. Grin like a fool into the mirror, to see where the apple of your cheek appears.
3. Dip your blush brush into the powder, shake off the excess, and brush it lightly over the apple of the cheek, moving toward the ear, with short, up-and-down vertical movements.
4. Then blend it in with one soft horizontal stroke on top of the vertical strokes, and blot a tissue on top to remove the excess, or cover lightly with powder.
5. If you're feeling particularly washed out, you can brush a light stroke of blush across your forehead up by your hairline *or* just above the brows where the sun would hit your face. (But don't overdo it.)

If you use a cream or cheek gel, dab a tiny bit on the apple of each cheek and gently rub it in with your fingers. (It's best to start with too little and layer on more later.) Make sure to blend very, very well. Many makeup artists use a sponge or brush to apply cream blush, as well as foundation and powder to help blend it. Take a tiny bit on the tip of the brush or sponge and stroke upward gently. (If the idea of using a brush on liquid formulations seems foreign, remember that artists paint with brushes, not sponges or powder puffs. And painting your face is an art.)

GO FOR A GLOW

LIQUID OR CREAM: Chanel Base Lumière, Clinique Allover Face Lustre Cream, Nars Multiple Sticks, Prescriptives' Cheekbuds Creamy Cheekcolor, Trucco's Alive Creme Blush.

GEL: Prescriptives Rosy Rouge Cheekcolor; Benetint, a blush-stain from Benefit; Chanel Fruit Gelée, Origins Pinch Your Cheeks.

POWDER: Bourjois Pastel Joves, Nina Ricci Powder Blush, Chanel Powder Blush, Lorac Blush, Clinique Beyond Blusher, Lancôme Blush Subtil, Bobbi Brown Essentials Blush, Yves Saint Laurent Blushing Powder.

moisture to your skin, and give it a natural, fresh look. Because cream blushes contain oils, they are also good for dry skin.

And one crucial bit of advice to avoid the Bozo the Clown look: apply color cosmetics in natural light whenever possible. A dimly lit bathroom will not give you the look you want in public.

Tip **A**pply a very light coat of powder before—and after—applying blush. The powder makes it go on more smoothly and prevents the blush from grabbing on to oily spots on your skin.

Contouring

Contouring is a technique that uses blush and bronzing powder to give the contours of your face—and your bone structure—better definition. It's a way to make your cheekbones look more prominent, your eyes look deeper, and emphasize your chin. Contouring is based on a principle that any painter learns in art school: dark colors recede (shading), light colors come forward (highlighting). Here's where a good brush comes in handy. It can help finesse all sorts of illusions that you couldn't begin to accomplish with a flimsier tool.

Makeup artists do a lot of contouring, because it enhances the depth and prominence of models' features in fashion photographs. At a press presentation several years ago, Carol Shaw, the makeup artist and founder of Lorac cosmetics, used my face to demonstrate the techniques of contouring, and I couldn't believe what a huge difference it made. Suddenly my cheekbones were transformed into Michelle Pfeiffer's, and the line of my jaw has never looked as strong. Because it is so dramatic—and takes patience and precision—you're not going to want to do this on a daily basis, but it's fun to experiment with it. Try the techniques in private, and hone your special effects for a special evening.

Shading can create or exaggerate a hollow and add depth to shadowy areas. The darker the powder, the deeper the contour. Use a bronzing powder or blush in a brown shade, about two shades darker than your skin.

How To: shade and highlight

▓ To hollow out the area under the cheekbone, suck in your cheeks and stroke a shade of light brown or dark beige powder (a slightly darker, more neutral shade) from the middle of the cheek outward and up on your temples toward the top of the ear. Blend extremely well, then cover lightly with your face powder.

▓ If you want to attract attention to the center of your face, apply the powder on the cheeks against the side of the nose and slightly outward in a triangle that runs from the bottom of your nose to the corner of your eye.

▓ If you want your chin to look more prominent, stroke some bronzing powder on the ball of your chin and outward in both directions. Blend extremely well with a brush, dry sponge, or your fingers, and "set" with face powder.

Highlighting opens up an area you want to emphasize and brings it forward. You can use a slightly shimmering powder to highlight.

Whether you are shading or highlighting, the powder should go on *after* you apply foundation—or without foundation.

Powder

Powder is another worthwhile splurge. Like foundation, it's easy to justify because powder, too, lasts a long time—up to three years. And the finer the powder, the more flawless the finish. A light dusting of powder will absorb oil and eliminate shine, which is why it's particularly good for oily skin or the T-Zone area. It will also set your makeup and give it a more polished look, filter out UV light, and make the skin look smooth and even.

For a sheer finish, choose a translucent powder. Loose, translucent powder has the lightest texture, and it looks wonderful, but it's also the messiest to work with. Pressed powder is portable and gives a more matte finish. It also gives an excuse for gorgeous compacts and the elegant gesture involved in powdering your nose. Loose or pressed powder can be a nice, sheer substitute for foundation. But don't pack on too much, especially if your skin is dry, or it will look cakey, exaggerate any little lines and crinkles, and make your skin look tight. Your powder should match your skin tone as well as your foundation does. If the color's off, powder will look pasty and theatrical. Custom-blended powders are an option if you have hard-to-match skin, but I'm not a big fan of them. They're overpriced, and there are enough ready-made versions for almost everyone.

Iridescent powder adds a little shimmer to the brows, jawline, and décolleté—an especially pretty look for evening. Bronzing powder is great for shading and contouring (see page 123), and a dusting of blush over bronzer warms the face. It will give you a bit of extra color when you need it: in the transition from

How To: apply a finishing touch

1. If you use loose powder, dip your powder brush into the powder. Shake or tissue off the excess.

2. Dust the face lightly in upward strokes.

3. Wipe the brush on a tissue, and then use it to remove excess powder from your face.

Apply pressed powder with a circular velour or sponge in light, upward strokes. Your velour or sponge won't last as long as the powder. If your applicator looks shiny and caked, or if hardly any powder comes off on your face when you glide the velour or sponge across, it's time to wash it or get a new supply. Otherwise, the oils from your skin will build up on the powder to create a shiny, hardened film. In that case, scrape off the surface with a knife, and the powder will be as good as new.

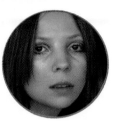
Eye Makeup

Eye makeup should emphasize both the shape and the natural color of the eyes. Use eyeliners or pencils for contour, shadow for shading and shaping, and mascara to elongate and thicken the lashes. Eye shadow can add depth to your eyes or simply help you look wide awake. When it comes to tricks of light and shadow, eye makeup can create illusion better than any other cosmetic.

Remember, the eye area tends to be naturally dry because of a dearth of oil glands. So before you do anything else to your eyes, make sure that you use an eye cream daily, faithfully. In 10 or 20 years, you'll thank me. Also, eye makeup is not going to look its best if you look

spring to summer, to boost your tan during the summer, or to hold on to it when summer moves into fall. It's also terrific for women of color because it evens out your skin tone, especially in winter.

When you use bronzing powder, keep the face powder to a bare minimum, and don't forget to blend a light sweep of bronzing powder on the neck as well. And forget about liquid bronzer: it not only looks as fake as a bad self-tanner but also inevitably comes off on your collar.

I've done more than my share of models coming off the red-eye," says makeup artist Bobbi Brown. "When you're tired, your skin gets dehydrated," she adds. "Drink a lot of water. Moisturize. Choose makeup with hydration. Go with less, not more. When you're tired, your skin looks one shade paler. Warm it up with a bronzer or blush. And don't forget your undereye concealer—preferably one to two shades lighter than your makeup."

Trade Secret

The Powder Room

*A light dusting of powder
will give any face a fine finish.*

Even Baudelaire—a man—understood the value of a good face powder. Of course, makeup was more universally unisex in those days, because of the need to cover smallpox scars and the results of rampantly poor hygiene. But powder is also a pleasure. "I like the way a beautiful foundation or powder slides on," a friend once said. "It heightens your sexuality. Makeup can make you look sexier, stronger, softer, or vampier than usual. And you can play along." Like Baudelaire, my friend is a sensualist. She, along with many women, finds a beautiful compact "enchanting," "charming," "bewitching." She goes for the drama of the gesture—pulling an elegant jeweled compact out of her little evening bag and putting a touch of shimmer to her cheeks.

A fine powder smells soft, feels silky to the touch, and smoothes over anything. Here are some of the most appealing loose, pressed, and shimmery powders.

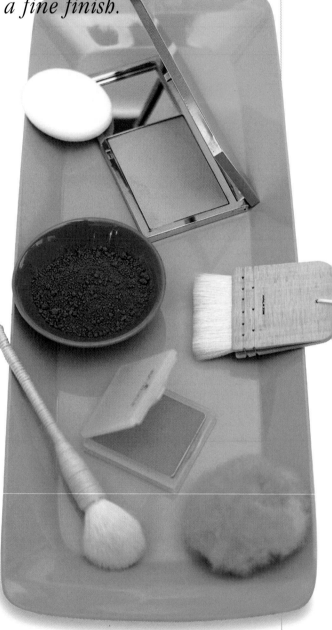

*W*ho can fail to see that the use of rice powder, so fatuously anathematized by innocent philosophers, has as its purpose and result to hide all the blemishes that nature has so outrageously scattered over the complexion, and to create an abstract unity of texture and colour in the skin, which unity, like the one produced by tights, immediately approximates the human being to a statue, in other words to a divine or superior being?

—CHARLES BAUDELAIRE, "In Praise of Makeup"

Trade Secret

Makeup artists stock up on 12-packs of soft, dry cellulose sponges. They use them to press powder onto the face, especially right up under the eyes, where a brush can leave clumps.

Make sure to remove any excess powder with a brush, so that you don't leave a cloud of dust in your wake like a member of the court of Louis XIV.

Best loose. Stila Illuminating Powder, Christian Dior Translucent Powder or Dior Light Oil-Free, T. Leclerc Poudre Compact, Guerlain Loose Powder, Prescriptives All Skins, Bobbi Brown Essentials Face Powder, La Bella Donna Mineral Makeup, Iman Luxury Loose Powder.

Best pressed. Shiseido Pressed Powder, T. Leclerc Poudre Compact (especially the "banane" color if you're a "warm"), Shu Uemura Face Powder, L'Oréal Feel Naturale Pressed Powder, Chanel Natural Finish Pressed Powder, Bobbi Brown Essentials Face Powder, Lancôme Ombre Subtile, M•A•C Matte. Less expensive, good choices: Neutrogena Healthy Skin Powder, Cover Girl Clean Pressed Powder.

Best shimmers. It makes sense that theatrical makeup companies have mastered the art of developing a shimmery powder. For the best shimmer powders, go to Stila, M•A•C, Alcone, and Make Up For Ever, a line started by a French makeup artist who began her career in the theater. Honorable mention: Benefit Kitten.

Best bronzers. In 1984, Guerlain created the first bronzing powder, called Terracotta, which is still one of the best. Other good ones are Laura Mercier Bronzer, Chanel Perfecting Bronzer, Vincent Longo New York Odalisque, and Bourjois Pastel Joues.

If you like colored eye shadow, apply it with great restraint. "Just a hint of a color won't look cheap," says makeup artist Laura Mercier. "And a darker color close to the lashes, with brighter colors kept further away, makes for a softer and more modern look."

The art of applying eye shadow may appear more complicated than for other cosmetics, because there are so many colors, textures, tools, and techniques to choose from. For a polished look, you're often juggling two shades—a darker one to make the eyes look deeper and a lighter one to open them up. It's enough to make you want to skip the whole thing and proceed directly to lipstick.

But experimenting with eye shadow is a fun way to indulge your latent inner artist— the one who may not have seen the light of day since you were five years old. In the privacy of your own home—or with a couple of trusted friends—try playing around with some of the techniques on the following pages. None of them is complicated—all you need is the adventurousness to try and a little practice in applying.

tired or dry in the eye area. So if you suffer from any of the Big Four problems—puffiness, crepeyness (papery dryness), dark circles, or fine lines—there are a few beauty Rxs to help you (see page 130).

Eye Shadow

Too much added color detracts from your eyes, even if it matches your eye color. In fact, although you may think blue shadow will bring out the blue in your eyes, many shades of blue will actually have the opposite effect. And that's why neutral eye shadows are the best. But neutral isn't restricted to brown. (Let's face it, brown can get a little boring.) By "neutral," I mean soft colors found in skin (browns, vanillas, mauves, beiges) or in the subtle undertones of skin (golds, olives, pale purples, blues, grays). Neutrals are easy to work with, because they meld well with one another and complement your skin tone.

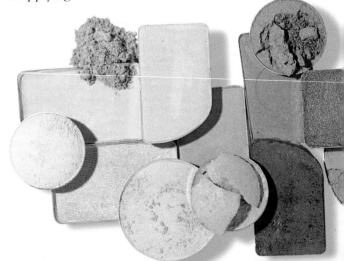

How To: use eye shadow or eyeliner to create illusion

A few simple techniques using eye shadow or eyeliner can dramatically affect the look and shape of your eyes. An eye pencil can be used instead of eyeliner for the same effect.

To make your eyes look . . .

closer together.
Stroke a light or medium neutral shade of eye shadow on the inner corner of your eyelids. Or use eyeliner to draw the line a bit thicker on the inner corner of the eye and stop the line where the outer corner of the eye stops.

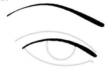

farther apart.
Take a matte shadow in a darker shade and stroke it outward and slightly upward, on the outer corners of the top and bottom lids. Or use eyeliner and start the line just a bit away from the inner corner of your eye. Make it slightly thicker toward the outer edge and extend it in a slightly upward curve.

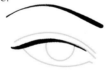

bigger.
Remember, light tones protrude, so you want to bring light to your eyes. Stroke a neutral shadow in a light shade in the crease of your lid above your iris. If you want color, stroke the neutral on first—bone, vanilla, taupe—and then layer the color on top. It lights up the eye as if there were a lightbulb behind the lid. Or stroke a light color on the lids, with a darker color in the crease and along the upper and lower lash lines. Or use eyeliner to follow the natural shape of the eye and draw a fine line at the base of the upper and lower lashes to give your eyes more definition.

rounder.
Put eye shadow all around the edges of the upper and lower lids to make your eyes look rounder. Or use eyeliner to outline the eyes at the base of the lashes. As you move toward the outer corner, thicken and "wing" the line upward ever so slightly.

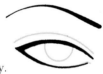

more oval.
Draw a fine line at the base of the lashes. Thicken it slightly in the middle of the lid, and draw it toward the outer corner to make your eyes appear more oval.

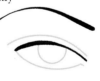

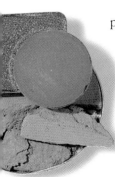

Eye shadows come in creams, powders, and pencils. Creams are the hardest to control. They can look beautiful, but they also tend to slip into the little creases on your lids and around the corners of your eyes. Pencils are easy to use, as long as you remember to smudge and soften the line as you go.

Powder is my all-time favorite because you can use it either wet or dry and it's the easiest to control. But because it can look drying, you need to find a powder that feels creamy. Dab your fourth finger in the tester color. Rub your thumb together with your fourth finger. If it feels smooth and emollient, it will look that way on your eyes. If your finger "gets stuck," the powder is too dry.

WHAT TO DO IF YOU HAVE . . .

Puffiness. Avoid salty foods and oily, creamy skincare products, which make puffiness worse. Stick to gels, which firm and tighten, for use around your eyes. If oil is one of the first five ingredients in your eye cream, it's too oily for you.

Crepeyness. If your eye pencil bumps and grinds across your lash line instead of drawing a smooth line, or if your top lid looks "puckery," your skin is "crepey," or overly dry. Don't overcleanse, and avoid products with SD alcohols and talc, a common ingredient in powder eye shadow. Dab a bit of cream concealer on your eyelids before you apply powder shadow. It will ease the dryness and help avoid "seepage."

Fine lines. Be extremely gentle when you touch the area around your eyes (not easy to do if you wear contact lenses!). And apply a good eye cream in the morning.

Dark circles. Dark circles are, to some extent, hereditary, but there are certain things like stress, unhealthy eating habits, vitamin and mineral deficiencies, smoking, and hangovers that darken circles even more. Circles seem to darken as you age because the thin skin gets thinner (a dwindling estrogen supply doesn't help) and the force of gravity pulls your face down, making the circles appear bigger. Try an eye cream with Vitamin K or one of these products: Avon Lighten Up Undereye Treatment, Peter Thomas Roth AHA Kojic Under Eye Brightener, M.D. Formulations Vit-A-Plus Revitalizing Eye Cream.

According to traditional Chinese medicine, there is a link between the undereye area and the body's elimination function. Western medicine has also acknowledged a connection between kidney function and undereye circles. Ask your doctor.

Redness. If your eyes are tired—or if they simply *look* tired—and your eyelids look red, pink, or brown, you'll want to neutralize that color first, before you put on eye shadow. Dab some concealer on your eyelids to even out the tone, or try Magic by Precriptives Red Neutralizer (a cosmetic concealer that gets the red out).

Techniques: Highlighting and Smudging

First, throw away that silly little foam applicator that comes with so many shadows. It's too stiff to maneuver, and it's why so many women walk around with streaky, clumpy, or jagged-edged eye shadow. Applying eye shadow with an angled natural brush helps you even it out in the socket area. A brush is also nice when you moisten powder shadow and use it to outline your eyes, because it will give you an even and precisely drawn line. But if you want your eye shadow to look soft, subtle, smudgy, smoky, or shadowy (all good choices, depending on your mood and the occasion), you probably don't want the perfect and distinct line you'll get with a brush. That's the time to use your invaluable fourth finger to soften the line.

Highlighting. Highlighting is the best way to open up the space between your eyes and eyebrows. Here's a handy little trick that makes almost every woman's eyes look bigger, more open, and wide awake.

1. If you want to make the space between the eye and the brow look roomier, dust vanilla or ivory powder on the browbone—the space directly below the arch of your brow—or use a shimmer stick there.

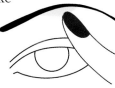

2. Blend well. For evening, try something with a pearl or a shimmer, but be careful: if you're at all crepey or wrinkly around the eye, the shimmers will highlight that, too.

Smudging. This is a simple way to emphasize your eyes and give them depth. (For a more subtle look, skip step 1.)

1. Smudge a bit of matte shadow in deep neutral or earth tones —brown, deep green, charcoal, navy, plum —in the center of the lid, softly out to the sides, and into the socket directly above the iris.

2. An eye pencil will give the outline of the eye a stronger look. Sharpen your pencil—black or brown —but don't sharpen it too much. You want a soft, rounded ball. (For a softer look, use powder and a brush, or smudge with your finger.)

3. Draw a line out from the center of the upper and lower lash line, and smudge gently with your fourth finger or hard-pressed Q-tip just enough to soften the line. If you choose a

MOD COLOR

Trade Secret

The 1960s craze of sugary acid greens, candy-coated corals, magenta reds, and brassy baby blues may look striking when resurrected in the fashion pages of *Vogue* or *Harper's Bazaar,* but in real life, it causes most sophisticated women to bolt. As well it should—it's not an attractive look. Unless you're an actress, a teenager, or a drag queen, or you're doing your Cher imitation, you probably don't want a pop art palette on your eyelids.

What about that old perennial, blue eye shadow? Blue eye shadow had its beginnings in the Victorian period, when a bluish tinge to the eyelids was considered beautiful and the sign of a weak and innocent heart. If you're fair-skinned, with black or platinum blond hair and brown or gray eyes, or very dark-skinned, it may look gorgeous on you. But even then stick to shades like pale blue, silver blue, or navy.

However, if you're up for some fun, try a makeup artists' favorite: Yves Saint Laurent Mascara Moiré, a colored mascara that comes in purple, forest green, bronze, copper, midnight blue, or gold. It's much more subtle than you may think. It catches and reflects the light beautifully as it hits your lashes, for extra glamour in the evening.

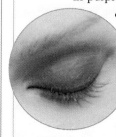

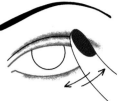

colored pencil—deep violet, navy blue, or green-gold instead of black—it will look even softer. Try to draw the line right up against the edge of your lid.

   4. Apply mascara.

Eyeliner

On women with medium to dark skin and a steady hand, eyeliner can look beautiful and dramatic. But if you want a softer look, put your liquid liner aside and use a pencil or shadow, says makeup artist Laura Mercier. To draw a precise line, hold the lid in place with your fingers, but don't stretch it—you'll only distort the shape. Apply eyeliner from the inner corner of the upper lid, and draw a line aross the base of the lashes in one stroke. If you're tired or hurried, forget about using eyeliner; your hand won't be steady enough. Besides, eyeliner calls attention to tired eyes. Instead, rub some soft brown or charcoal shadow into the lash line. Good lines: Revlon Jetliner, Yves Saint Laurent Eyeliner Moiré, Prestige Liquid Eyeliner (the point is thin, which makes it easy to apply).

Mascara

State-of-the-art mascara claims to do just about everything for your lashes that you'd do for the hair on your head: protect from dryness and breakage; create a style (smooth or curly—it's your choice!); last forever; and reduce irritation, especially if you wear contacts or have sensitive eyes.

How To: make lashes lush

Mascara contains a lot of wax, and the wax can develop crystal formations that prevent it from going on smoothly. Using a thinner brush can help, because it's more precise and makes it easier to get into the corner lashes while avoiding the clumps. A short wand is better than a longer one, because it gives you more control.

1. To avoid clumping and smudging, always wipe the mascara wand lightly with a tissue before you apply it.

2. Apply upward, from below the upper lashes, in parallel strokes, starting in the middle and moving out to the edges.

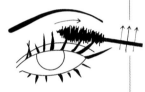

3. Give a few coats to the edges, which is where you want to concentrate your efforts, by blinking onto the brush. Use very little—even none!—on the lower lashes to avoid smearing.

4. If your mascara clumps, use a clean old toothbrush to "comb" through your lashes and remove them. Sometimes mascara smudges beneath the eyes because it's attracted to oily concealer or eye creams. If you don't use mascara because it always smudges, try these suggestions. Pat a bit of powder under your eye before you apply mascara. Always remember to wipe the mascara wand first.

Mascara Moments

The way that women shape their brows, shade their eyelids, and lengthen their lashes provides an eye-opening look at shifting styles—and sensibilities—through the years. Each look below defines a decade. Q: Can you guess whose eyes these are?

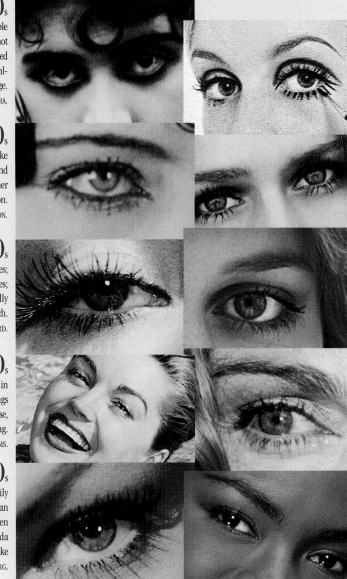

1910s
Before mascara was available commercially, beads of hot wax were sometimes applied to the tips of each lash. Kohl-rimmed eyes were the rage. A: THEDA BARA.

1920s
Silent-film stars spoke volumes with their eyes and set the trend for heavy liner and lots of lash definition. A: GLORIA SWANSON.

1930s
Smouldering bedroom eyes; sultry, long, leggy lashes; pencil-thin brows perpetually raised in a quizzical arch. A: JOAN CRAWFORD.

1940s
Waterproof mascara comes in handy for weddings, screenings of *Casablanca*, and, of course, synchronized swimming. A: ESTHER WILLIAMS.

1950s
Thinly plucked, heavily penciled brows. Italian bombshells Sophia Loren and Gina Lollobrigida inspired obvious falsies (fake lashes). A: ANITA EKBERG.

1960s
The Carnaby Street mods ushered in an era of upholstery fringe, with lashes so long and thick they resembled wigs. A: TWIGGY.

1970s
Lashes were hand-twisted and embellished, hair by hair, to fill in what nature left out. A: LAUREN HUTTON.

1980s
Short, full lashes created a wide-eyed effect, enhanced by lots of no-nonsense clear or black mascara. A: PRINCESS DI.

1990s
Thick brows framed a wild-eyed, vixenish, ultra-eyelash-curler look. Colored mascaras in blue, purple, and green were trendy. A: MADONNA.

2000s
Impeccably groomed, beautifully shaped brows. New "curling" mascaras bring out an eye-opening curl. A: LAURYN HILL.

Classic Eye Looks

Four easy ways to open up your eyes . . .

Soft

Natural eyes look great with a strong or subtle lip color.

1. Brush a light or neutral shade—vanilla, suede, pale lemon—on your upper lids and into the crease.

2. Stroke on black or brown mascara.

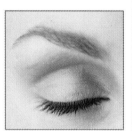

Shimmery

Contrast a polished, shimmery eye look with a matte or sheer lip color.

1. Brush a light shadow with a hint of bronze, copper, or silver onto your upper lids and into the crease.

2. With a darker shadow or pencil, press a line across the base of the upper lids and along the outer corner of the lower lids.

3. Gently smudge with a hard-pressed Q-tip.

4. Stroke on black mascara.

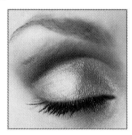

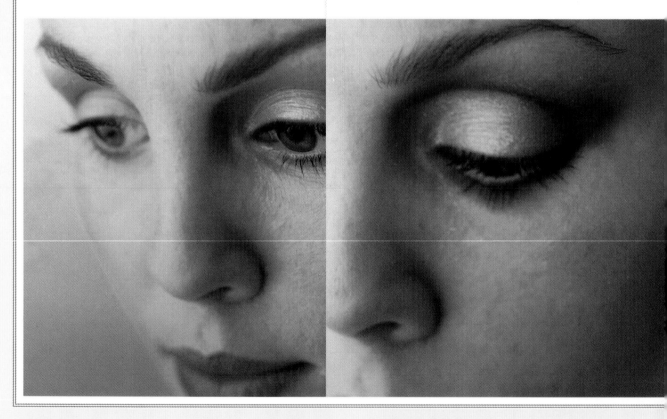

There is only one good reason for the existence of eye shadow: to bring focus to your eyes. A neutral shade will quietly attract attention. Something shimmery makes eyes gleam and sparkle. Dark, smoky shades set a dramatic tone. And light tones make your eyes bright. A word on color: remember, opposites attract. Choose an eye shadow color that contrasts with the color of your eyes—blue shadow on brown eyes, or lavender on green—and they'll really pop.

Smoky

Dramatic eye makeup works beautifully with glossy lips.

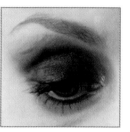

1. Brush a deep shadow on your upper lids and into the crease.

2. Draw a line out from the center of the lower lid with a pencil and smudge gently in each direction with a hard-pressed Q-tip.

3. Offset the dark with light: a stroke of vanilla, off-white, or bone shadow under the arch.

4. Apply black mascara.

Stylized

A graphic, gamine eye pairs up perfectly with simple matte red lips.

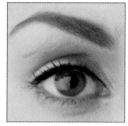

1. Apply a wash of light, pale shadow to your upper lids.

2. Draw a smooth line with black pencil or eyeliner on the upper lash lines.

3. Highlight under the arch with a stroke of vanilla, off-white, or bone shadow.

4. Apply black mascara.

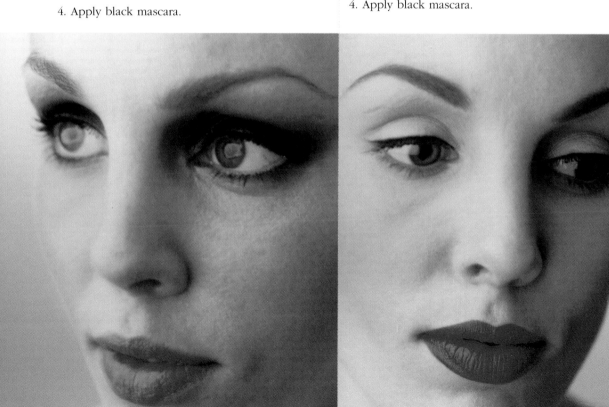

But the bottom line is that it's just not worth it to spend a pile of money on mascara, especially since you have to throw it out a few months after opening. Mascara is easily contaminated by bacteria, which you definitely don't want in your eyes. Plus, as mascara gets older, it also gets clumpier and eventually dries out. Discard mascara after four months, max.

There are two basic types of mascara—waterproof and regular—and unless you're a swimmer or you cry a lot, stick with the regular, because the waterproof version is hard to remove. Maybelline Great Lash, in the hot pink and chartreuse tube, is still one of the best—and cheapest—around. It's also the one that makeup artists and models use, consistently, backstage at designer fashion shows.

Most women prefer black mascara, for good reason. Black is basic yet sophisticated, and, like the little black dress, it works well on almost anyone. But if you're blond or simply want a more natural look, try brown. And if mascara in any shade is too dark for your lashes, try "clear," which, by the way, is not a waste of money. Clear mascara lifts and separates the lashes, for a subtly enhanced look. Of course, you can use that old standby Vaseline to do the same thing, but it can get goopy. Always apply mascara in a stationary position. This is no joke. *Never* apply mascara on a moving subway, train, bus, or in a car. If you poke yourself in the eye (and it happens all the time), you can scratch your cornea.

Lash curling. If you want to give your eyes a more open, wide-awake look, you may want to curl your lashes before applying mascara. (Never curl after applying or your lashes could

UNDER $10

BE$T BUYS

Top of the line cheapies: Maybelline Great Lash Mascara, Maybelline Volume Express Mascara, L'Oréal Lash Out, L'Oréal Le Grand Curl Mascara, Revlon Color Stay Extra Thick Lashes, Revlon Everylash and the curling version of Everylash, Neutrogena Full-Length Defining Mascara, Sephora Mascara (no clumping). M·A·C Mascara costs a bit more, but it comes with a built-in antibacterial warning system: the rosewater scent dissipates after three months. Once that goes, so should your mascara.

If you have sensitive eyes, spend the extra money for a sensitive-eye formulation, which contains less wax than most other mascaras. Wax can be an irritant and also makes mascara tougher to remove. Sensitive-eye formulations bind more gently to the lashes with a silk protein powder. For sensitive eyes try Chanel Cils Caresse Fragile Lash Builder, Princess Marcella Borghese Superiore/State of the Art Mascara, and Bobbi Brown Essentials Mascara (a thinner, less tenacious formulation than most, it goes on fairly sheer and is easy to remove).

break off.) To use an eyelash curler: open the scissorlike apparatus, rest your upper lashes in the little trough, close the curler, and hold for about 30 seconds. Avoid curling your lower lashes, because they are more vulnerable.

Eyebrows

Even if you never touch another cosmetic again, buy a good pair of tweezers and develop the skill to use them. Because no makeup trick on the planet will make you look better than a pair of beautiful brows.

"A well-groomed brow will frame the eye and give the face a polished look," says Eliza Petrescu, waxing director and eyebrow designer at the Avon Centre Spa and Salon in New York City. "Eyebrow Designer"? That raised my eyebrows, too, especially when I heard that Eliza charges $65 to work her magic. But among fashion and beauty insiders, Eliza's work is universally considered wizardry and she's so much in demand that Avon has opened the country's first "eyebrow boutique" on the spa's mezzanine.

Well. I went, I interviewed, I had my brows done. My conclusion? We all have a lot to learn from Eliza.

"People tend to tweeze too much," Eliza says. Her most important advice is to be careful about the distance between the brows and the length of the brows. To get it right, she suggests: Look in the mirror, hold a pencil vertically against the highest bone on the side of the nose, and note where it meets the brow. (If you need to, draw a line as a guide.) Do this on both sides of the nose. Pluck only in between. To determine the end of your eyebrow, extend a pencil (or tweezer) diagonally from your nostril, over the outer edge of your eye toward the brow. Where it lands is where your brow should end. Whatever you do, says Eliza, don't pluck the top of the brow. "If you pluck it, it will become fuzzy, and then you won't be able to create or contour an arch."

How To: groom your brows

If your brows are sparse or spotty and you want to fill them in, there are several ways to do it.

1. Take an angled eyeshadow brush and press just a bit of eye shadow to the brow (medium or dark brown for brunettes, taupe for blondes or redheads, charcoal for silver or gray hair). Follow the direction of the brow and extend the brushed-on shadow to the edge of the eye.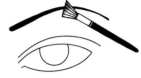

2. Pat a tissue on top to blot up any excess.

If your brows are really thin, you can pencil them in slightly thicker, but it's difficult to make this look natural. Take an eye pencil under the brow and follow the brow line out to the edge of the eye. Use your powder sponge to press some powder on top, very gently, to soften the line. Then use a brush to lightly fill it in with shadow.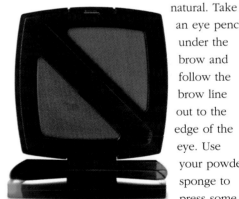

Tip Chanel's Perfect Brow Compact is an all-in-one brow kit. It costs a fortune, but it's terrific. Eliza's Eyebrow Essentials (the travel size is all you need) will also give your eyebrows everything they need.

If your brows are messy on top, have a facialist wax them. But make sure to talk to her first about the shape that you want. Obviously, you can choose any shape you like, from a perpetually quizzical arch to a thin Marlene Dietrich line. For me, the most elegant brow is elongated, clean, and simple.

My advice: if you've never plucked your eyebrows before, see a professional the first time because it's possible that once hair is tweezed, it may never grow back. It's rare, but in case this happens to you, you'll want to get it right the first time.

Eyebrow Plucking. Some women prefer to moisturize before they pluck; they say it hurts less that way. I prefer to pluck when my skin is dry because I can be more precise with the tweezer. But if that's painful for you, try putting a dab of Anbesol on the area to numb it, or hold a cold washcloth to the brow for a few seconds before you start. A tweezer with a pointed or slanted tip will grip the hairs best.

Always pluck *below* the brow line, so the hair won't grow back in a scraggly-looking line, and follow the natural arch of your brow. Use the top of the brow as a guide on how to shape the bottom. Pluck the hairs out toward the ears, in the direction in which they grow. Remove stray hairs, but don't pluck too much at once.

Pluck a few hairs and then stop. Look in the mirror, step back, and see how you're doing. You can always take out more later, but once you've overplucked, you'll have to live with that thin, artificial line until the hair grows back.

Eyebrow Tinting. Lightening your brows can lighten the look of your face. Obviously, you can darken them if you want them to stand out more, but this isn't a great look for most people. To get a rough idea of how bleaching will look, take a light brown or taupe eyeshadow and rub it on your brows. Because of potential damage to your vision, always have your eyebrows tinted by a professional.

Lipstick

No cosmetic has the power to transform like lipstick. Even women who don't wear makeup wear lipstick—and say they feel naked without it. According to a Simmons Market Research Bureau study, over 40 percent of women apply lipstick more than four times a day, and 67 percent of 30,000 women surveyed by Avon said that lipstick is the one cosmetic they can't live without. A necessary part of dressing, the ritual stroke of color on the lips is often the last thing a woman will do before she leaves the house. Another beauty paradox: why do naked lips seem so naked and painted ones so normal—and so desirable?

Like a new pair of shoes, a new lipstick holds a promise—the promise of change, romance, instant glamour. Lipstick leaves an indelible mark and makes a lasting impression. A suggestive slash of red or a pretty pink literally opens up a woman's mouth: it makes her feel gutsy, sexy, and self-assured. No other cosmetic is easier to apply. If you can color in a coloring book, you can color in your lips. With enough practice you won't even need a mirror. But there are some lipstick tips and tricks that can improve any technique (see pages 142 and 144).

Lip Service

Lipstick is composed of pigment, which determines its color; emollients or oils, which moisturize and carry the color; and wax, which gives lipstick its shape. (In the old days, fish scales were added for shimmer. Today, beetle carcasses are a main source of pigment!) The ratio of these ingredients to one another determines how the lipstick looks and feels on your lips. The more pigment, the more drying. The five basic formulations are sheer, shimmer, cream, matte, and long-lasting. Mattes contain the most pigment, sheers the least.

The lips are an extremely vulnerable part of the body, and lipstick should provide protection: a good lipstick will moisturize the lips and shield them from the sun. The softest, most moisturizing lipsticks are the ones with the smallest amount of pigment, because pigment is drying. Around World War I, the emollient used in lipstick was olive oil, which would turn rancid on the lips. These days, the most lubricious lipsticks contain moisturizers like Vitamin E, collagen, and amino acids, and some contain sunscreens for protection—although a matte lipstick will offer sun protection merely because of its opacity. (A University of California study concluded that men were seven times more vulnerable to lip cancer than women, because lipstick protects women's lips.)

Most makeup artists double up on products, which is a fun and economical thing to do: using lipstick as blush or eye shadow to fill in sparse brows. **warning** But NEVER PUT FOUNDATION OR BLUSH ON YOUR LIPS. Not only can it dry your lips, but if you ingest it, it may be carcinogenic. Foundation and blush contain certain D (drug) &C (cosmetic) dyes made from coal-tar additives. Some D&C dyes are restricted "for external use only" by the FDA and cannot be used on lips or around the eyes, where they are readily ingested or absorbed. There is an ongoing controversy about the use of *any* coal-tar dyes in cosmetics, partly because they trigger allergies in some people, and they've also been shown to cause cancer in lab mice, although the FDA says the cancer risk is minimal. But they're cheap, and they're still the best source of color available. If you want D&C-free lipsticks, look for Aveda, Aubrey Organics, Dr. Hauschka, Ecco Bella, Kiss My Face, and Paul Penders brands.

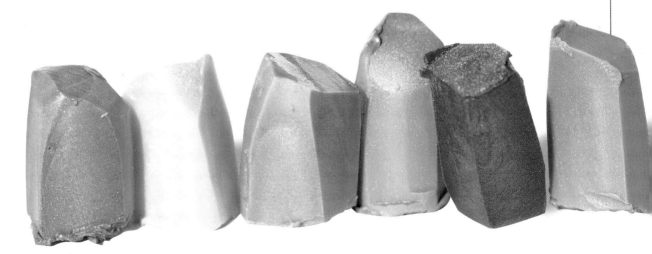

L I P S T I C K   L E X I C O N :

	THE SCOOP	THE LOOK	THE FEEL
SHEER	Sheers, also known as stains, tints, and glosses, contain minimal pigment and offer minimal coverage. They're so sheer, you don't need a mirror to apply them.	A natural, understated wet look with a hint of color and varying degrees of shine	Sheers are light and slippery, and they don't last long on the lips.
SHIMMER	Shimmers, formerly known as frosted, are more beautiful and subtle now. They look heavily metallic, pearly, or opalescent in the tube, but on the lips, the coverage is soft and subtle.	Shimmers catch and reflect light so that the lips shimmer	Shimmers contain bits of mica, a light reflector. The current versions feel lightweight, smooth, and creamy.
CREAM	A matte look without the heavy matte feel, creams contain more oils and conditioners than mattes, which makes them lighter. They're also known as moisturizing lipstick, hydrating lipstick, and lip rouge.	Not quite as deep as matte, but velvety and dewy-looking	Creams are smooth and lubricious, like richly colored lip balm.
MATTE	Mattes last longest (except for long-lasting lipsticks), because they contain the most pigment, and pigment makes a lipstick last. But mattes can be drying. Lighter mattes are known as demimatte or semimatte.	Provides deep color with a flat, opaque, nonshiny surface	Until recently, mattes made the lips feel dry, powdery, and chapped. Current formulations contain added moisturizers, but don't expect moist from matte.
LONG-LASTING	Many work on a time-release principle. The heat of the lip stimulates continuous release of color. Ingredients like porous silica seal it in, and cetyl octoanate (common in foundation) makes it last.	Deep and rich, they do not easily fade	These can last from five to eight hours. They feel like a creamy matte going on, but at the end of the day they can feel drying.

the way they look, the way they feel

THE BEST PRODUCTS	LIP TIP
M•A•C Lipgloss, Chanel Glossimer, Yves Saint Laurent Rouge Pur Transparent, Christian Dior Marshmallow Gloss, L'Oréal Rouge Pulp Liquid Lip Color, Kiehl Lip Gloss, Clinique Almost Lipstick, Trucco Lipstains, Stila Lip Polish, Clarins Sheer Lipstick, Max Factor Ultralucent Lip Polish, Origins Lip Gloss, Lancôme Sheer Magnetic Lipstick, Lorac Lip Gloss, Laura Mercier Healthy Lips	*Color in the lips with a light or nude pencil before you apply sheer lipstick and it will stay on longer.*
Lancôme Rouge Absolu, Prescriptives Mattina, Origins Frost Bites, Origins Shimmer Sticks, Laura Mercier Lip Colour, Stila Allover Shimmer, Chanel Rouge Lumiére, Bobbi Brown Essentials Shimmer Lip Gloss, Hard Candy Lip Gloss Cubes (metallics)	*If you want deeper color or longer-lasting shine, layer a shimmer on top of a matte.*
Prescriptives Extraordinary Lipstick, Origins Lip Crayons, L'Oréal Colour Riche Hydrating Lipcolour, Bobbi Brown Essentials Lipstick, Prestige Creamy Matte Lipstick Crayon, Princess Marcella Borghese Lumina Lipstick, Clinique Re-Moisturizing Lipstick, Yves Saint Laurent Rouge Pur, Clinique Chubby Sticks, Shu Uemura Lipstick, Chanel Hydrabase Creme	*If you outline the lips with a nude or light pencil, a creamy lipstick won't feather.*
M•A•C, Shiseido Matte Variations, Shu Uemura Powder Lipstick, Iman, Princess Marcella Borghese La Moda Matte Lip Color, Orlane Rouge Extraordinaire, Christian Dior Très Très Dior, Neutrogena Plush Lipcolor, L'Oréal Crayon Grand Lipcolour, Nars Matte or Semi-matte Lipstick	*If you like a matte look but find it drying, slick a layer of Hudsalva (Swedish, all-natural cocoa butter stick) or Vitamin E stick over lipstick.*
Clinique Long Last Lipstick, Revlon Colorstay, L'Oréal Colour Supreme Longwearing Lipcolour, Lancôme Rouge Magnetic	*Make sure to condition your lips every so often by piercing a Vitamin E capsule and rubbing it on, or dabbing on some shea butter.*

Lipstick Tips

■ Store lipstick—and perfume—in the refrigerator. It'll last longer.

■ Never use a tester on your lips—it's unhygienic. Test lipstick on your fingertips instead of the back of your hand: the color and texture are closer to those of your lips.

■ If you want your lipstick to last, use pencil first as a base. Outline and color in your lips with pencil (nude, if your lipstick shade is light), and slick your lipstick on top.

■ Your lips will also look softer, "smudgier," and less defined if you don't use pencils or lipliners.

■ To avoid lipstick on your teeth, run your index finger through the middle of your lips and pull it back out. The excess will come off on your finger, not your teeth.

■ In a pinch, your lipstick can double as blush. (But *never* use blush on your lips; see page 139.)

■ Outline your lips in pencil before you apply lipstick or gloss if you don't want your lipstick to feather.

■ Women over 50 usually look better with a cream lipstick rather than a matte or gloss. Every bit of moisture helps.

■ If your lipstick shade turns out to be brighter than you thought it would be, color in your lips with a pencil a few shades darker than your lipstick (for instance, brown pencil under dark red lipstick) and layer the lipstick on top. Or coat the lipstick with a darker lip gloss, which will turn down the heat.

Color

Designer lipsticks do generally last longer, hold better, and bleed less. But the main thing you're paying for in a designer lipstick is designer color, which, when it comes to that perfect Chanel shade, may be well worth it. More than other cosmetics, lipstick most closely follows fashion, and the most fashion-conscious companies usually have the most stylish lipsticks because they best understand the nuances of color. In the 1920s and 1930s, lipstick came in three choices—light, medium, and dark—the small, medium, and large of the time. By the 1950s, Revlon brought out new shades every six months, and women got hooked on color trends, just as they became hooked on fashion trends. Today, there are approximately 250 new color cosmetics launched each season. Whoever said "a kiss is just a kiss"?

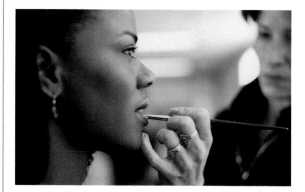

Although most women don't change lipstick shades the way they change earrings, they do carry a small stash of lipstick choices in their bags for different occasions, outfits, and moods. If you're toying with the idea of a darker or more daring shade, try it first in a gloss or sheer. The effect is much more subtle than a matte, but you'll get to try the color on for fit.

Lip Lines

Just as certain styles in fashion became emblematic of an era, certain lip lines, colors, and contours came to define a decade. Q: Can you guess whose lips these are?

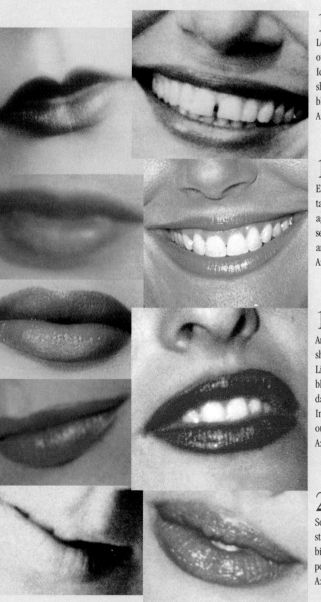

1920s

Think Betty Boop. Flappers drew Cupid's bow, bee-stung lips in deep maroon or burgundy. Very matte, soap based, and extremely drying. Average cost: 10 cents. A: CLARA BOW.

1930s

Slightly more natural, curvy, sensual shape, but still highly stylized. Satiny texture. A: INGRID BERGMAN.

1940s

Romantic heart shape in true red with the upper lip drawn in two heaving humps. A: BETTY GRABLE.

1950s

Arfully drawn, full-bottomed shape in bright fuchsias, pinks, oranges, and corals chosen to match one's dress. A: NATALIE WOOD.

1960s

Mod makeup in revolutionary colors: white, beige, pearly, frosted, silver, and gold. Voluptuous, pouty shape. A: MARY QUANT.

1970s

Longer, thinner shape, outlined for contrast. Icy, berry shades; wet, shiny gloss; the first black lipstick. A: LAUREN HUTTON.

1980s

Elongated shape with tapering edges. The beige age: glossy, "natural" or seminude browns; blue- and brick-reds. A: CHRISTIE BRINKLEY.

1990s

Anything goes. Glossy, shimmery, matte, or creamy. Light or dark, brownish rose, blood red, "vamp" black-red, dark purple, or lavender. Immaculate, oversized, outlined in pencil. A: LINDA EVANGELISTA.

2000s

Soft, smudgy lip rouges, stains, shimmers. The bigger the better: plump and possibly surgically enhanced. A: ANGELINA JOLIE.

If you're a fan of Chanel lipstick, stock up on Bourjois at Sephora. It's made at the same place, and it seems like the same gorgeous stuff—at half the price. When in Paris, do as the Parisians do: shop at the discount stores Monoprix and Prisunic for Arcancil, another inexpensive French substitute for couture color.

If there's one thing women want, it's a lipstick that makes a long-term commitment, one that won't waffle, feather, or fade away and won't stray where it doesn't belong—onto teacups and shirt collars. In the old days, long-lasting lipsticks were made with bluish or purplish pigments that would temporarily "dye" —and also overdry—the lips. In France, Rouge Baiser, a deep bluish red, was a cult classic until it was taken off the market because it was so hard to remove. Ever since Hazel Bishop developed her tenacious No-Smear Lipstick in the 1950s, every major cosmetics company has come out with its own kiss-proof version. Many work on a time-release principle in which the heat of the lip stimulates a continuous release of color (see pages 140–141). Those "everlasting lipsticks" sold on infomercials will keep your lipstick on, but they contain shellac and resin, both questionable substances to have on your lips.

The Lip Pencil

There's nothing like an old-fashioned, inexpensive lip pencil. Pencils keep lipstick within bounds, on your lips, where it's supposed to be, and they keep it on longer. However, the new push-up pencils are frustrating. They're expensive,

How To: use lip pencil to create illusion

To make your lips look . . .

bigger: Use a pencil to draw your lips slightly wider on the top and bottom, and then layer on lipstick. Or dab a little concealer in the middle of your lips, on top of your lipstick. It lightens the lipstick one shade in the center, opens up the lips, and makes them look bigger.

smaller: Use a pencil to draw them a bit inside the lip line, then layer on lipstick. Or dab a slightly darker shade of lipstick in the middle of your lips, on top of your lipstick. Be sure to blend, and use only a dab.

stronger: Outline your lips with a pencil that's the same color as your lips for more polish, shape, and definition.

softer: Use a light-shade pencil to outline the lips and fill them in with the same color of gloss.

poutier: Outline and color in your lips with pencil, then dab some gloss or shimmer in the middle of your lower lip.

they break, the color gets stuck, and you never know how much you've got left until you run out. Stick with the old-fashioned pencils, and make sure you have a sharpener always on hand. The cheaper you can find them, the better. So stock up on Wet 'N Wild and Duane Reade Lypstique. When shopping for a pencil, draw a line on your hand and rub it lightly with your finger. If it smears, it's too greasy. If it flakes and pulls your skin back and forth as you rub, it's too dry.

Putting It All Together:

THE LOOKS

These are real women. They are friends, acquaintances, and coworkers, people you might see in your everyday life. I worked with professional makeup artists to create the looks shown on the following pages. They each understood and embraced a concept of simple, healthy, natural beauty, which I believe most women want. Unlike traditional makeovers, these are intended to enhance a woman's look, not transform it. The faces have not been airbrushed, retouched, or altered except through the use of makeup. Any of these looks can be pumped up or toned down; I also offer five-minute versions, makeup tips, and more dramatic transformations of "the look" for evenings out. To me, this is what real beauty looks like. And this is what makeup can do for you.

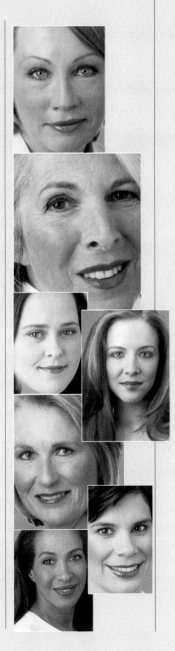

The Look FRESH:
soft lips, rosy cheeks

THE IDEA: Patty is an outdoorsy type, so we gave her a natural, bloom-of-the-rose look.

THE LIPS: Pretty in pink

THE EYES: Strong and bright

THE FACE: Healthy flush on cheeks

THE ESSENTIALS: Pink blush (powder or gel), rose lipstick, pale pink and sable (mauvy-brown) shadow.

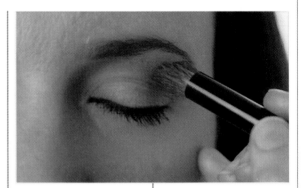

1. Since Patty's skin is dry and a bit blotchy, makeup artist Suzette Rodriguez used cream foundation to soften it and even it out. TIP: For lighter coverage, you can use a tinted moisturizer instead.

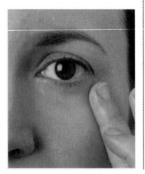

2. She dotted concealer under the eyes with her fourth finger and down the bridge of Patty's nose to make it look thinner. (Because fingers are warm, the concealer melted in and gave lighter coverage than if applied with a brush.) Then she set it with loose powder.

3. Using an angled eye shadow brush, she brushed light shadow on the lids to open up Patty's eyes. To give them depth, she brushed dark shadow into the crease, stroking up and out toward the brow.

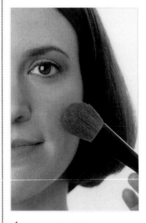

4. Then Rodriguez had Patty smile to find the apple of her cheek. She brushed blush only on that area to emphasize the cheekbones.

5. Lipstick applied with fingers gave a softer look.

LIP TIP

If your lips are on the thin side, dab a bit of white lip gloss onto the center of your lower lip to give the illusion of a fuller, poutier lip.

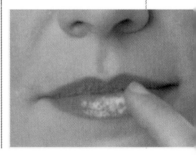

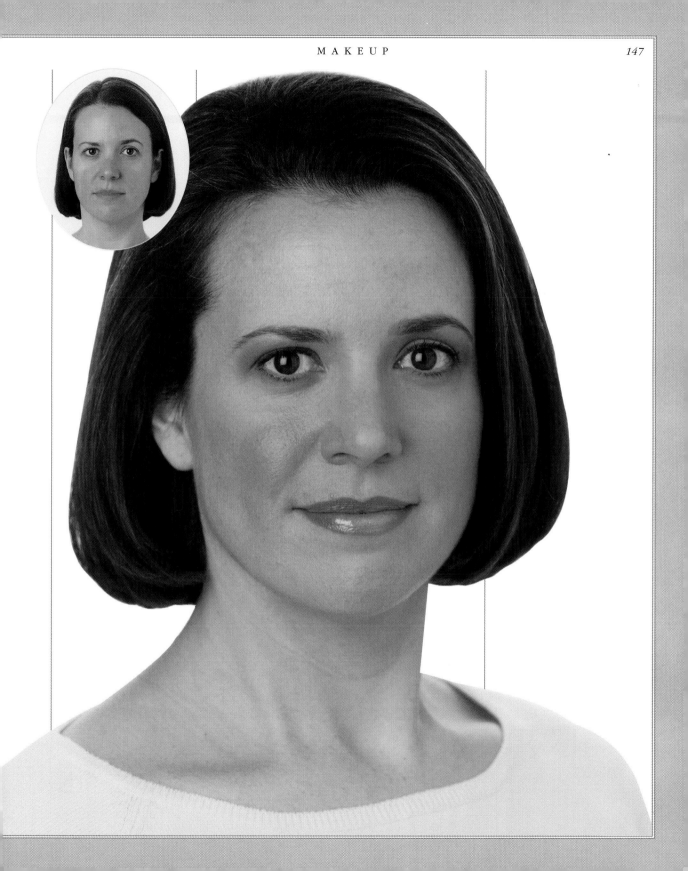

The Look UNDERSTATED GLAMOUR: *a bronzy glow*

THE IDEA: Luisa is confident with makeup, and we wanted to spotlight her beautiful eyes.

THE LIPS: Reddish-brown

THE EYES: Light bronze and brown

THE FACE: Skin as if lit from within

THE ESSENTIALS: Black eye pencil or eyeliner, pale bronze shimmer shadow, bronzy blush

1. Before she began, makeup artist Hiromi Ando tweezed Luisa's eyebrows. She kept the thickness but gave them a more defined shape.

2. After applying a cream foundation, Ando applied concealer to the undereye area and blended it with a light tap of her fingers. Then she set it with powder— just a tiny bit—so the eye pencil wouldn't seep into it.

3. She smudged a dark brown powder shadow in the crease of Luisa's eyelids. On the edges of the lids, Ando brushed a light bronze shimmery shadow, which opens up the eyes and

attracts the light. She applied a pencil eyeliner as close to the lashes as possible and brought the line out past the corner to accentuate the almond shape of Luisa's eyes.

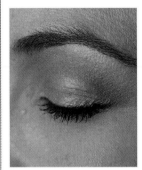

4. On the apple of Luisa's cheek, Ando stroked on powder blush. Then she dusted on powder— a translucent gold that let the skin show through and wouldn't look muddy.

5. Finally, Ando applied a cream lipstick (a reddish-brown) and blended it with a brush for a soft, pouty look.

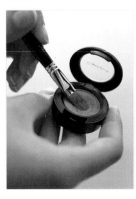

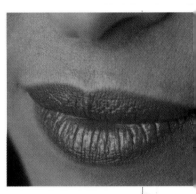

PENCIL TIPS

The sharper the point, the subtler the look. For a full line (like Luisa's), keep the tip rounded. Start at the inside corner of the eye and try to draw the line in one continuous stroke. Light pressure draws a thinner line; firmer pressure a thicker one.

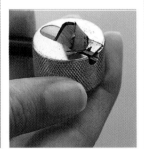

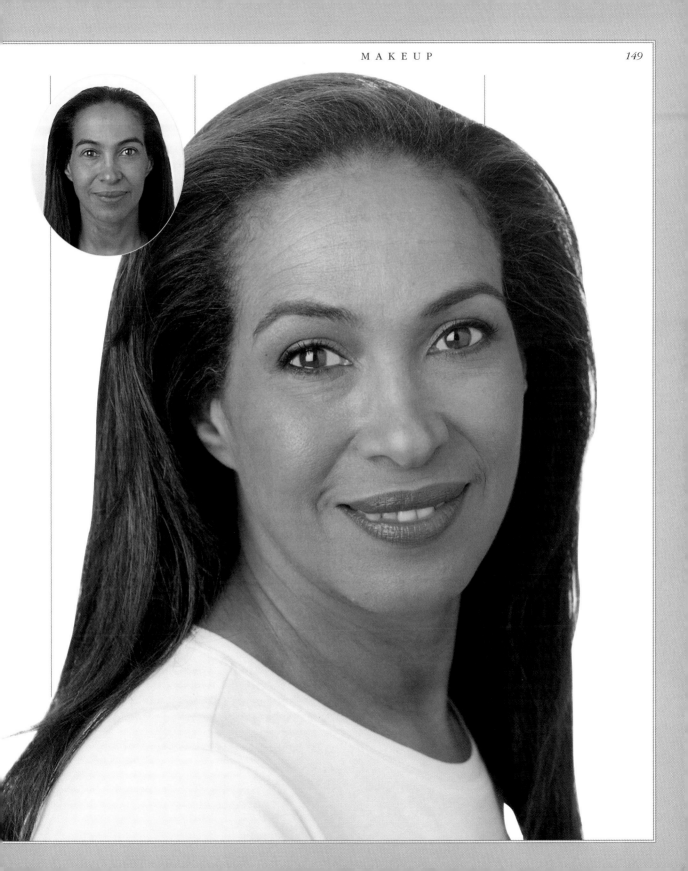

The Look STRONG:
sheer textures, rich colors

THE IDEA: Ellen's strong but simple style called for a makeup look to match.

THE LIPS: Rich, ruby red

THE EYES: Deep

THE FACE: Natural, healthy skin

THE ESSENTIALS: Bronzer, light-reflective foundation, cream lipstick, eye cream

1. Ellen's olive skin isn't overly dry, so makeup artist Suzette Rodriguez started with a light lotion. Next, she applied a light-reflective liquid foundation—a nice option for mature skin that's still moist, because it minimizes pores.

2. Instead of concealer, Rodriguez applied foundation under the eyes. (Concealer is heavy and can settle into lines and emphasize them.)

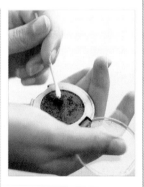

3. Even strong brows can grow sparse. Rodriguez used a boar's-hair brush to fill them in with soft brown powder shadow. (It lasts longer and looks more natural than a pencil.) Rodriguez then brushed mahogany

shadow over the lids and into the crease, using a Q-tip to blend it. For eyeliner, she applied the same brow shadow.

4. A bronzer-as-blush was used to warm up Ellen's skin. A bronzing stick or cream bronzer looks more natural than powder on mature skin.

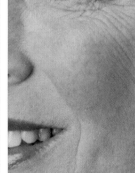

5. Color on the lips warms up the face, especially if you have white or gray hair. Rodriguez applied an almost sheer ruby red.

6. She stroked on black mascara, then

applied a dab of eye cream to plump up lines below the eyes.

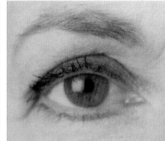

POWDER LINER

Put a dab of eye cream or water on the back of your hand and moisten a brush, then dip it into eye shadow. Dot it on the back of your hand, then draw a smooth line across your lash line. "Don't start in the middle," Rodriguez warns, "go from one end to the other." If you can't do it in a single stroke, use tapping motions, as if you're connecting dashes. Keep the shade tight to the lashes.

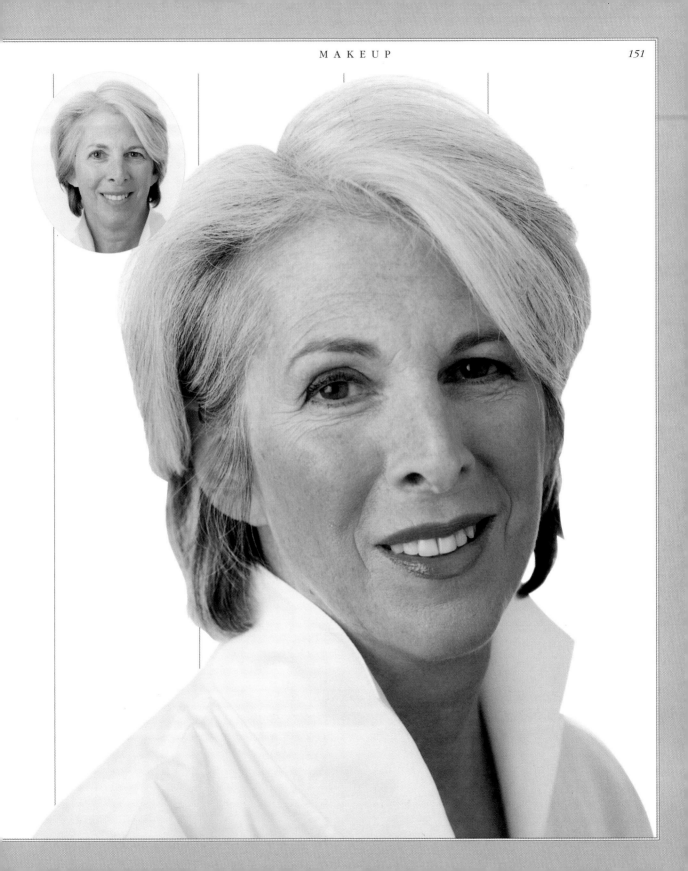

The Look NICE AND EASY: *plummy palette*

THE IDEA: Marion isn't adventurous with makeup, so we chose soft plums and mauves for an easy, everyday look.

THE LIPS: Berries and cream

THE EYES: Bring out the blue-green

THE FACE: Golden-pink glow

THE ESSENTIALS: Tinted moisturizer, cream blush, black mascara, mauvy lipstick, and plummy-brown shadow

1. Cream concealer is a good way to camouflage red, ruddy patches and broken capillaries. We dabbed it by the sides of Marion's nose, into the inner corner of the eyes, and under the iris.

2. Marion doesn't wear foundation, but because her skin has become drier recently, we applied a tinted moisturizer. It provides minimal coverage, along with moistness and sun protection.

3. We misted her face with water and blotted it with a tissue to give

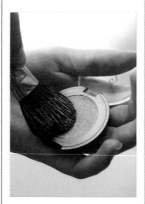

her skin a fresher look. We then applied pink-gold cream blush with a brush, which blended it well into

Marion's skin. The warm gold brightened up her face.

4. Next we brushed a sheer plummy-brown shadow onto her lids to bring out the blue-green in her eyes. We dabbed a silvery highlighter on the inner corner of the top lids and followed with black mascara.

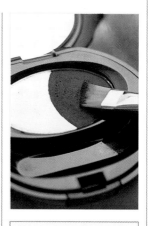

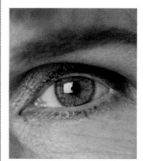

5. We brushed on a light, creamy mauve lipstick and finished with a tiny dab of gloss on the center of the bottom lip to add fullness.

FOR MATURE SKIN

Use tinted moisturizer instead of foundation. Too much foundation looks cakey and chalky. Never use concealer where there are lines or wrinkles; it'll seep right in. Use only sheer eye shadow; opaque makes lids look crepey. Lashes fade as you get older, so mascara can make a big difference. Or run a black or brown eye pencil back and forth across your lashes.

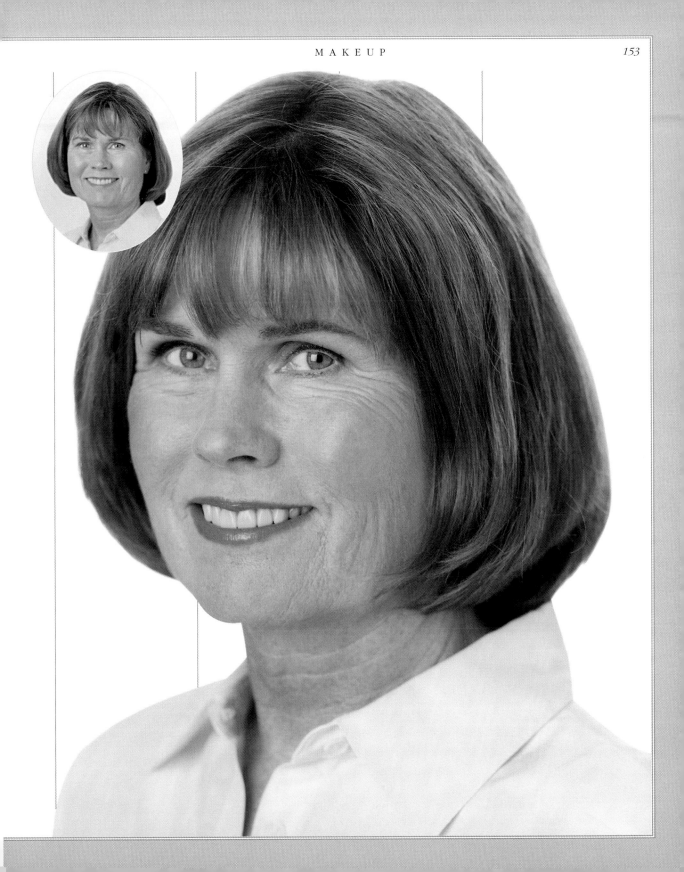

The Look SMOKY:
light lips, dramatic eyes

THE IDEA: Cameron likes to go out, so we gave her a sultry evening look.

THE LIPS: Soft and slick

THE EYES: Smoky

THE FACE: Glossy, healthy sheen

THE ESSENTIALS: Cream eye shadow, powder, mascara, cream blush

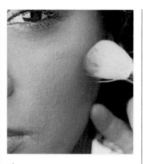

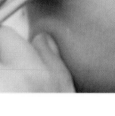

1. Since the focus was on the eyes, makeup artist Hagan Linss started there with a smoky gray-purple shadow on Cameron's eyelids. For depth and a sexy sheen, she layered a green cream shadow on the crease. She brushed a brown-pink cream shadow under the arch to attract light.

2. Linss then drew a line inside the eyelids with black eyeliner and stroked on several coats of black mascara to balance the lashes with the rest of the eye.

4. A red cream blush was used to match the reddish undertones in Cameron's skin. It was followed with a light dusting of powder to matte the blush.

5. For a soft lip look, Linss outlined the lips with a neutral pencil, then mixed a clear gloss in her palm with a light pink lipstick and stroked it on with a brush.

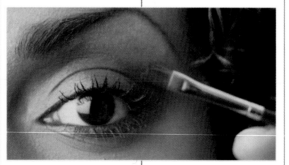

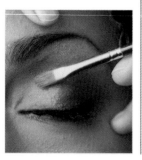

3. Because Cameron has oily skin, the foundation was an oil-free liquid. It wasn't sheer, because Linss wanted full coverage.

SOFT SHEEN

Makeup artists stock up on a drugstore balm called "Rosebud Salve," which adds subtle sheen to the cheekbones, browbones, and forehead, and keeps the skin looking juicy over a long evening. Another trick: Carry a small atomizer and mist a light spray of water on your face when it feels dry. Then, blot gently with a tissue.

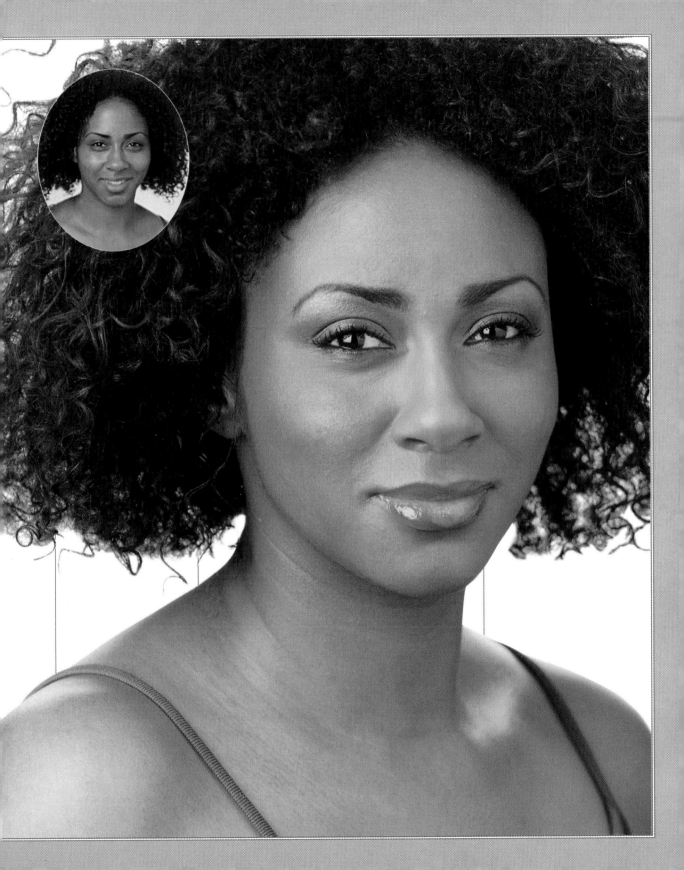

The Look ROMANTIC:
a soft, natural look

THE IDEA: Rosie hardly ever wears makeup, so we wielded the brush with a light touch and simply enhanced her natural beauty.

THE LIPS: Sheer, pale pink

THE EYES: Dovelike

THE FACE: Creamy, porcelain skin

THE ESSENTIALS: Translucent powder, black mascara, an eyelash curler, and tweezers

1. Makeup artist Hiromi Ando began by tweezing Rosie's eyebrows. She left them full but gave them a clean line. Good makeup artists become expert tweezers, because they know that a well-groomed brow opens up the eyes.

2. Because Rosie's skin is dry, Ando applied an alabaster cream foundation onto a sponge and dabbed

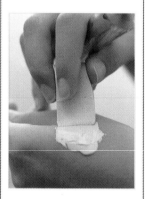

it lightly on her sensitive skin.

3. She brushed taupy mauve powder shadow onto the crease of the eyelids and along the lash

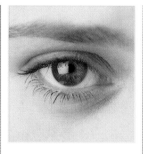

line, then blended the two. No eyeliner and no pencil: "I want to keep it soft," says Ando, "and not have too much contrast." The taupe shade brought out the gray in her eyes.

4. Rosie's lashes are so straight that an eyelash curler was the tool du jour. Curled lashes focus extra attention on the eyes. Black mascara was then applied practically one lash at a time, so it wouldn't look heavy.

5. Ando dipped a brush into a pot of rosy pink gloss and stroked it on. Gloss always looks darker in the pot

than it does on the lips, but it was so sheer, it was almost transparent.

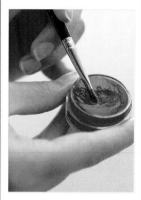

6. A light dusting of translucent powder made Rosie's skin look even more flawless.

DAY TO NIGHT

To turn the heat up a few notches, you can add shimmer to your repertoire. In Rosie's case, a silvery or pink-gold highlighter would catch the light beautifully under the arch of her brow or on her lash line, lower lip, or cheek.

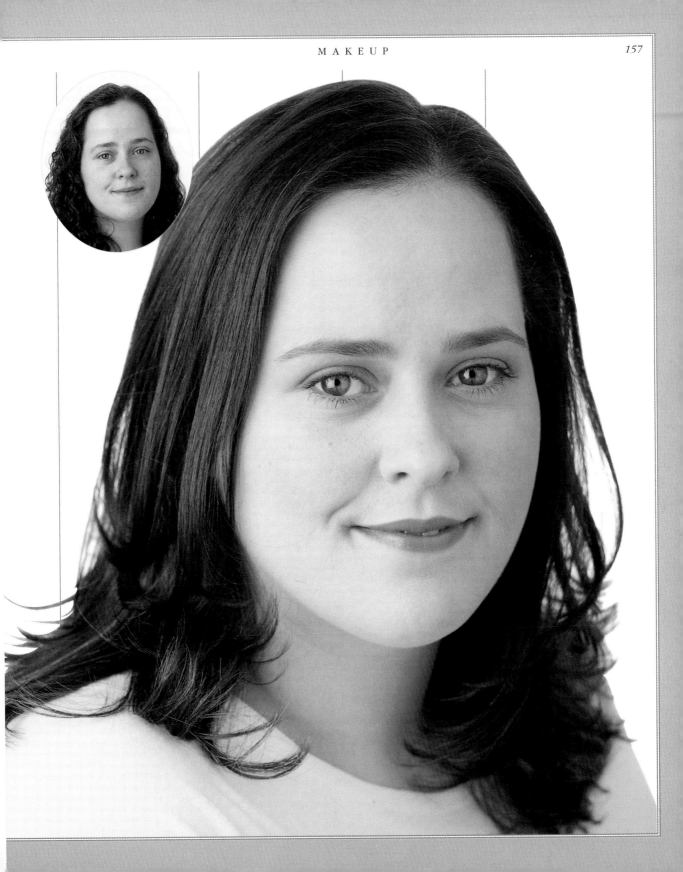

The Look POLISHED:
a notch above neutral

THE IDEA: Pat is a busy executive who wants to get the most out of the least amount of time and products.

THE LIPS: Natural, slightly peachy

THE EYES: Soft and warm

THE FACE: Healthy

THE ESSENTIALS: Sheer liquid foundation, lip pencil, silvery lavender-taupe eye shadow

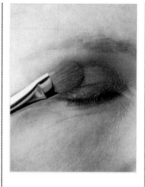

1. Makeup artist Sue Devitt applied a rich moisturizer all over Pat's face, except for the T-Zone, then blotted the excess with a tissue. Moisturizer before makeup softens lines and plumps up

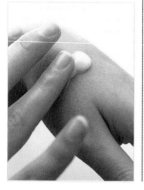

dry skin. Then, she applied sheer liquid foundation. "If you're over forty, stick with liquid, not cream," says Devitt.

2. After a dab of concealer, Devitt brushed a silky powder eye shadow onto Pat's upper lids and into the crease. Ash blondes need warmth with their makeup—especially around the eyes. Good shades: lavender-silver and silvery taupe (used here). Bad ones: green

and yellow tones. Then Devitt pressed a chestnut brown shadow into the lash line on the upper and lower lids to contour and define the eyes. TIP: If you're older, use powder, not a pencil, to line your eyes.

3. Because Pat's lashes are fair, Devitt put on a brown mascara.

4. She used a beige lip pencil to outline Pat's lips, then softened it with her fingers before layering a peachy cream lipstick on top.

LIP LINES

If you've got vertical lines around your lips, use a lip pencil—even a nude shade—as a sealant to prevent the lipstick from slipping into the grooves and feathering. Hold the pencil at an angle to get a wider nib instead of a thin line. Then cover it with a cream lipstick or gloss. Remove any excess with a lip brush.

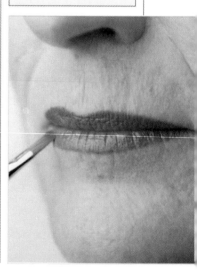

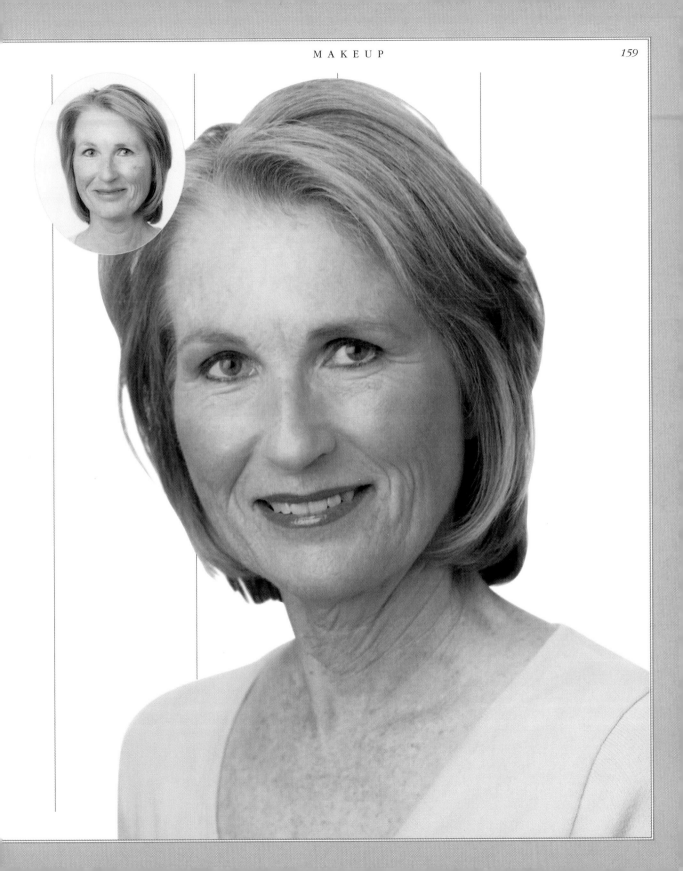

The Look SHIMMERY:
opalescent eyes, pearly lips

THE IDEA: Giema has the perfect face for shimmery makeup.

THE LIPS: Pearly soft

THE EYES: Shimmery color

THE FACE: Minimal foundation

THE ESSENTIALS: Black eye pencil, shimmery powder eye shadow, black mascara, lip gloss

1. Makeup artist Gigi Hale brushed a silvery blue powder shadow on Giema's lids,

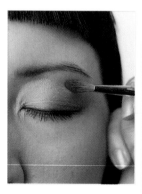

starting with the inner corner and working up and out. She stroked it past the corners and on the outer edge of the lower lid.

2. Hale drew a line with black pencil against the upper lash line and blended it with fingers to soften it. If you have high cheekbones, it's harder to wear pencil or dark shadow on the lower lids, because your cheeks push the skin up against them and smudge it. We used powder shadow rather than cream on the lower lid because it sets better.

3. For the same "cheeky" reason, she applied black mascara to the top lids only

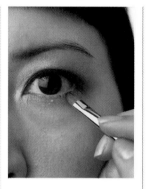

and, using an angled brush, filled in Giema's brows with brown powder shadow.

4. Hale dotted liquid foundation in a few places to even out Giema's skin tone and used a bit under the eyes as concealer. She used a pink-apricot cream blush and blended it well with her fingers.

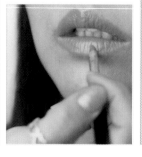

SUBTLE SHIMMER

Pearls and shimmers on the lips or eyes are a little risky. If you want to tone it down, go for either one or the other. To emphasize the lips, layer a dab of pearl or shimmer lipstick in the center of your mouth, on top of a matte lipstick, and keep your eyes matte. Or keep your lips matte and stroke a pearl or shimmer shadow on the lids or under the arch of the brow. Another easy option: simply dust your cheeks and browbone with shimmery powder.

5. She filled in the lips with a neutral pencil and slicked a pearly pink gloss on top.

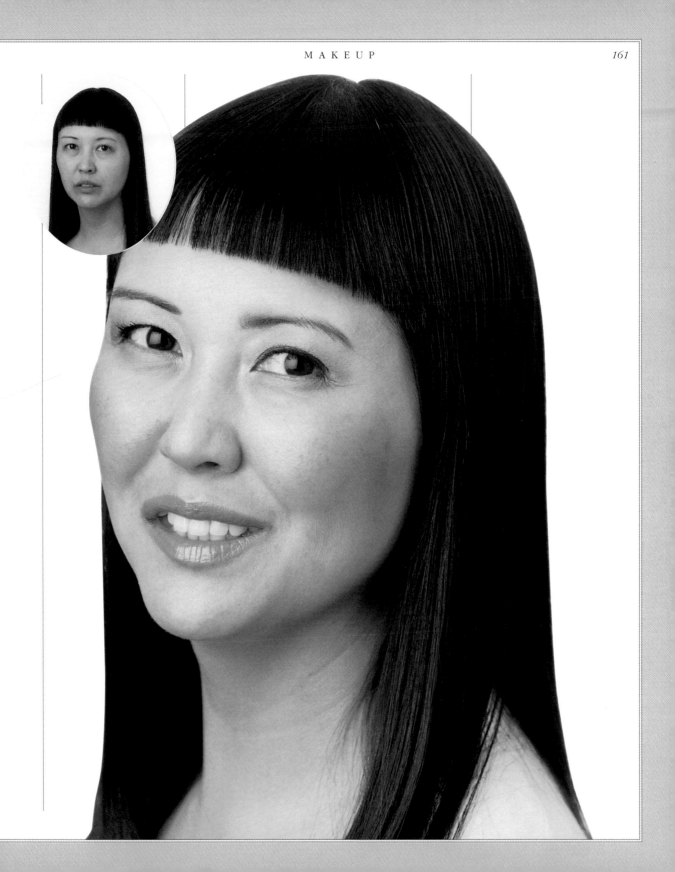

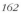

The Look TRENDY: *monochromatic color*

THE IDEA: Lara could go as trendy as she likes, but to bring out her rich coloring, we chose a soft apricot wash.

THE LIPS: Peachy

THE EYES: Terra-cotta

THE FACE: One color family

THE ESSENTIALS: Concealer, eyelash curler, same shade blush and eye shadow

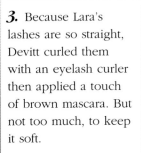

1. Makeup artist Sue Devitt applied a pale ivory liquid water-based foundation. She used a cream concealer to camouflage a minor breakout. "You can always look good with very little makeup, as long as you've got concealer," says Devitt.

2. She brushed on apricot powder blush to warm up Lara's cheeks, then applied a matte terra-cotta apricot powder shadow to her top lids and brought some around to the lower lash line. The rich shade pulled together eyes, lips, skin, and hair.

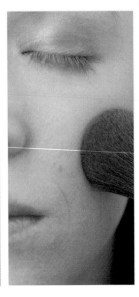

3. Because Lara's lashes are so straight, Devitt curled them with an eyelash curler then applied a touch of brown mascara. But not too much, to keep it soft.

4. She brushed on a deep peachy lip gloss with lots of shimmer, and Lara was ready to go.

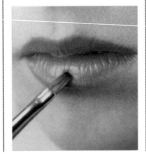

FOR REDHEADS

Because redheads have thin, delicate skin, they should avoid heavy makeup formulations. Sheer foundations will downplay freckles but not hide them. Sunny eye shadows like peach and terra-cotta brighten up the hair and the eyes. If you want to go darker, coppery shades are beautiful, too. Look for sheers or silky mattes.

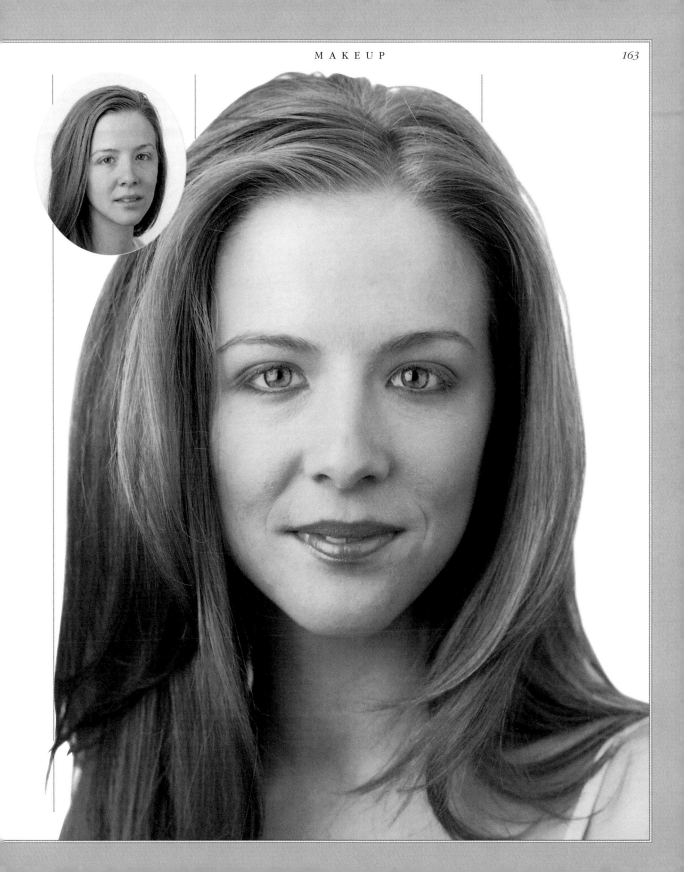

The Look PROFESSIONAL: *shades of bronze*

THE IDEA: Margot is a working mom who has no time for makeup. Here she looks natural but polished.

THE LIPS: Red-brown

THE EYES: Shades of neutral

THE FACE: Bronzy

THE ESSENTIALS: Cream bronzer, lipstick, black mascara

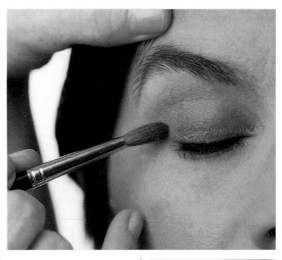

1. Makeup artist Hagan Linss massaged two coats of moisturizer into Margot's dehydrated skin. She let them absorb for a moment, then applied water-based foundation (for extra moisture) all over her face with a sponge.

2. She applied cream concealer with a brush and blended it into the inner corners, by the sides of the nose and eyes, and up into the top of the lid.

3. To give Margot's olive skin a bronzed glow, Linss chose a bronze cream blush a shade darker than the foundation and used it to contour the cheeks. That was followed by a light, translucent powder.

4. With a soft brush, Linss applied a wash

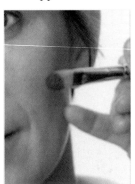

of browns to Margot's eyes: a light ocher toward the inner corner and a darker khaki brown on the lid and toward the outer corners. She dabbed a glistening peach shadow under the arch of Margot's brow as a highlighter and lined the inside rim of her eyes with a dark brown pencil.

5. To pull it all together, she stroked a red-brown lipstick on the mouth and smudged it in.

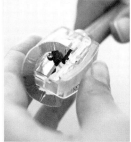

DAY INTO NIGHT

To look more dramatic for evening, add contrast by mixing textures. Work with your basic color palette, but mix sheer with shimmer or metallic with matte.

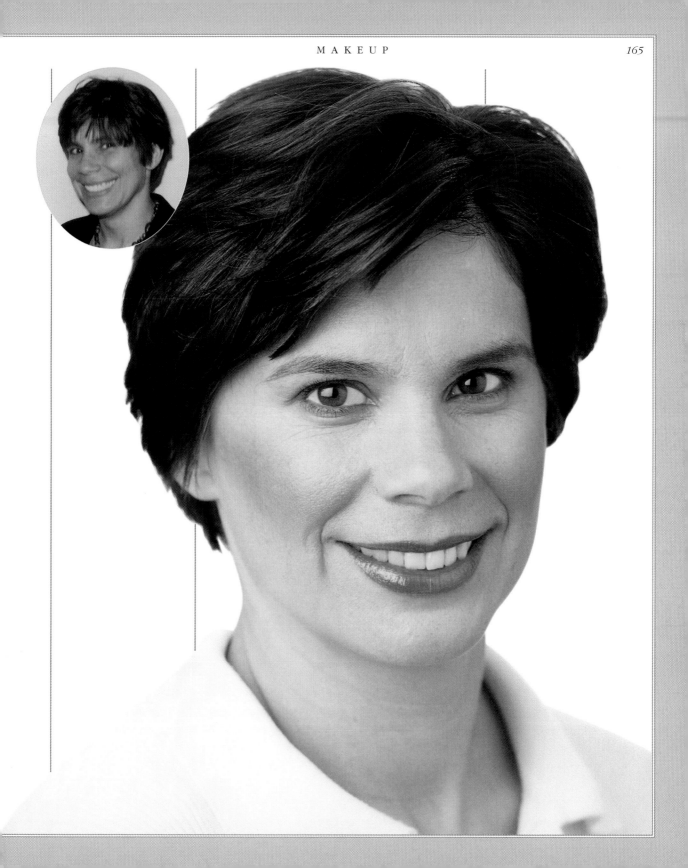

The Look SUNNY: *light and peachy*

THE IDEA: Mary Lynn is energetic and outgoing, so we gave her a warm, California-style glow.

THE LIPS: Apricot gloss

THE EYES: Light powder shadow

THE FACE: Light coverage

THE ESSENTIALS: Tinted moisturizer, brown eye shadow, lip gloss, and creamy lip pencils

1. Because Mary Lynn has good skin, makeup artist Suzette Rodriguez chose the lightest coverage: tinted moisturizer, just to even out a little random redness.

2. Cream concealer was applied under the eyes (with a brush and fingers) where Mary Lynn had dark circles.
TIP: If you have little lines around your eyes, don't use an oil-free or stick concealer. It's too dry for your skin.

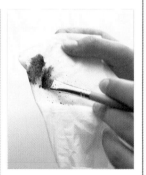

3. Rodriguez filled in the brows with light brown shadow, then stroked a light heathery vanilla powder shadow on the eyes from the lash line to the crease. Then she lined the top lash line by pressing the

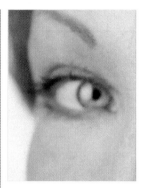

brush into the lash line so the powder was barely there. She finished with a light coat of black mascara.

4. When choosing the color of your blush, go with the color you turn when you're flushed. In Mary Lynn's case, it was a warm apricot.

5. Rodriguez used a brush to mix a few

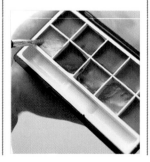

creamy lip shades on her hand, brushed it on the lips, blotted it with paper towel so that it was just a stain, mixed more on her hand with gloss, then reapplied it.

6. She finished with a dusting of translucent powder.

FIVE-MINUTE VERSION

Apply tinted moisturizer and concealer (if you need it). Stroke on a bit of pencil in the outer corners of your eyes, and smudge softly with your fingers or a Q-tip. *Or* touch the lids with an almost sheer, pale wash: silvery shimmer, heathery vanilla. Stroke on mascara. Slick on gloss or a sheer lipstick.

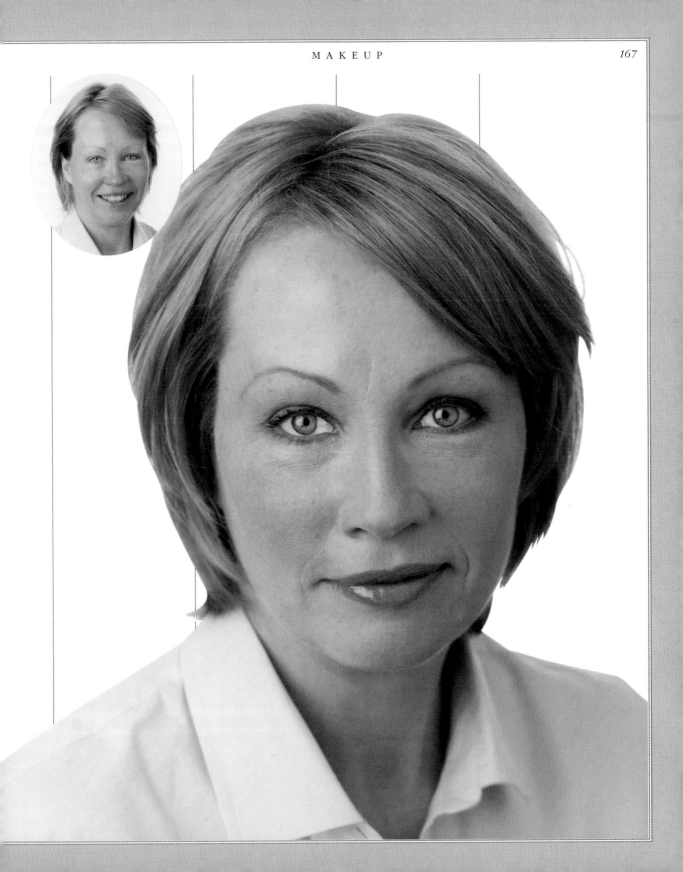

The Look RADIANT:
burnished glow

THE IDEA: Marjorie has beautiful skin, so we kept her makeup to a minimum.

THE LIPS: Rich color

THE EYES: Subtle shimmer

THE FACE: Luminous skin

THE ESSENTIALS: Black mascara, berry lipstick, powder, oil-free foundation

1. Marjorie's skin is a bit on the oily side, so makeup artist Hiromi Ando used an oil-free foundation. She applied it with her fingers to "melt" it into the skin.

2. She brushed on a bronzy cream blush, then dusted loose bronze translucent

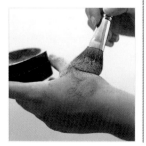

powder on her hand, shook the excess off the brush, and applied it lightly to the face, just enough to help absorb any remaining oil.

3. Ando chose a pewter powder eye shadow with a bit of shimmer. Shimmery beiges and deep metallic browns like copper, bronze, and pewter make dark skin look even more luminous, but make sure the texture is semi sheer. She brushed the shadow over the entire lid and pressed a tiny

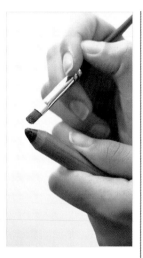

bit into the lower lid, and finished with a coat of black mascara.

4. Ando mixed several shades of clove and berry on the back of her hand and applied the blend to Marjorie's lips with a brush. She then outlined the lips

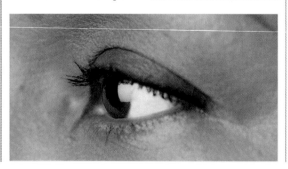

with a light brown pencil and smudged it with her finger.

BEST SHADES FOR DARK SKIN

When you pick foundation," says Ando, "avoid grayish tones, which can look ashy on the face. Gold tones work best for a wide range of dark skin tones." Strong berry lip shades—plum, blackberry, raspberry—look beautiful. Mocha, pink-browns, and burgundy are also good shades for dark skin. Avoid: oranges and bright reds.

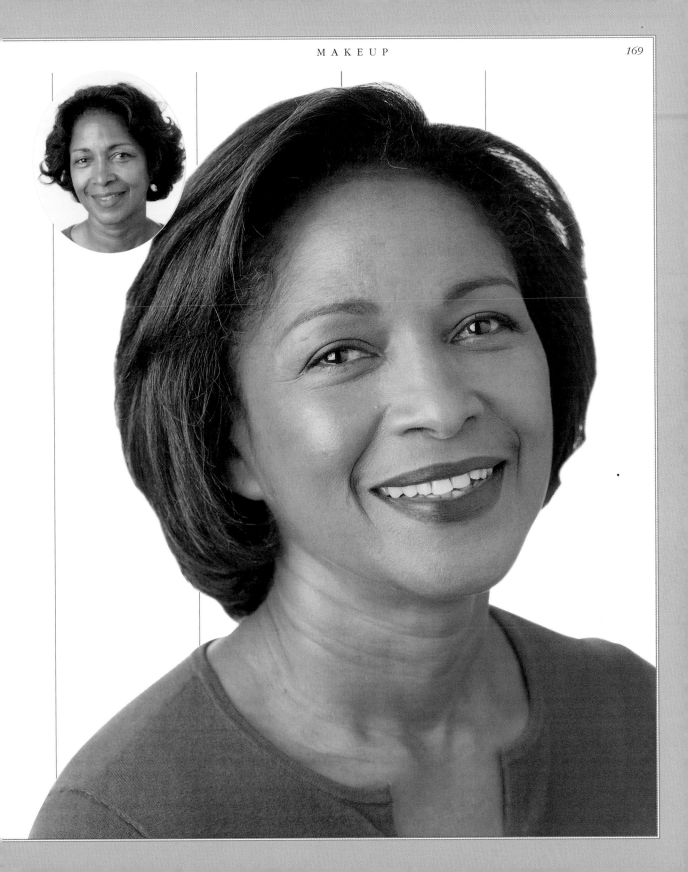

The Look GLAMOROUS:
a strong mouth, intense eyes

THE IDEA: Angela is used to a no-makeup look but wanted to see herself in something dramatic.

THE LIPS: Polished to a high-gloss

THE EYES: Strong and bright

THE FACE: Flawless

THE ESSENTIALS: Sheer lip gloss and garnet lipstick, white eye pencil, dark eye shadow, black mascara

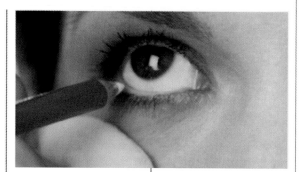

1. Angela has good, healthy skin, so makeup artist Suzette Rodriguez simply covered a few blotchy spots with a pale stick foundation and blended it with her fingers.

2. Because Angela's brows are sparse, Rodriguez filled them in with brown powder shadow. A deep mahogany shadow was chosen to intensify Angela's hazel brown eyes. Rodriguez shook the brush to remove excess and stroked the

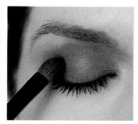

color on the lid and up into the crease. Then, she dabbed a bone highlighter under the arch.

3. To keep Angela's eyes looking deep but not too dark, Rodriguez took a creamy white pencil with a nubby point and ran it back and

forth on the inside of Angela's lower lids. This brought light to the eyes. A few coats of black curling mascara followed.

4. With a brush, Rodriguez stroked a peachy apricot cream blusher on the apple of Angela's cheek.

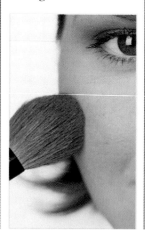

5. She applied a shimmery garnet lipstick with a brush, then layered on a coat of sheer lip gloss for a "patent leather finish."

TRAVEL LIGHT

For an evening out, find products that will fit into a tiny bag. Put a bit of lipstick on the tip of a retractable brush—it's lighter and more compact than a tube. Do the same with powder and a retractable mini powder brush, or carry a small sheaf of blotting paper instead of a compact.

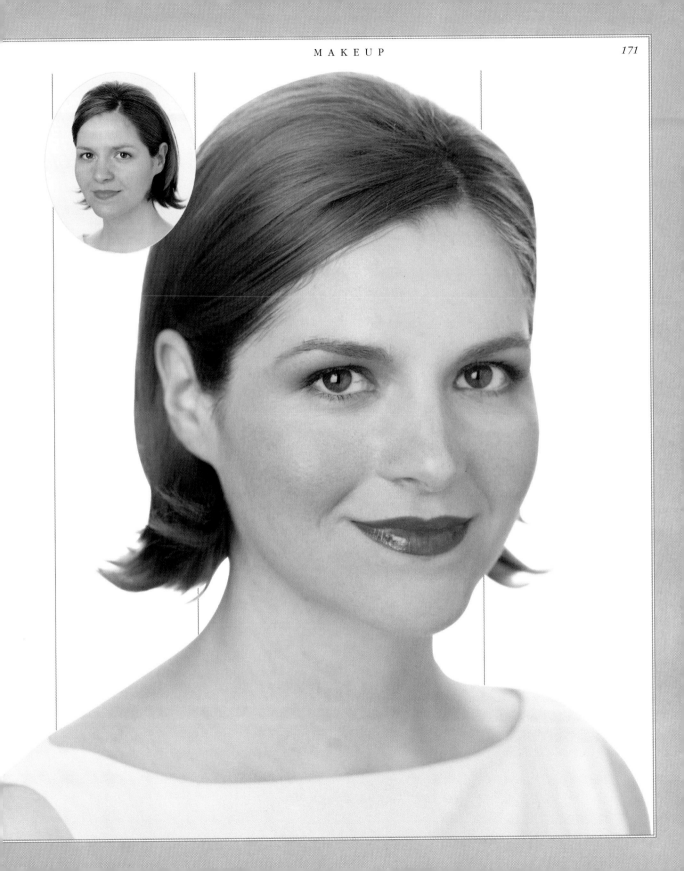

No-Brainer Beauty:

Lip, Cheek, and Eye Colors That Work for Almost Every Woman

Out of all the makeup colors in the universe (and we know they're endless), it's comforting to know there is a small handful that work anywhere, anytime, on almost any woman. Every makeup artist carries a stash of core cosmetics in her makeup bag, which she considers her foolproof few—the subtle shades that look great with any complexion.

"Makeup has changed so dramatically over the last few years," says makeup artist Liz Michael. "These days, there aren't as many standard colors around. Instead, you get more complexly blended—and more transparent—colors."

For example, the best new browns are no longer just brown. They also contain flecks of pewter, silver, copper, bronze, lavender, or mauve. "It's really hard now for people to look at a product and say, 'Oh, that's a plum,'" Michael continues. "But it's made it really easy for women to wear a wider range of colors that they wouldn't have been able to wear before."

The most versatile colors (like the ones on the facing page) have a bit of shimmer, transparency, or both. Just remember: The more transparent the product, the more you can experiment with a shade that wouldn't normally work for your skin tone, because it allows some of your natural color to come through. The same transparent color—lightly

CRACKING THE COLOR CODE

Zeroing in on a great eye shadow isn't brain surgery. Here are a few simple tricks that help narrow the field instantly. The first seems to defy logic, but here it goes: If your eyes are blue or green, avoid blue or green eye shadow. "Always go for contrast," says Michael, "because it makes the color of the eyes stand out." What you want is for the shadow to frame your eyes. Think about it: If you put a white picture in a white frame, it won't really frame the picture, will it?

Large eyes can stand up to darker shadow; with small eyes, stay light. Avoid flat, muddy-beige colors at all costs—they look dirty. Also avoid shimmery products on the face, period, if you have problem skin. For blue, green, or gray eyes: shades of brown with a hint of bronze, copper, silver. For brown eyes: silver-brown, pale lemony yellow, sandy honey-golden tones. Take care with shades of gray, which can look very cold.

applied or layered on with a heavier hand—looks completely different on each face but flatters all equally. An opaque matte won't do that. Also remember that colors look a lot darker in the tube or palette than they do on your face. So don't be scared away. Makeup should be fun and easy to use. No matter what your skin tone, eye color, or personal style, the products on the facing page will light up your face.

Shimmery: *A touch of Urban Decay YDK or Stray Dog (not pictured) will give you a glint of glamour.*

Striking: *Shu Uemura S 788 is a changeling; it looks slightly different on every lip but flatters all. Dab it on for a semi-sheer look or layer more on for intense color.*

Light: *Awake Alaskan Morn is a smooth, silky powder eye shadow that will make you look, well, more awake.*

Sheer: *Clinique Black Honey looks really dark—almost black— in the tube, but it's super sheer with a hint of color for lips.*

Polished: *Shu Uemura #945 looks like pewter and adds polish when worn alone, as a highlighter, or on top of another shadow. (Nars Ashes to Ashes is a similar but slightly less shimmery shade.)*

Gleaming: *Stila Gleam Lip Polish is almost nude—but not quite. (Stila Joan is a deeper, richer color, which also gleams.)*

Dark: *Aveda Raven black mascara—or any black mascara. It's as basic as a little black dress or a set of pearls.*

Sunny: *Stila Sun Eye Shadow is a light everyday shade that will brighten up your eyes, but it's so subtle that it's barely there.*

Transparent: *The multipurpose Nars Multiple Sticks in Malibu (pictured) or South Beach give a healthy flush to lips, eyes, and cheeks.*

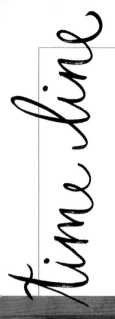

time line

the face

1600 B.C. Egyptians use a mixture of frankincense, cypress, and milk to try to remove wrinkles.

4000 B.C. In Egypt, eye makeup is used to protect against eye disease, repel flies, moisturize the skin around the eyes, and shield the eyes from harsh sunlight.

1500 B.C. Egyptians exfoliate with pumice or animal fat mixed with salt.

400 B.C. Babylonians darken their skin with hematite and red ocher, or lighten it with white lead. Egyptian women lighten their skin with yellow ocher.

4000 B.C. Women paint the upper lids and eyebrows black using galena, and the lower lid green with malachite. Kohl eventually replaces galena.

300 B.C. Greeks exfoliate with sand, ashes, and pumice. They use oil to dissolve dirt, then scrape it off with a sharp metal rod called a strigil.

3000 B.C. In Egypt, ointments prepared from vegetable oil or animal fat—and a dab of perfumed beeswax—protect the face and body from the sun, dust, and dryness.

First century A.D. Roman women wear beauty masks made of flour and water to bed. To soften their skin, Roman noblewomen sleep with strips of fresh meat— preferably veal— on their faces.

1760 B.C. Babylonian women wash their faces with boiled fat and ashes.

Second century A.D. Palestinian women mix starch, white lead, and crimson pigment to give their skin a pinkish glow.

Second century A.D. Galen, a Greek physician, invents cold cream. He uses olive oil and adds rose petals for scent.

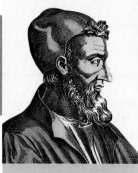

Third century A.D. Talmudic law forbids Jewish women to apply makeup on the Sabbath and requires husbands to give their wives 10 dinars for cosmetics.

Third century A.D. Cleansing masks are discovered in India when people put wet clay on their faces to protect the skin during steam baths and are pleased with the result.

Third century A.D. Japanese women cleanse by rubbing a bag of rice bran on their faces and use nightingale droppings to whiten the skin.

1300s. In Europe, cosmetics become popular among the aristocracy, and leeches are applied to the face to lighten the skin.

1400s. Upper-class Frenchwomen use white or beige water-soluble paste on their faces, and some make a concoction of asparagus roots, wild anise, and the bulbs of white lilies steeped in the milk of asses and red goats, aged in warm horse manure, and filtered through felt—to improve the skin.

1500s. Italian herbalists boil rosemary in white wine to make a complexion tonic. (They drink it, too.)

1500s. In the southwestern United States, Native Americans discover foundation: The animal fats they grease themselves with in winter to seal in warmth and in summer to protect against insects make an excellent base for ceremonial body paints.

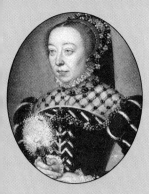

1550. Catherine de Médicis beautifies her skin with a mixture of crushed peach blossoms and almond oil.

Late 1500s. In Europe, "transparent skin" is the look. A bluish tinge is seen as the sign of a weak and innocent heart and considered beautiful. Women accentuate their veins with blue pencil.

1600s. French noblewomen wash in aged wine; their skin benefits from the tartaric acid.

1600s. In England, wealthy women wear ceruse, a pale base of egg white or lead and vinegar, to tighten the skin.

1603. Queen Elizabeth I is said to have died with an inch and a half of makeup on her face. In her day no one ever washed—they used makeup to conceal skin often deeply pitted by smallpox scars.

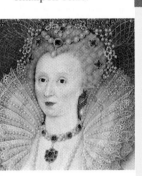

1633. To cure pimples, the English book *Gerard's Herbal* suggests eating cucumbers mixed with oatmeal and mutton.

Late 1600s–1700s. Patching is the rage in Europe. To temporarily camouflage pockmarked, pitted skin, "patchers" cut small bits of silk into fanciful shapes (crescent moons, flowers, stars) and glue them to the face.

1700s. In America, a lady's cosmetics bag might consist of cold creams, bleaches made from citrus fruits, astringent, oils, hair dye, false hair, kohl eye shadow, lotions, washes, and pomades. Use of makeup is considered a mark of gentility.

1770. The English Parliament passes an act that prohibits every woman "from trying to entrap any of His Majesty's subjects" with the aid of cosmetics. A woman so accused could be tried for witchcraft and her marriage declared void.

1789. During the French Revolution, cosmetics fall out of fashion; they are considered tools of the aristocracy.

1800s. In the United States, makeup is considered immoral because of its association with prostitutes and actresses.

1800s. "Enameling" the face with white lead salts is a fashionable—and sometimes fatal—practice.

1846. Pond's Extract, the first commercial cold cream, is introduced.

1850. Fowler's Solution, an arsenic-based cream, is marketed as a treatment for acne.

1850s. Victorian women ingest arsenic to improve their complexions, apply carmine to their cheeks for color, and use belladonna to brighten their eyes.

1860s. Victorians cleanse with lemon juice or cucumber mash.

1880s. Women consume prussic acid, corrosive sublimate, and caustic potash—all toxic substances—to improve their complexions.

1885. Chemist Robert Chesebrough (founder of Chesebrough-Pond's) is the first to use mineral oil as a moisturizer in a commercial product. The ointment he creates is the forerunner of Vaseline.

1886. In the United States, "skinning" treatments—using electricity and acid to smooth the skin—leave many near death from infection.

1886. Avon is founded by door-to-door book salesman David Hall McConnell after he realizes that his free perfume samples are more popular than his books.

1894. The Manufacturing Perfumer's Association (MPA) forms to curb taxes and combat government regulation. It's the forerunner of the Cosmetic, Toiletry and Fragrance Association (CTFA)—now a powerful industry lobby based in Washington, D.C.

1896. The first dental floss was made of the silk used for surgical sutures. During WWII, when silk was needed for parachutes, floss became nylon.

1900. The number of U.S. perfume and toiletries manufacturers has grown from 67 in 1880 to 262. Industry revenues have risen from $2.2 to $7 million.

1900. The "nose machine" is invented to force crooked, oversized noses into more socially acceptable shapes.

the face time line

1900. Rouge is now popular for daytime use, but still not considered respectable to wear at night.

1900. Entrepreneur Anthony Overton creates "High-Brown," the first commercial face powder marketed to African Americans.

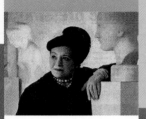

Early 1900s. Injections of carmine (a red substance derived from the cochineal insect) promise to recapture the "bloom of youth" but instead create bumps and pimples that, unlike the "bloom," never go away.

Early 1900s. Paraffin injections to reduce wrinkles and plump up sagging skin leave many women with lumps of wax in their faces.

1901. The first face-lift is performed in Germany.

1902. Helena Rubinstein opens the world's first modern beauty salon in Melbourne, Australia.

1904. Guerlain creates Crème Secret de Bonne Femme, now the oldest existing commercial beauty cream.

1906. The Pure Food and Drug Act is passed, prohibiting false marketing of cosmetics.

1908. During a facial, massages are commonly performed with an electric vibrator.

1909. Max Factor (below), a former theatrical face painter in Russia, opens his professional makeup studio in Hollywood.

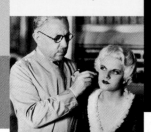

1909. Elizabeth Arden opens her Fifth Avenue salon, catering to society ladies.

1910. Sergei Diaghilev's Ballets Russes inspire an Orientalist trend; kohl becomes all the rage in the United States.

1912. The Sherley Amendment to Pure Food and Drug Act tightens ban on mislabeling.

1913. Women wear a "chin supporter" to conceal double chins and smooth out wrinkles.

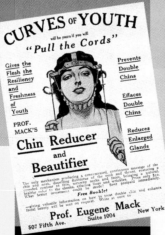

CURVES OF YOUTH
will be yours if you will
"Pull the Cords"

Gives the Flesh the Resiliency and Freshness of Youth

Prevents Double Chins

Effaces Double Chins

Reduces Enlarged Glands

PROF. MACK'S
Chin Reducer and Beautifier

The only mechanism producing a concentrated, continuous massage of the chin and neck, dispelling disfiguring flabbiness of the neck and throat, restoring a healthy contour to the cheeks, effacing lines and wrinkles. Prove only \$th. What better investment could be made?
Free Booklet—giving valuable information on how to treat double chin and enhance facial beauty will be sent on request. Write at once to:

Prof. Eugene Mack
507 Fifth Ave.   Suite 1004   New York

1914. The decline of French imports during World War I opens the way for beauty products made in the United States.

1914. Noxzema is invented by Baltimore pharmacist George Bunting, who peddles it on Maryland beaches, claiming it can soothe sunburn and "knock eczema."

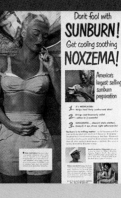

Don't fool with **SUNBURN!** Get cooling soothing **NOXZEMA!**

America's largest selling sunburn preparation

1914. T. L. Williams watches his sister Mabel apply petroleum jelly to her eyelashes and gets the idea for a mascara company, which he names after her—Maybelline.

1915. The first metal containers for makeup are invented by Maurice Levy.

1916. Film vamp Theda Bara starts the "cosmetic beading" trend by applying drops of hot wax to the ends of her lashes.

1917. *Vogue* endorses a nasal clamp for women with wide nostrils.

1919. The number of beauty product companies in the United States rises to 569, with revenues of almost \$60 million.

1920s. Hormone creams containing estrogen and progesterone become popular "antiaging" products.

1920s. Coco Chanel declares the suntan a "fashion accessory."

1920s. One acne "remedy" calls for the ingestion of Fleishmann's yeast cakes three times a day.

1920s. To simulate a tan, orange makeup is invented.

1920s. Portable makeup containers are marketed; fancy compacts increase cosmetics sales.

1920. Aziza Cosmetics is founded in Paris by Nina Sussman, who makes mascara in her kitchen.

1923. Kurlash, the first eyelash curler, is invented.

1928. Kleenex invented.

1929. Reported cases of skin disease increase 50 percent in the United States —a direct result of unsafe cosmetics ingredients and the growing popularity of commercial cosmetics.

1930s. Dr. Palmer's Almomeal Compound, an exfoliating mask, is found to contain traces of nitrobenzene, a chemical known to cause headaches, dizziness, and sometimes even death.

1930s. A by-product of turtle flesh is marketed as an antiwrinkle cream; it's heavily perfumed to hide the rank smell.

1930. Elizabeth Arden invents Eight-Hour Cream, an all-purpose salve and a best-seller to this day.

1931. Almay promotes itself as the first manufacturer of "ethical" cosmetics.

Late 1930s. South African chemist Gordon Wulff invents Oil of Olay, initially used during WWII to prevent dehydration of burn wounds on British Royal Air Force pilots.

1932. Charles Revson, Martin Revson, and Charles Lachman launch Revlon with their first product, nail enamel.

1932. French novelist Colette (right) creates her own line of beauty products and opens a salon.

1933. *100,000 Guinea Pigs* is published, followed in 1938 by *American Chamber of Horrors.* Both these sensational exposés of the beauty industry help to bring about tighter FDA regulation.

1935. Students at cosmetology school learn facial techniques (above left).

1936. *Mademoiselle* magazine publishes the first "makeover" —transforming a reader into the "Made Over Girl."

1937. Pan-Cake, the first water-soluble cake foundation, is created by Max Factor, originally for use in films.

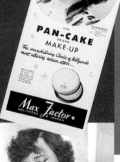

1938. Actress Mary Pickford starts the short-lived Mary Pickford Cosmetics, Inc.

1938. American women buy 52,000 tons of cleansing cream, 18,000 tons of nourishing cream, 27,000 tons of skin lotion, and 20,000 tons of complexion soap.

1938. A half-hour facial at the Elizabeth Arden Salon in New York City costs $2.50.

1938. After a woman claims to have been blinded by Lash Lure eyelash dye, Congress approves the Food, Drug and Cosmetic Act, restricting the use of dangerous substances by cosmetics manufacturers and establishing legal definitions for cosmetics. The Wheeler-Lea Amendment strengthens the ban on misleading advertising.

1940s. Hollywood stars like Merle Oberon use chin straps and Scotch tape behind the ears to smooth out wrinkles.

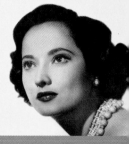

1942. In July, the War Production Board classifies cosmetics as "inessential" and limits production. In October, the board reverses its position, citing the importance of cosmetics for morale.

1943. Estée Lauder launches her company with a line of six products.

1944. The first pressed powders appear on the market.

1946. Red is hot! American women buy $30 million worth of red lipstick.

1946. Estée Lauder introduces the "free-gift-with-purchase" concept.

the face time line

1950s. Synthetic substances like cortisone and Mercurochrome are first used in skincare products.

1950s. Women adopt the heavily lined "doe-eyed look" from stars like Sophia Loren.

1950. Chemist Hazel Bishop invents the indelible lipstick that "stays on you, not on him."

1951. European aristocrats Michel and Hubert D'Ornano found Orlane cosmetics.

1952. Revlon's sexy ad campaign for "Fire and Ice" —a full-throttle red lipstick—is a sensation. It markets makeup for those "who love to flirt with fire, who dare to skate upon thin ice."

1953. Ava Gardner is one of the first movie stars to endorse a cosmetic—Max Factor's Cream Puff pressed powder.

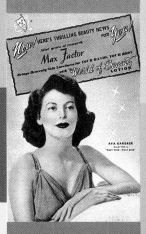

1954. Max Factor introduces Erace, the first cream concealer.

1955. Vitamin A is found to increase the number of live cells in the epidermis, giving the skin a healthy glow; Frances Denney includes it in her Vita Super Masque, an early retinoid formulation.

1955. The popular "Mandarin look" features pale skin, plucked brows, and the eyes extended with liner into an almond shape

1957. 99.7 percent of American college girls regularly wear lipstick and 79.4 percent use face powder.

1958. "Undercoating," a technique using colored face powders to even out the skin's undertones, is popular. A more natural shade of powder is applied on top.

1958. The Delaney Clause, restricting the use of any substance found to cause cancer in laboratory rats, is added to the Food, Drug and Cosmetics Act.

Late 1950s. The first "sheer" foundations appear on the market.

1960. Aubrey Hampton founds Aubrey Organics, the first organic hair- and skincare company.

1960. The Color Additive Amendment requires that coloring ingredients in cosmetics (as well as food and drugs) must be tested for safety and approved by the FDA.

1962. Helena Rubinstein offers the first "Day of Beauty," consisting of an exercise class, massage, lunch, facial, shampoo and hairstyling, manicure, pedicure, and makeup session—all for $35.

1963. Texan Mary Kay Ash spends her life's savings to develop her skincare formula; six years and millions of dollars later, she rewards her top sales directors with pink Cadillacs.

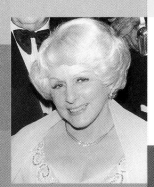

1963. Retin-A, developed by Dr. Albert Kligman of the University of Pennsylvania, debuts as a prescription acne treatment. Twenty-five years later it becomes popular as an anti-wrinkle cream.

1965. Flori Roberts launches the first major cosmetics line designed especially for women of color.

1965. The "pale look" is trendy—pale lips, no blush, bleached eyebrows, lots of dark eye shadow, mascara, and false eyelashes.

1965. Pablo—one of the first celebrity makeup artists—introduces "fantasy" and "bizarre" eye looks incorporating jewels, flowers, and op art designs.

1966. London's Mary Quant creates the mod look—lots of bold colors and geometric designs— in fashion and makeup.

1967. Estée Lauder launches Clinique, a company that downplays glamour and stresses "scientific" skincare. Salespeople wear lab coats, and products are packaged in antiseptic green.

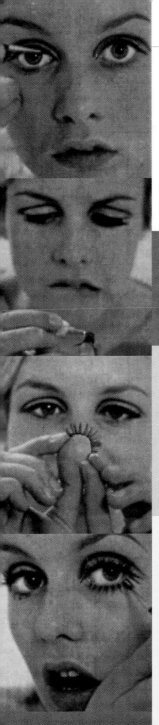

1968. African-American model Naomi Sims appears on the cover of *Life,* and black models Bethann Hardison, Toukie Smith, Pat Cleveland, and Grace Jones hit the fashion runways in New York and Paris.

1969. Biba store opens in London, selling dramatic makeup in shades of purple, plum, and turquoise.

1970s. Temple University dermatologists Van Scott and Ruey Yu pioneer research on alpha-hydroxy acids and use them to treat icthyosis, an extreme dry-skin condition.

1972. With Congress pushing for increased regulation by the FDA, the CTFA decides to regulate itself. By 1976, it sets up the Cosmetic Ingredient Review (CIR) to centralize safety information and data on cosmetic ingredients.

1967. Supermodel Twiggy's look is all the rage. She draws lashes around the eyes with a pencil and applies multiple layers of false lashes and mascara.

1972. Glam rules! David Bowie releases *Ziggy Stardust* and inspires women—and men—to wear glitter on their faces.

1973. The Fair Packaging and Labeling Act (FPLA) mandates that cosmetic ingredients be listed on the outer label, in decreasing order according to the amount in the product.

1974. Lauren Hutton is the first model to sign an exclusive contract with a cosmetics company; Revlon pays her $100,000.

1974. Beverly Johnson graces the cover of *Vogue;* she is the first African-American model to be on the cover of an American fashion magazine.

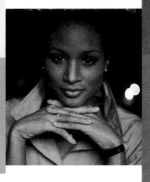

1975. Chanel launches its beauty line.

1975. The FDA attempts to regulate use of the term "hypoallergenic" but is blocked in court by cosmetics manufacturers, leaving them free to define it as they please.

1978. The FDA allows the claim that certain sunscreens "prevent premature aging."

1978. La Prairie, the Swiss makeup line based on "cell extracts," is founded.

1979. Estée Lauder launches the Prescriptives line, which custom-blends foundation to match a broad range of skin tones.

1980. AHAs achieve popularity in Europe when Guerlain uses them in its Issima line.

1981. In response to pressure from animal rights groups and public opinion, The Johns Hopkins Center for Alternatives to Animal Testing is established and funded by the cosmetics industry.

1983. Joe Lewis of M.D. Formulations develops Aqua Glycolic Lotion, the first AHA product for the general consumer market in the United States.

1984. Guerlain creates Terracotta, the first bronzing powder.

Mid-1980s. Revlon's Ultima division introduces "The Nudes," a sheer, subtle, natural look in makeup.

1985. Model Paulina Porizkova is paid $6 million to become "the face" of Estée Lauder.

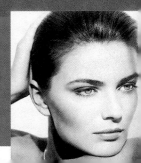

the face time line

1985. M·A·C (Makeup Art Cosmetics) is launched by makeup artist Frank Toscan. Its image is colorful, progressive, and theatrical.

1986. California passes Proposition 65, which requires consumer warnings on products containing chemicals known to cause cancer and birth defects.

1986. In the United States, annual skin cream sales reach $1.9 billion.

1988. L'Oréal buys the Helena Rubinstein company.

1988. In the United States, aging baby boomers are responsible for a 69 percent rise in cosmetic surgery.

1988. Dr. Alastair Carruthers, a Canadian dermatologist, is the first to use botox cosmetically after his ophthalmologist wife notices wrinkle reduction on patients who've been treated for spasms around the eyes.

1990s. Makeup artists' cosmetics lines—M·A·C, Bobbi Brown, Lorac, Nars, Laura Mercier, and Stila—dominate the decade's makeup trends.

1990s. Dermatologists begin to use lasers to zap wrinkles.

1990s. Sales of age-repair elixirs go from $325 million to $3.6 billion.

1990. Makeup artist Bobbi Brown revives the natural-looking makeup craze by launching 10 shades of neutral-colored lipstick.

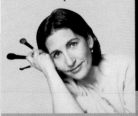

1991. Cellex-C—a Vitamin C derivative developed at Duke University—is the first product that claims to deliver L-ascorbic acid to the skin and allow it to penetrate.

1991. Naomi Wolf publishes *The Beauty Myth,* a controversial, best-selling book about images of women in the media that is highly critical of the beauty industry.

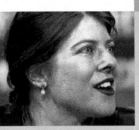

1991. Prescriptives introduces "All Skins," and Maybelline launches "Shades of You," cosmetics lines for women of color.

1994. 44 percent of American women wear makeup every day; 55 percent go without it on the weekend.

1995. Vamp, Chanel's new black-red shade for lips and nails, becomes an instant classic.

1995. M·A·C signs drag queen RuPaul as its spokesmodel.

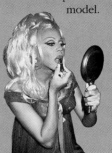

1996. Independents Bobbi Brown and M·A·C are bought by cosmetics giant Estée Lauder.

1996. The FDA approves Renova, the first prescription skin cream marketed specifically to reduce facial wrinkles and brown spots.

1996. Marcia Kilgore opens the luxe Bliss spa in New York City, which specializes in facials for the fashion cognoscenti. Three years later, Bliss sells for a reported $30 million.

1997. Inspired by supermodel Claudia Schiffer's pearly whites, baby boomers flock to cosmetic denistry for veneers, laser whitening, or power bleaching.

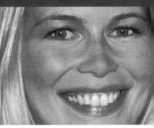

2000. Natural, alcohol- and dye-free "mineral makeup"—made from pulverized minerals like titanium dioxide, iron oxide, and mica—becomes popular for use after laser surgery.

2000. *The New York Times* reports that women who wear makeup earn 30 percent more than women who don't.

2000. Department stores no longer dominate cosmetics sales. Boutiques, the Internet, and specialty shops such as the Body Shop, Origins, and Sephora chip away at their dominance.

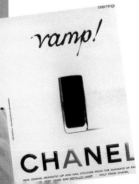

vamp!

CHANEL

PART TWO hair

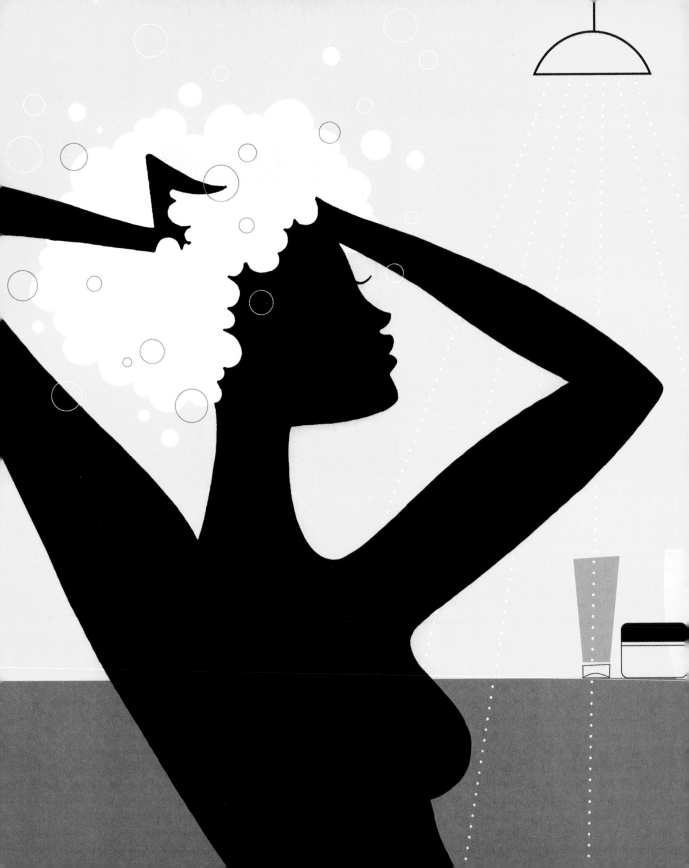

CHAPTER SEVEN

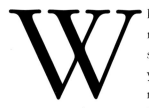

haircare

Eventually I knew precisely what hair wanted:
it wanted to grow, to be itself . . . to be left alone by
anyone, including me, who did not love it as it was.

—ALICE WALKER

When you finally do manage to free yourself from bondage to your hair and find the right style, cut, conditioner, or color, it's as though a huge psychological burden has been lifted. In Alice Walker's case, relief came naturally. But for most women, the answer is harder to come by. That's why when we search for a hairstylist, we're really looking for much, much more: a confidante, a therapist, someone who can disentangle our thoughts about our hair. A woman and her hairdresser have the ultimate codependent relationship, or as Vidal Sassoon says, "If you don't look good, we don't look good."

When you come right down to it, what purpose does hair really serve? Does it keep us warm? Hardly. Does it protect us? No. At least not in the literal sense. In fact, it is precisely its lack of function that gives hair its meaning. Hair is a decoration, a genetic marker, an erotically tinged pillow for the head. Ironically, style is what gives hair substance.

Throughout history, hairstyles have been a mirror of social change. In the 1920s, as women shed their corsets, went out to work, and took up the male vices of cigarettes and drink, their short new bobs telegraphed their newfound freedom. During the 1950s, restrictive styles like the stiff bouffant (helmet hair) reflected women's tightly bound and circumscribed lives. In the rebellious 1960s, African American women freed their hair and went natural, instead of straightening or relaxing it to conform to a white standard of beauty. In the 1960s and 1970s, men and women literally let their hair down; the Beatles wore theirs girlishly long, while Twiggy wore hers boyishly short. Today, rebellious, gender-bending teens flaunt their angst (and confuse their parents) by shaving their heads, weaving in extensions, or streaking their hair fuchsia.

Whether you color it like Courtney Love, cut it in a curt coif like Diane Sawyer (anchor hair), or let it just "be itself" as Alice Walker did, your hair says something about who you are, how you want to be seen by others, and how you see yourself.

From biblical times to the present, a woman's hair has been her crown and glory. But you can't expect your hair to take care of itself. Good hair, like good skin, is the result of a tricky balance of good genes, good care, smart shopping, and a healthy lifestyle. You can't do much about your genes, but there's a lot you can do to give the hair you were born with the chance to be its softest, springiest, and shiniest. This chapter will give you some of the basics you need to know to make your hair "the beauty, the splendor, the wonder," as the musical *Hair* proclaimed it was meant to be.

Heads Up

Hair is made of keratin, the same protein that forms the base of nails, teeth, and, of course, skin. The hair root starts deep in the dermis and grows up through a follicle and out through the scalp—at which point it's called a shaft. Though the scalp lies hidden for most of us, the health of our hair depends on a healthy scalp. Too much oil (sebum) on the scalp can clog the follicle and inhibit healthy hair growth. If there's too little, the scalp is dry and flaky. And if you don't keep your scalp clean, excess sebum and sweat will clog the hair follicles and inhibit healthy hair growth. Children don't start producing oil on their scalp until they're about

SPLITTING HAIRS

- Each of us is born with all the hair follicles we'll ever have.

- The average number of hairs on your head is 140,000 if you're blond, 100,000 if you're brunette, and 90,000 if you're a redhead. (No one knows why, but if it's any consolation to brunettes and redheads, blond hair usually has less body.)

- Hair grows approximately one-half inch each month (faster in warm weather).

- On average, a healthy person loses between 75 and 100 hairs per day.

- Each strand is 97 percent protein, 3 percent moisture.

- The only living part of the hair is the root or bulb, which is invisible—unless you pull it out.

- Each hair has a life cycle of one and a half to seven years. In the shedding stage, which lasts about three months, the hair falls out to make room for a new hair, and the cycle starts again. So periodically you'll see lots of hair on your brush or in the sink. Don't freak out—it's normal. If you see thinning spots on your scalp or notice a dramatic change in the amount of hair loss, see page 201.

four years old, which is why their scalps are often flaky. Toward the other end of life, sometime in our 70s, we stop producing sebum, and the scalp dries out once again. In between, we do our best to maintain happy, healthy, and, of course, "meaningful" hair.

Like clear skin and strong nails, soft, shiny hair is an indicator of good health. Understandably, the body feeds its essential organs, the

HAIR SHAFT

❶ The cuticle, or outermost layer, is made up of overlapping scales, as on a fish. Healthy cuticles lie down smoothly and reflect light, which gives hair its shine. A conditioner can help smooth the cuticle. Most women can tell whether they need conditioner by the way their hair feels: dry, brittle, broken ends. Here's a test to find out whether your cuticle is damaged. Shampoo and condition your hair, then comb it out. If the comb sticks in your hair down toward the ends, your cuticle is damaged, and you need a deep-moisturizing conditioner.

❷ The cortex, the bulk of the hair strand, makes up 90 percent of its weight. It gives the hair texture, strength, elasticity, and color because it contains melanin, or pigment. Some leave-in conditioners with protein actually penetrate the cortex and build up the hair from the inside out. (When you use permanent hair color, it needs to penetrate the cortex in order to "take.")

❸ The medulla is the light, air-filled core. We don't know just what it does, and some people with fine hair don't have it.

heart and brain, first. Whatever is left at the bottom of the feeding trough goes to the extremities, which is why dull, lank hair can often signal a vitamin deficiency or illness. But there's no doubt that chemical processes, product abuse, and overzealous styling can also render hair lackluster, weak, and lifeless. A healthy lifestyle—and intelligent haircare—will lead to healthy hair, the same way it leads to healthy skin.

Basic Haircare Regimen

1. Shampoo. Keep your hair clean. The sebaceous glands that lie at the base of each hair shaft secrete oil. As the sebum makes its way down the shaft, it coats the hair with a greasy layer that not only lubricates and softens the hair but also attracts dirt and airborne debris. Shampooing the hair cleans the hair and scalp and lifts dirt and oils.

2. Condition. Not everyone needs to condition her hair, and those who do don't need to condition each time they wash. There are three main reasons to condition your hair: to moisturize it, to add shine, and to make it softer and easier to comb. Conditioners coat the hair shaft with emollients that remain on after you rinse: they help reduce tangles, static electricity, and flyaway hair, and they smooth the hair cuticle so that it reflects light better and thus has more shine. Conditioners are like moisturizers for the hair. Apply conditioner from the middle of the strand to the ends, *not on top,* or it will flatten your hair. If your conditioner makes your hair

WHAT'S YOUR HAIR TYPE?

To take the best care of your hair, you need to know what type of hair you have.

HAIR TYPE	CHARACTERISTICS	CAUSE	RX
OILY	Greasy, clumps together at the root, gets dirty quickly	Genetics, over-stimulation of oil glands due to stress, vitamin deficiency, poor diet, sweat	*Shampoo often, with a gentle, "frequent-use" shampoo.*
DRY	Dull, breaks easily, frizzy, prone to split ends, stiff	Genetics, environ-mental factors (sun, salt, chlorine), scalp deficient in fatty acids or other nutrients, overprocessing (perms, straightening, relaxing, blow-drying, aggressive styling products, and hair coloring)	*Use a moisturizing shampoo (look for wheat germ oil on the ingredients list) and conditioner, along with an intensive conditioning treatment once a month or, if super-dry, every two weeks; cut back on your use of the blow-dryer; look for gentler products (relaxers without lye; low-ammonia, low-peroxide hair color); and simplify your hairstyle, so you won't need to manipulate your hair as much.*
NORMAL	Strong, soft, shiny, full of body, easy to handle	Genetics, well-balanced diet, gentle haircare	*Keep doing what you're doing: shampoo every couple of days or daily with a gentle, "frequent-use" shampoo.*
OILY SCALP, DRY HAIR	It happens: you can have hair that's greasy at the root and dull, lackluster, stiff, and brittle on the ends	Overprocessing	*Shampoo every other day with a shampoo for normal hair, and concentrate on the scalp. Alternate once a week with a purifying (clarifying) shampoo; use a moisturizing conditioner from midstrand down to the ends and a deep conditioner once a month.*

flat anyway—wax, silicone, and balsam ingredients sometimes do—switch brands.

3. Brush and/or comb. Brushing at the end of the day removes dirt and debris. It also helps spread the oil down the hair shaft. But if your hair is curly, brushing will flatten out the curl, so don't do it, except right before shampooing. Brushing with a natural-bristle brush helps get the blood flowing on your scalp. If you *don't* brush, be sure to massage.

4. Massage the scalp. The scalp is thickest at the nape of the neck, but scalp skin, overall, is thick skin. It has an intricate microvascular system, however, and because the scalp is the only part of your skin that doesn't move much on its own, it needs all the help it can get. Massage stimulates the flow of blood and oxygen to the bulb of your hair, which feeds it and helps it grow and thrive. (Bad circulation can result in thinning hair.) So before you go to sleep, take one or two minutes to massage your scalp. Starting at the base of the skull, gently rub upward and outward in small, circular movements. You won't see results overnight, but in the long run, your hair will be healthier if you massage regularly. And it feels great!

Shampoo

There was a time, not too long ago, when shampoo meant Prell and conditioner meant Tame Creme Rinse. Indeed, I have vivid childhood memories of torturous Saturday mornings spent in the bathtub, my mother and my grandmother working half a bottle of Tame through my long, tangled mass of curly hair. Back then,

How To: shampoo

Wash your hair in warm water (neither very hot nor very cold), because it opens the cuticle.

1. Pour a dime- or nickel-sized dab of shampoo in your palm (it's enough, even if you have long hair).

2. Rub your hands together, and massage the shampoo into the scalp with your fingertips (never use your fingernails!).

3. Then work your way out to the ends, because this is the direction in which the hair cuticle lies. If your hair is apt to tangle, don't clump it together too much as you work the shampoo into the hair.

4. Rinse in cool water, which closes the cuticle and stimulates circulation to the scalp.

5. After rinsing, gently blot the hair dry with a towel—don't rub. Rubbing can rough up and wear away the cuticle, weaken the hair shaft, and yank out your hair.

(At a salon, they might shampoo twice because it feels so great, but at home, once is enough.)

shampooing once or twice a week was generally considered often enough—and if your hair was dry, once a week would do, because less oil attracted less dirt.

These days, the pendulum has swung in the opposite direction, and Americans overdo it with hair hygiene—shampooing once a day, twice if we go to the gym. But shampooing every day is not necessarily good for your hair—unless it is naturally very oily or you're in your teens and your oil glands are going crazy. Curly hair or fine African American hair tends to be on the dry side, because it takes longer for oil to make its way down a curly hair shaft. If you shampoo curly hair more than two or three times a week, the ends will dry out.

When you shampoo too often, you strip the hair of its sebum (oil) and perspiration—which is, obviously, what you want to get rid of when you wash. But sebum also seals and smooths the hair's cuticle, which in turn reflects light better and makes the hair look shiny. (When hair is overprocessed or broken off, the scales stick out like flaps on a rock-climbing wall, they don't reflect light, and your hair looks flat. So don't overdo it.)

On its own, hair is naturally shiny. If you want healthy, shiny hair, shampoo in moderation and restrict your portion of gels, creams, mousses, and balms to a dime-sized dab. And if you shampoo daily, dilute your shampoo (cup your palm, and mix in one capful of shampoo to one capful of water) or alternate your regular shampoo with a mild shampoo (look for "frequent use" or "everyday use" on the label) or *gentle* children's shampoo (not all are).

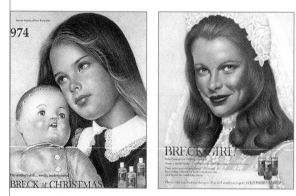

In 1908, Breck became the first commercial shampoo in the United States. The company was an advertising innovator, too, with the 1946 debut of the Breck Girl. Breck "It" girls numbered close to 300 and have included Kim Basinger (right), Brooke Shields (left), Christie Brinkley, and Cybill Shepherd.

SHINE ON

In Hawaii and Australia, women use the oil from crushed macadamia nuts to make their hair shine. Native Americans use jojoba oil or bear grease. Italians use olive oil. African women use shea butter, from the nut of the karite tree, and Mexicans use avocado oil. Actually, "the secret to shiny hair is to rinse your hair very well," says Frédéric Fekkai, owner of Beauté de Provence salon in Manhattan. Shampoo residue dulls the hair. Fekkai recommends his grandmother's rinse: "Mix a tablespoon of vinegar or lemon juice into a glass of cool water, and then rinse through your hair." Because the treatment is so acidic, says Fekkai, it closes the hair cuticle, which allows it to reflect light "like a mirror." And go easy on the goop; remember, "a little dab'll do ya."

Here are some shampoos that make hair shine: Alterna Hemp Seed Shine Shampoo, Back to Basics Beer Shampoo, Finesse, Neal's Yard Rosemary & Thyme Shampoo, Rio Vista Equine Shampoo, Frédéric Fekkai Gentle Use Shampoo.

DECODING A SHAMPOO LABEL

Most shampoos are similar to the detergents that you use in the laundry. Would you treat a delicate fabric this harshly? Note that almost half of the ingredients (below) on this typical shampoo bottle help to keep the product together rather than do anything for your hair.

INGREDIENTS:

WATER	Accounts for 60 to 75 percent of your sudsy stuff
AMMONIUM LAURETH SULFATE	Drying synthetic detergent that breaks up dirt so it can be rinsed away
SODIUM LAURYL SULFATE	The harshest detergent; try to avoid if possible
COCAMIDOPROPYL BETAINE	A milder detergent, to balance the harsh ones
LAURAMIDE DEA	Creates the foam and lather consumers expect—but nothing else
SODIUM CHLORIDE	Salt; adds viscosity to the product
CITRIC ACID	Binds to dirt so it will wash away, inhibits too much foam, adjusts pH
FRAGRANCE	This stuff must smell really bad for a synthetic fragrance to be this high up on the list; whatever mint or jasmine (see below) you smell comes from this chemical
PALMITIC ACID	Gives shampoo its smooth texture
TETRASODIUM EDTA	Prevents shampoo from altering or breaking down
PANTHENOL	Vitamin B complex; really does make hair feel thicker and smoother
ALOE VERA GEL	Moisturizer; too far down on the list to do any good
PROPYLENE GLYCOL	Moisture-absorbing ingredient that gives hair body and fullness
DMDM HYDANTOIN	Used as a preservative. May release formaldehyde; try to avoid
IODOPROPYNYL BUTYLCARBAMATE	Preservative
BALM MINT	Similar to Balm of Gilead, but here, it's too little, too late
JASMINE EXTRACT	Not enough for any benefit; just an excuse for herbal label touting
FD&C GREEN NO. 3, D&C YELLOW NO. 10	Coloring that contains coal tar, a suspected carcinogen

Sulfates can make the eyes sting, strip the natural oils from scalp and hair, and irritate, inflame, and dry the scalp. But they do foam up nicely, cleanse thoroughly, and hold together well, and so they're almost impossible to avoid. The gentlest shampoos balance the sulfates with milder detergents like cocoamides, which, unfortunately, are more expensive. Looking at the order of ingredients on the label will provide a clue as to how gentle the shampoo is. Shampoos that list a cocoamide before a sulfate are gentler. Sodium lauryl sulfate is generally considered the harshest sulfate; sodium laureth sulfate is gentler—look for it on the label.

Although it sounds like a ploy to make you buy more shampoos, it is actually important to rotate your shampoo, so a residue doesn't build up on your hair. Besides, hair gets bored with the same old shampoo after a while, and it just doesn't work as well as it once did. Play the field, and alternate different shampoos, especially if you color, perm, straighten, or otherwise process your hair.

Choosing the Right Shampoo

Most soap shampoos went out in the 1940s and have been replaced by shampoos that cleanse with "surfactants" or "sulfates"—synthetic detergents that emulsify and remove dirt. Surfactants became popular in the 1940s and 1950s because they were cheap and didn't flatten the hair, but they were also harsh and drying. Soon afterward, conditioners were developed to undo the damage.

Obviously, the most important thing is to choose a shampoo that's right for your hair type. Most shampoos are labeled for "dry," "oily," "normal," or "fine" hair—and that's actually a fairly reliable guide. Because shampoos must clean your scalp as well as your hair, choose a formula that works for both—which is usually not difficult, though it is possible to have an oily scalp with dry, chemically processed hair. The needs of your hair change as the seasons change and as you grow older. Like skin, the hair becomes drier with age, and if you're also coloring it more often, it makes it even drier. Remember to judge your hair the way it is now, not the way it was 20 years ago.

Once you've narrowed the category down, read the ingredients. Look for shampoo labels where plant extracts, such as sweet almond oil, jojoba, avocado, tea tree oil, peppermint oil, carrot extract, horsetail extract, lavender, rosemary, kelp, and wheat proteins are listed before the halfway mark. Wheat germ protein and keratin add body and coat the hair shaft; hydrolyzed soy protein repairs broken hair; and panthenol or pro–vitamin B_5 really does strengthen the hair. Shampoos with high enough levels of plant extracts buffer moisture loss and keep your hair from drying out, making it look, feel, and stay healthy.

ACID OR ALKALINE? THE pH TEST

In the 1960s, Jheri Redding, an Illinois farmboy-cum-cosmetologist, founded four haircare companies that are now household names: Redken, Jhirmack, Nexxus, and Jheri Redding Products. Besides founding one of the first companies that sold haircare products through salons, Redding revolutionized the salon industry when he first marketed "pH-balanced shampoos." Like P. T. Barnum, he traveled around the country, dramatically demonstrating that the most desirable shampoos were more acidic (pH below 7) than alkaline. As part of his sideshow, he'd dip a piece of litmus paper into his shampoo, which came up a glowing orange, pink, or gold. Then he'd dip into a competitor's product and it would come up a nasty purple or black.

For the next 10 years, "acid-balanced" shampoos were extremely popular throughout the industry, until the whole craze died down. But most cosmetic chemists now agree that a low pH is good for any hair—especially treated hair. Redding was right.

Condition

Conditioners make the hair smoother and add body and shine. Most conditioners are made of large molecules that literally stick to the outside of the hair and make combing easier, which prevents the hair from snarling and breaking. (Hair tangles when the cuticle doesn't lie flat and the hairs can't slide by one another with ease.) Because they coat the hair, conditioners make it look shiny and protect it from sun damage or drying styling aids. But with so many on the market, how do you know which one to use?

Today, conditioners come with a lot of different names—"revitalizers," "reconstructors," "finishing rinses," "elixirs," "untangling balms," and "hair masks"—but there are basically three different types: (1) *rinse-through,* which you leave on for less than a minute and wash right out; (2) *treatment or repair* (aka deep conditioners), which you leave on for anywhere from 10 to 20 minutes; and (3) *leave-in,* which you comb through but don't rinse out. Here's a thumbnail gloss on the ingredients you see on many conditioning labels. Conditioners often contain silicone, a highly reflective—but heavy—substance, along with moisture-binding humectants. The ceramides and complex lipids act as glue and make the scales lie flat. Emollients reduce frizz, and synthetic polymers bulk up the hair. Some treatment and leave-in conditioners contain proteins, which penetrate to the cortex and reinforce the structure from within.

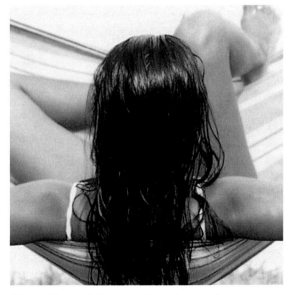

To avoid overdrying your hair, let your hair dry naturally in the sun whenever possible instead of using a blow dryer.

SPIN CYCLE OF HAIR ABUSE

Too much SHAMPOO and CONDITIONER can leave a buildup of product residue on the hair shaft. So to cut through the buildup, you use a CLARIFYING SHAMPOO, which overstrips the hair and leaves it dull. Then you'll be in the market for a SILICONE GEL, which promises to bring back the shine. It does, but it can also make the hair limp. And you'll cycle back to SHAMPOO and CONDITIONER. But conditioner can also make the hair limp, and you'll find yourself layering on MOUSSE or GEL to create the volume and curl you just conditioned out of your hair.

If you use a gentle shampoo and a little conditioner *only* when you need it, you won't get caught up in this cycle in the first place.

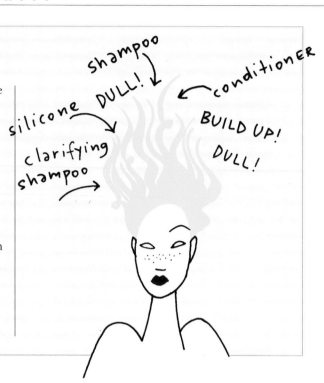

If your strands are thick, coarse, or curly, conditioning will take the nightmare out of combing your hair. Use a protein-rich conditioner regularly, with an occasional repair or leave-in conditioning treatment. (If your curly hair is also fine, you'll have to experiment until you find a conditioner that's not so heavy that it weighs down your hair.) If you make structural changes to your hair on a regular basis—color, perm, or other processing—it will need conditioning to soften it and bind in moisture. Use a moisture- and protein-rich conditioner regularly, with an occasional repair or leave-in conditioner.

Otherwise, use conditioner sparingly. If your hair is of medium texture but you like the way conditioner makes it feel, go ahead and use a rinse-through or detangling conditioner. But use only a dime-sized dab and keep the conditioner at the ends of the hair. If you blow-dry your hair, alternate a rinse-through conditioner with a leave-in cream conditioner once a month. Apply to towel-dried hair and style.

Before conditioning, squeeze excess water from your hair so it will absorb better. Spread conditioner through your palms before you work it into the hair. Use only a tiny bit and work it through the middle of the hair and down through the ends. Or comb the conditioner through—from middle to end—with a wide-toothed comb. If your hair tangles, comb from the bottom up, a little bit at a time, as if you were climbing a ladder.

"Conditioner shouldn't be used on short, fine hair—ever," says Frédéric Fekkai. "There's no need for it, and it makes the hair flat." If you need to detangle, Fekkai suggests using a light-weight detangler or a cream rinse—it detangles without weighing the hair down. And if your fine hair is shoulder-length or longer, look for a lightweight, volumizing conditioner.

Hair Products

There is very little distinction between most mass-market shampoos and conditioners, especially those manufactured by huge conglomerates. For example, when one mass-market manufacturer bought a famous salon line, the formula was changed to become just like all its other haircare lines, even though it is still marketed under the salon label. The company knows the salon franchise sells—and as we all know, marketing rules.

But are salon products generally better than drugstore brands? And does it pay to spend more on something that you are literally going to wash down the drain? Unfortunately—because they certainly cost more—in most cases, yes. Salon products generally have a lower pH than most drugstore brands, and they're gentler and more emollient. They tend to be specifically targeted to salon clients, who are using more products on their hair, or else they wouldn't be there. The good news is that many fine salon lines are available at some cosmetics supply houses (try Sally's Beauty Supply Co.) for a fraction of the price, but because they're not "officially" available there, stock up when you see your favorite, because you may not see it the next time. All of the products on the chart on pages 194–195 are gentle, well formulated, and of excellent quality.

At-Home Hair Packs

In the old days, homemade conditioning treatments were pretty straightforward stuff—lemon juice, beer, or mayonnaise—none of which, actually, puts moisture back into the hair, although they do add shine and softness. If you have a lazy Saturday morning and your fridge is stocked, pamper yourself with one of the super-rich hair packs below and on page 197.

COMING UP ROSES

Gil Gamlieli recommended this gorgeous, sweet-smelling, banana-rose conditioner for dry hair and dry scalp. The honey is full of Vitamins A, B, and C; the bananas contain potassium; the almond oil is a terrific lubricant. It feels and smells so good, it'll send you into a state of sybaritic bliss.

> 1 cup water
> ½ cup milk
> 1 cup dried rose petals
> 2 bananas
> 2 tablespoons honey
> 2 tablespoons almond oil

SHEA BUTTER: A NUTTY IDEA?

Shea butter (or karite) is one of the best moisturizing ingredients for extremely dry, frizzy, coarse, or damaged hair. Products containing shea butter are especially good conditioners for African American hair. Use regularly until the condition of the hair improves, and then alternate with your regular shampoo or conditioner. Best products: Mode de Vie Karité Shea Butter Shampoo or Conditioner, René Furterer Karite Nourishing Conditioning Cream, Philip B. Shea Butter Shampoo, L'Occitane Shea Butter.

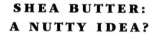

BEST SHAMPOOS

TYPE OF PRODUCT	WHAT IT DOES	WHO SHOULD USE IT	RECOMMENDED PRODUCTS
EVERYDAY	Washes hair with the gentlest possible ingredients	Those who wash their hair daily; anyone with a sensitive scalp	PENNY ISLAND WILD LAVENDER SHAMPOO (H), AVEDA ALL SENSITIVE SHAMPOO (S, D), ABBA COMPLETE SHAMPOO (S), PAUL MITCHELL AWAPUHI SHAMPOO (D), BEAUTY WITHOUT CRUELTY DAILY BENEFITS SHAMPOO (H), NEUTROGENA EXTRA MILD FORMULA WITH SUPERIOR RINSABILITY (D)
MOISTURIZING	Restores moisture; strengthens the hair shaft; adds volume and increases elasticity	Those with dry, brittle, damaged, or overprocessed hair	MODE DE VIE CREAM SHAMPOO WITH SHEA BUTTER AND VANILLA (H), FINESSE (D), OUIDAD CLEAR SHAMPOO—curly, frizzy hair (S, I), ABBA CRÈME MOIST SHAMPOO (S), MOLTON BROWN REMEDY (B, D), PHILIP B. BOTANICAL VOLUMIZING SHAMPOO (S, I), MASTEY ENOVE VOLUMIZING CRÈME SHAMPOO (D)
BALANCING	Washes away excess oiliness	Anyone with oily hair and scalp	ESSENTIEL ELEMENTS WAKE-UP ROSEMARY MINT SHAMPOO (B), MOLTON BROWN ROSEMARY SHAMPOO (B, D), PENNY ISLAND CITRUS SHAMPOO (H), DiCESARE TEA TREE OIL SHAMPOO (D), KIEHL'S CONCENTRATE SHAMPOO FOR OILY HAIR (B, I)
CLARIFYING	Contains an acidic ingredient such as cider vinegar to cut through product buildup that flattens hair; increases shine	Those with frequently conditioned, green, limp, or lackluster hair	ORIGINS NO DEPOSIT SHAMPOO (B), PANTENE PRO-V CLARIFYING SHAMPOO (D), PURE HORIZONS CLARIFYING SHAMPOO (H), FRÉDÉRIC FEKKAI APPLE CIDER CLEARING RINSE (S), NEUTROGENA CLARIFYING SHAMPOO (D)
FOR SWIMMERS	Prevents overdryness; increases shine	Anyone whose hair is frequently exposed to chlorine, salt water, and sun	L'ORÉAL KIDS SWIM SHAMPOO—good for grown-ups, too (D), AVEDA HAIR DETOXIFIER (D), PAUL MITCHELL SHAMPOO THREE (D), MASTEY SWIMMER'S SHAMPOO (D), BODY DRENCH DECHLORINATING SHAMPOO (D)

CODE: (S) = SALON, (I) = INTERNET, (D) = DRUGSTORE, (B) = BOUTIQUE, (H) = HEALTH FOOD STORE

BEST CONDITIONERS

TYPE OF PRODUCT	WHAT IT DOES	WHO SHOULD USE IT	RECOMMENDED PRODUCTS
RINSE-OUT	Reduces tangles; increases shine; smoothes the hair cuticle; softens the hair; reduces static	Anyone with hair that's dry, brittle, or frizzy from chemical processing, heat styling, sun, salt water, or chlorine	PANTENE PRO-V CONDITIONER (D), EMERALD FOREST BOTANICAL CONDITIONER (H), MODE DE VIE SHEA BUTTER CONDITIONER (H), PHYTEROSE (S, D), PAUL MITCHELL SUPERCHARGED CONDITIONER (D), VIBRANCE ORGANIC CARE CONDITIONER (D), ABBA MOISTURE SCENTSATION (D)
LEAVE-IN	Protects hair from sun and heat damage	Those who heat-style frequently or whose hair takes a lot of sun exposure	JOICO ALTIMA PROTECTIVE LEAVE-IN RECONDITIONER (D), NEXXUS LEAVE-IN CONDITIONER (D), RENÉ FURTERER KARITE NOURISHING CONDITIONING CREAM (D), SENSCIENCE INNER REPAIR LEAVE-IN CONDITIONER (D), AUSSIE REAL VOLUME SHAMPOO AND LEAVE-IN CONDITIONER (D)
DEEP-CONDITIONING OR REPAIRING	Restores moisture; bolsters the hair strand by spackling proteins and moisturizers into the cracks characteristic of damaged hair	Those with dry, overprocessed hair; brittle hair; or split ends	CHARLES WORTHINGTON RESULTS HAIR HEALER (D), OUIDAD DEEP TREATMENT FOR DAMAGED AND FRIZZY HAIR (S, I), KIEHL'S LECITHIN AND COCONUT ENRICHED HAIR MASQUE WITH PANTHENOL (B, I), PANTENE PRO-V DEEP FORTIFYING TREATMENT (D), L'ORÉAL HYDRAVIVE DEEP HYDRATING MASQUE (D), SEBASTIAN THICK ENDS CONDITIONER (D)
VOLUMIZING	Makes hair appear fuller; binds proteins, balsams, and polymers to the hair shaft	Those with limp or thin hair	TIGI ESSENSUALS THICKENING CONDITIONER (D), SENSCIENCE INNER CONDITIONER FOR FINE HAIR (D), ABBA BOTANICAL HIGH THICKENING CONDITIONER (S)
DETANGLER OR CREAM RINSE	Smoothes and detangles	Those with fine hair that snags	JOHNSON & JOHNSON SPRAY DETANGLER (D), MUSTELA SPRAY DETANGLER (D), PHILIP B. BOTANICAL DETANGLER (S, I), RENÉ FURTERER LIGHTWEIGHT DETANGLING CRÈME RINSE (S), THICKER FULLER HAIR WEIGHTLESS CONDITIONING RINSE (D)

HAIRCARE Q & A

Q. **All-in-one shampoo-conditioners are easier to use and more economical, but are they as good?**

A. *I don't recommend shampoo-conditioners for the simple reason that they build up quickly and they weigh down the hair. Plus, they should never be used on oily hair. One notable exception is Finesse.*

Q. **Why shampoo twice?**

A. *Some experts claim that the first rinse removes dirt, oil, and product buildup and the second adds volume. But it's really not necessary to lather twice if you do it well.*

Q. **Are special shampoos for colored, permed, or processed hair really necessary?**

A. *Yes, they are. Chemically processed hair has special needs. Shampoos for color-treated hair won't strip the color out the way many other shampoos will, and they contain ingredients that are gentle and moisturizing. (See page 223.)*

Q. **What is a clarifying shampoo, and what does it clarify?**

A. *Clarifying shampoos contain an acidic ingredient, like apple cider vinegar, to cut through built-up residues left by styling products and shampoos. If one is used before you color, perm, or relax your hair, the treatment will absorb better and go on more evenly. However, they're too drying to use every day.*

Q. **What is a volumizing or body-building shampoo?**

A. *These contain proteins that bond to the hair and literally add volume, strand by strand. But if used too often, they can build up a residue that weighs down the hair. If your hair is flat or fine, these work well to create volume, but be sure to alternate them with a regular shampoo.*

Q. **What does a highlighting or color-enhancing shampoo do?**

A. *These shampoos are designed to keep your color from fading and add tone to the hair. They can work beautifully to extend the life of your color. They will also add shine to gray hair and help reduce the yellow; and they are good to use after a perm because the peroxide in the neutralizers can lighten the color of your hair.*

Q. **Do I need sun protection for my hair?**

A. *Even though studies conducted by René Furterer, a French haircare company, show that after three days of unprotected UV exposure, the scales pull away from the hair shaft and make the hair brittle, styling aids and your regular conditioner will coat your hair and give it sufficient protection without additional SPF products.*

If you spend a lot of time in the sun, do wear a hat to protect your scalp—you should wear one anyway, especially if you color your hair, because the sun will oxidize it and your color will fade.

1. Put the water, milk, and rose petals in a saucepan and simmer for 15 minutes. Remove from the burner and cool.
2. In a blender, mix the bananas, honey, and almond oil. Blend on low and pour into a bowl.
3. Gently fold the cooled rose petal mixture into the banana mixture.
4. Massage into scalp and hair.
5. Cover with a plastic shower cap and leave on for 25 or 30 minutes.
6. Rinse with warm water and shampoo.

TROPICAL BREEZE

When my hair feels as dry as a bed of straw, I use this heavenly treatment created by Richard Córdoba, a colorist from Bogotá, Colombia, who recommends it for dry or damaged hair and oily scalp. It'll keep hair soft and silky for two weeks.

> *4 sprigs rosemary*
> *1 cup boiling water*
> *2 teaspoons almond oil*
> *½ papaya*
> *½ avocado*
> *¼ lemon*

1. Steep the rosemary in the boiling water. Let it cool.
2. Massage the scalp with the almond oil.
3. Mash together the papaya and avocado, and squeeze in the lemon.
4. Put the rosemary tea in a spray bottle.
5. Apply the fruit mixture to the hair.
6. Spray the tea on the hair.
7. Cover with a shower cap and leave on for 15 minutes.
8. Shampoo.

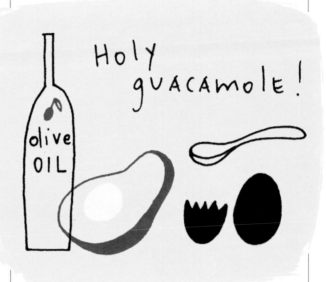

HOLY GUACAMOLE!

This is a deliciously simple, Vitamin E–rich protein pack for overprocessed hair.

> *½ avocado*
> *1 tablespoon olive oil*
> *1 egg*

1. Mash the avocado, and mix in the other ingredients.
2. Spread throughout your hair—don't forget the ends.
3. Cover with a shower cap, and leave on for 15 to 20 minutes.
4. Rinse with cool water. Shampoo.

Tip To intensify any treatment: after applying conditioner, wrap your hair in Saran Wrap, wring out a towel soaked in warm water, and wrap it around the plastic wrap.

Brush and Massage Scalp

In the days when women with waist-length hair sat in front of their vanity tables at night and began their nightly beauty ritual, they would lean over, begin at the nape, and brush 100 strokes with a flat, wide, boar's-bristle brush. Vigorous brushing is no longer considered a good idea for everyone—it can break hair when wet and can make oily hair oilier—but moderate brushing will help keep your hair healthy.

The right brush will massage the scalp, help stimulate circulation, and moisturize the hair by distributing the oils down to the ends. It also helps remove dust and grime; aerates the hair, which gives it more volume; and eliminates loose hair, clearing the way for new hair growth. A flat, natural-bristle brush is still the best for basic, everyday haircare.

Natural bristles are the most porous, which makes them best at picking up the scalp's natural oils and carrying them down to the ends of the hair. Many natural-bristle brushes are rubber-based or rubber-nubbed. The nubs enable the bristles to penetrate even the thickest hair. They also help reduce static and flyaway hair. And because the rubber base is flexible, it doesn't pull at the roots. The longer your hair, the larger the surface of the brush should be. The thicker your hair, the denser the bristles you need.

HAIR DOs (AND DON'Ts)

DOs

- Massage your scalp for a minute—or have someone do it for you—every night before you go to bed to stimulate the blood flow to the roots of your hair.
- After shampooing your hair, rinse with cool water. This makes the hair cuticle lie flat, and your hair will look shinier.
- When you shampoo, don't scrub the ends too much. Excessive scrubbing dries them out and makes them brittle.
- Since chlorine and salt water dry out the hair, apply a little conditioner to the hair before swimming.
- Blot—don't rub—your hair dry. Rubbing hair can cause the strands to snag and tangle.

DON'Ts

- Don't apply conditioner or styling products to the scalp; they can clog pores and cause flaking. Restrict these products to the hair only, especially the ends.
- Don't wash or rinse your hair in hot water. Hot water dries hair just as it dries skin. It also opens the hair cuticle, which makes it more absorbent. This is a particularly bad idea if you use styling aids—gels, creams, mousses—because they will absorb into the hair, weigh it down, and make it look greasy. Stick to a warm or tepid temperature.
- Don't pull your hair back in tight ponytails, braids, headbands, or combs for long periods of time because they can break the hair and even cause "traction" alopecia, a type of hair loss.
- Don't brush your hair too much when it is wet. It will snap and break.

To avoid breakage, brush hair in steps, starting at the bottom and working your way up. For extra body, turn your head upside down and brush—gently—from the nape of the neck forward. Then brush from the sides toward the crown, and finally turn your head right side up and brush front to back. This stimulates the blood flow to the root and helps get rid of dandruff.

With curly hair, however, brushing tends to flatten the curl, snare the hair, and make it look frizzy. If your hair is curly, stick with a wide-toothed comb, but do brush whenever you don't care how your hair will look immediately afterward: before you wash your hair, for example, or before you go to bed. And be sure to massage your scalp regularly to make up for the fact that you're brushing less.

To massage your scalp, start at the nape of the neck and massage upward with your fingertips spread apart, moving in slow, circular rotations. Next, put your fingers together, one hand on each side of the top of your head, and zigzag back and forth from the forehead to the crown.

Flaking Scalp

It probably doesn't matter much to you whether your problem is dandruff, dry scalp, or seborrheic dermatitis. What does matter is that you're afflicted with a flaky, itchy, tight, or inflamed scalp, and you just want to fix it.

Dandruff and dry scalp are both considered forms of dermatitis. Dandruff is often mistaken

> *Tip* **M**assage dandruff shampoo into your scalp and leave on for a couple of minutes before you rinse, so that it can be absorbed by the scalp.

for a dry scalp, but it can afflict an oily scalp just as easily as a dry one. It's believed that dandruff is caused by an overgrowth of yeast that's found in moderation even on healthy scalps. The yeast, *Pityrosporum ovale,* irritates the oil glands below the surface, and the scalp responds by accelerating the cell turnover. Dandruff results when the skin cells divide and multiply at such an accelerated rate that they reach the surface before they die and clump there. These flakes of white, scaly skin look bad, and they *itch*.

Sometimes, what's believed to be dandruff is simply shampoo residue from sloppy rinsing or flaking from that gel you're hooked on. Or it could be dry scalp caused by dry indoor heat, harsh shampoos, too-frequent shampooing, conditioners or gels applied directly to the scalp, hair processing, or a too-hot blast from a blow-dryer.

If you've been coloring, perming, relaxing, or straightening your hair, your scalp can become oily, flaky, and inflamed, which may mean that you have a more severe form of dermatitis called seborrhea. One common mistake is to treat seborrhea with a harsh dandruff shampoo—that only makes it worse. So, first of all you need to know what kind of problem you have. Here's how you can tell.

Dandruff Test

Turn your head upside down and brush or vigorously rub your scalp back and forth with fingers over a sheet of dark paper. If you see tiny, dry, powdery bits, you have dry scalp. If the flakes are larger and look slightly moist or greasy, they're dandruff. If you have large greasy flakes and your scalp is irritated and red, chances are you have seborrhea. If the scales stick to the scalp, it may be psoriasis, and if it doesn't clear up, consult a dermatologist.

If what you have is dry scalp, first use a clarifying shampoo with cider vinegar to remove any buildup of shampoo or conditioner on the scalp. Then try an oil treatment or scalp cream designed for dry, itchy scalp: Kiehl's Enriched Massage Oil for Scalp, Phyto Therathrie Phytopolleine, or René Furterer Carthame Intensive Oil Supplement for Dry Hair & Scalp.

Although dandruff is generally believed not to be caused by microbes, most antidandruff shampoos are germicides. Go figure. Most contain one of five ingredients approved by the FDA for fighting dandruff: salicylic acid, zinc pyrithione, sulfur, selenium sulfide, and coal tar. All of these ingredients will really dry out your scalp and your hair along with it, which puts you in the front seat of the beauty roller coaster: you got rid of your dandruff, all right, but now your hair looks like straw. Why go through all that when you can prevent dandruff in the first place?

Dandruff is seasonal, occurring more frequently and more severely from October to March, when your hair is exposed to dry indoor heat. So use the following simple rinse every couple of weeks to stay on top of the flakes.

BEATING DANDRUFF THE GENTLE WAY

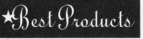

Tea tree oil is an herbal antiseptic that many physicians now believe fights bacteria and yeast buildup. Try a tea tree oil shampoo like Desert Essence Keep-the-Clean Wash Shampoo, Nature's Gate Rainwater Herbal Tea Tree Oil Shampoo, or Terrain Tea Tree Shampoo. Alphaworks by ABBA is a little stronger, because it contains AHAs along with the tea tree oil. You can also mix two drops of tea tree oil in your palm with your regular shampoo. Try this three times a week for three weeks and see if it helps.

Other herbal shampoos that work for dandruff: Penny Island Wild Lavender Shampoo, Beauty Without Cruelty Aromatherapy Daily Benefits Shampoo, Ecco Bella Dandruff Therapy Shampoo, and, for the cheapest alternative, try Dr. Bonner's Peppermint Pure Castile Soap (it will flatten your hair, but it will also squelch your dandruff).

For stubborn dandruff, try René Furterer Melaleuca Shampoo (tea tree oil with zinc pyrithione—it's strong), Avon Controlling Dandruff Shampoo, or Phyto Therathrie Phytocyres, Philip B. Anti-Flake.

DANDRUFF-DEFYING RINSE

A few sprigs of rosemary
2 cups water

1. Boil the rosemary in the water and cool.
2. Rinse through the hair and massage into the scalp.

Antiseptic botanicals like tea tree oil (aka melaleuca) are terrific alternatives to harsh dandruff shampoos. But they remain a big secret because they're not FDA-approved for use as "dandruff shampoos." Nonetheless, gentle shampoos that include tea tree oil, rosemary, or sage can really work to control dandruff, and they won't dry out your scalp or hair. If your flaking is severe, you may need a true dandruff shampoo. In that case, alternate your dandruff shampoo with a gentle herbal shampoo to go easier on your hair and scalp. It's worth the splurge for a better-quality dandruff shampoo, especially since it will last longer because you won't use it for every shampoo.

If none of the above treatments works, see a dermatologist, because you may have seborrhea or psoriasis, which mimic dandruff but often require medical treatment.

Beauty Comfort Food. Oatmeal is comfort food for the skin and hair as well as sustenance for a hardy spirit on a cold winter morning. Oatmeal soaps and scrubs are a practically prehistoric means of sloughing off dead, scaly skin cells and soothing dry, itchy skin, dry hair, and dry scalp. For fine hair, hydrolyzed oat protein is also an effective volumizer. The oat protein penetrates the hair shaft, reduces flyaway hair, conditions, and makes combing easier. Penny Island Oat Amino Complex (a health-food-store line) and Aussie's 3-Minute Reconstructor are both good oat products.

Hair Today, Gone Tomorrow

When Princess Caroline of Monaco went bald several years ago (her hair has since grown back), the world became aware of alopecia areata, aka hair loss or baldness. Alopecia areata starts with one or more small round bare patches on the scalp. Sometimes alopecia sufferers develop marks on the nails that look like tiny pinpricks, and sometimes the nails become more grossly distorted. Depending on the cause, the hair may grow back naturally within a year or may respond to treatment. Sometimes it won't. Though no one knows what causes alopecia, current research suggests that something triggers the immune system to constrict the hair follicle.

Typically considered a male problem, thinning hair, which can refer to actual hair loss or thinning in the diameter of the hair shaft, is not uncommon in women age 35 and over. In fact, it's a hidden epidemic that affects two million females in the United States, according to the National Alopecia Areata Foundation (NAAF).

If you suffer from hair loss, take heart. According to Dr. Zachary Zerut, at New York City's Albert Einstein Medical Center, "Now that we've discovered how to grow hair in a test tube, in a few years, we'll have a cream or a pill that will grow back hair on your head." And since cloning is commonplace, nothing seems too far-fetched to me.

Prevention

If you're genetically predisposed to hair loss, here are some guidelines to help you prevent it.

▇ Eat the recommended daily allotment of protein.

▇ Eat sulfur-rich foods like beans, milk, dairy products, fish, and eggs. Cysteine, one of the

rona's hair remedies

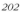

At the root of it, most hair and scalp problems can be solved quite simply. Sometimes the problem is seasonal; sometimes it's the wrong shampoo or conditioner or the result of styling aids that are too heavy for your hair, and a quick fix is all that's needed.

PROBLEM	CAUSES	SOLUTIONS	PRODUCT TYPE
DRY, DULL, STRAWLIKE HAIR	*Overprocessing (from coloring, perms, straightening, relaxing); heat damage; salt water; sun exposure; chlorine*	■ Steam your hair in a warm shower for a few minutes to open the hair cuticle. Then use a conditioner for your hair type. ■ To protect against heat damage, apply a heat-activated product before exposing hair to heat. ■ After shampooing, rinse with cool water, which makes hair look shinier.	**THICK OR COARSE HAIR:** hair masks, hot oil treatments, leave-in conditioners **MEDIUM HAIR:** deep-conditioning treatments **FINE HAIR:** protein packs
FLAT HAIR; NO VOLUME	*Overconditioning; product buildup; heavy conditioner*	■ Cut the amount and frequency of conditioning in half. Switch to a lighter conditioner. ■ Every two weeks, alternate your shampoo with a clarifying shampoo to cut through the buildup. ■ Use a volumizing shampoo. ■ Use volumizer only at roots. ■ Reverse tactics: condition first, rinse, *then* shampoo.	Volumizers or thickening sprays
FRIZZY HAIR	*Humidity; overprocessing*	■ Keep hair conditioned, shampoo every three to five days, and rinse in between with conditioner, *not* shampoo. ■ Mix a dime-sized dab of gel in your palm with an equal amount of cream and scrunch through your hair. ■ In dry climates, use a curl rejuvenator to bring curls back to life. ■ Most important, dry your hair *completely* before you go out into humid weather.	Gels, spray gels, creams, curl rejuvenators
FRAGILE, BRITTLE HAIR	*Chlorine; excessive sun exposure; chemical processing*	■ Use a deep conditioner with keratin or plant proteins like wheat and soy. ■ African American hair responds well to a light oil (see page 240). ■ Sleep on silk or satin pillowcases—cotton fabric can snag hair!	Deep conditioners, oils

PROBLEM	CAUSES	SOLUTIONS	PRODUCT TYPE
SPLIT ENDS	*Rough treatment with brush, blow-dryer, hair accessories, or hands; under-conditioning; overstyling; overprocessing*	▨ To really get rid of split ends, cut them off and treat your hair more gently next time. Hair that tends to split at the ends should be trimmed every 4 to 6 weeks. ▨ Switch to a moisturizing shampoo and conditioner, like Sebastian Thick Ends Conditioner. ▨ Before styling damp hair, work conditioner into ends or use pomade to "glue" ends together.	Pomades, moisturizing shampoos and conditioners
FLYAWAY HAIR	*Static, especially in winter*	▨ Spray a water-based hairspray (*not* an aerosol) on a comb and comb it through the hair. ▨ Finger-comb a light pomade or gel through the hair, or rub some between your palms and pat lightly on hair, especially the ends. ▨ Use Bounce in the dryer to reduce static on clothes, or run a sheet through your hair. ▨ If your hair is so static that it literally stands on end, spray Static Guard on your comb or brush and run it through your hair. ▨ At the roots, use a pomade, wax, or stick styler to slick hair down (if you're out of hair goop, substitute lip balm or body lotion). ▨ Comb damp hair with leave-in conditioner and let it dry naturally. ▨ Don't overbrush—use your fingers instead.	Water-based hairsprays, leave-in conditioners, oils, pomades, or wax
LICE	*They spread from head to head by direct or indirect contact, as any parent of elementary schoolchildren well knows*	▨ If you prefer a homeopathic remedy, mix 8 drops of sabadilla into a palmful of citricidal (you can find these ingredients at health food stores), massage mixture into wet hair, leave on for 5 to 10 minutes, and rinse thoroughly. ▨ Have someone pull the lice out of the hair at least once daily. ▨ Wash hair with tea tree oil (lice hate the smell). ▨ Coat hair with olive oil (lice slip off) or spray generously with hairspray. ▨ To prevent: spritz hair with a mixture of lavender and water.	A commercial pesticide shampoo like Nix
SWIMMER'S HAIR OR GREEN HAIR	*Chlorine; salt water; exposure to sun; blond hair reacting to chlorine or copper salt*	▨ Wear a bathing cap. ▨ Wash hair immediately after swimming; dilute shampoo with club soda. ▨ To correct green hair, use a clarifying shampoo or cleansing treatment.	Swimmer's shampoo; clarifying shampoo

building blocks of the hair shaft, is made of sulfur-rich amino acids.

▒ Take your vitamins (make sure you're getting a good B-complex that includes biotin, and Vitamins A and C).

▒ Take flaxseed oil in liquid or capsules. According to Dr. Andrew Weil, author of *Eight Weeks to Optimum Health,* flaxseed is a source of omega-3 fatty acids that "improve the circulation, which is what you need to feed the hair root." Wheat germ oil and gourd seed oil, both rich in Vitamin F, also provide essential fatty acids to build the hair.

▒ Season your food with cayenne pepper and ginger, both of which aid circulation.

▒ Avoid excess sugar and caffeine.

Treatments

See your doctor or dermatologist as soon as you notice hair thinning. Your dermatologist will offer several standard treatments. None is a sure bet, but each works some of the time. In some cases, early intervention offers the best hope of success.

Cortisone. This steroid medication is most effective in mild cases, in which it works roughly one-third of the time. There are four methods: (1) applying a topical cream, (2) injecting the scalp, (3) injecting through the muscle, and (4) taking prednisone, an oral medication.

Rogaine. The FDA has approved a 2 percent Rogaine medication for men and women and a 5 percent version for men alone, though many

CAUSES OF HAIR LOSS

Genetics. Males whose mothers' fathers went bald probably will go bald, too, and there's not much they can do about it, except take Rogaine or Propecia, which will help hold on to whatever hair is left. Women can also have a genetic predisposition toward thinning hair, but Propecia is not an option for them, though Rogaine does work well in some cases. Talk to your dermatologist.

Hormonal imbalance. Raging hormones triggered by the birth control pill, pregnancy (postpartum alopecia), cessation of breast-feeding, and menopause can all cause hair loss. In the first three cases it grows back within six months to a year; in the latter it may never grow back.

Medical conditions. Thyroid conditions or autoimmune diseases (like lupus) can cause temporary hair loss. Your doctor can tell with a blood test whether you have a medical condition that's causing hair loss.

Medications. Chemotherapy, of course, is the most obvious example. But thyroid, blood pressure, antidepressant, and antiseizure medications can also cause hair to fall out.

Nutritional deficiency, excessive dieting, or eating disorders.

Major life stresses, such as death or illness in the family, work trauma, relocating.

Environmental exposure to toxic chemicals.

Chemical processing. It's rare, but too much in too short a time may account for hair loss.

Hairstyles. The constant pulling of styles like ponytails, tight braids, or extensions can break the hair and damage the follicle, leading to hair loss.

Trichotillomania (see facing page).

women have very good results with either or both. Ask your doctor.

Contact irritants. A dermatologist applies chemicals to the scalp that set up an allergic reaction. Apparently, this interferes with the immune response and disrupts whatever that response was doing to stop hair growth. Side effects include rash, severe irritation, and, in some cases, swelling of the lymph nodes.

PUVA. This psoriasis treatment relies on a combination of psoralen, a medication that makes the skin extremely sensitive to the sun, and UV light.

Coverups and sprays. Products such as Couvre temporarily darken the area to camouflage the skin in spots of thinning hair. It's messy, but if your problem is mild, it may help you feel better.

HAIRPULLERS ANONYMOUS

Even though it's estimated that 8 to 10 million people in the United States suffer from trichotillomania, it was considered rare until recently, because most sufferers are too ashamed to seek help. Trichotillomania is the repetitive urge to pull out one's hair; the pulling is usually restricted to hair on the head, scalp, eyebrows, and eyelashes, though, in some cases, body hair is also pulled.

A lot can be done to treat trichotillomania; behavioral therapy alone or in combination with certain antidepressant drugs seems to be the most effective. Other treatments include hypnosis, dietary restrictions, 12-step programs, support groups, traditional therapy, and acupuncture.

For information, contact the Trichotillomania Learning Center (TLC), a national nonprofit support group: 1215 Mission Street, Suite 2, Santa Cruz, CA 95060. Phone: 831-457-1004; fax: 831-426-4383; Website: www.trich.org; e-mail: trichster@aol.com.

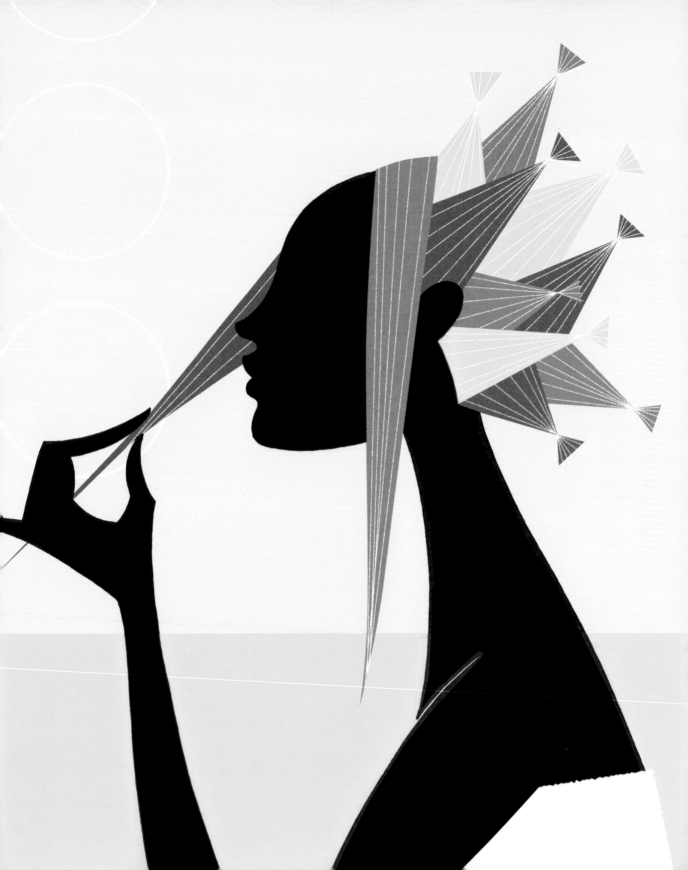

hair color

Does she . . . or doesn't she?
Only her hairdresser knows for sure.

—CLAIROL SLOGAN, 1955

In the 1950s, Clairol's provocative ad campaign suggested it was now acceptable for women to color their hair—as long as they didn't talk about it. And heaven forbid if your roots were showing—you'd never live it down. In those days, women changed their hair color for basically two reasons: to cover gray or to go directly to blond.

Today, few women feel beholden to the hair color they were born with. In fact, more than 50 percent of women in the United States color their hair. Thanks to hair-color chameleons like Linda Evangelista, who changes color like Cher changes wigs, it now seems a lot easier—and more acceptable—to play around with the color of your hair.

Coloring your hair is not only quick and easy in the 21st century, but the chemicals in products are much less caustic to the hair. Yesterday's brassy bottle blonde and the spooky Morticia Addams brunette are entirely avoidable, which has certainly helped to change women's attitudes about hair color. And in any case, shades have become so rich and subtle that nowadays no one will know if you "do" or you "don't"—unless you choose to make it obvious.

Beautiful and natural-looking color is, of course, as sought after as ever. And since the right hair color—like the perfect lipstick—can bring out your eyes and make your skin glow, it's no surprise that top colorists like Christophe (for Catherine Deneuve), Brad Johns (for Claudia Schiffer), Sharon Dorram (for Meg Ryan), Christopher-John (for Madonna), and Louis Licari (for everyone else) now make almost as much as the CEOs of small companies—and it's almost as impossible to snag an appointment with them. Smart women know that finding a good colorist, especially in the beginning, is the secret of soft, richly hued hair.

Choosing Your Color

If you're thinking about coloring your hair for the first time, book a consultation with a colorist, or talk to a colorist at the salon where you have your hair cut. The consultation will be quick but free, and even if you decide to do the job yourself, the advice of a professional will help. Before you start, ask yourself what you want to change about your hair. Do you want to brighten your natural-born mousiness? cover gray? make a dramatic change? Your reasons for coloring will determine which products you should use, the best techniques, and whether or not you can do it yourself. I strongly recommend that you get your hair colored at least once by a professional. A good colorist will lay out your options and tell you how to achieve the look you're after with the least damage to your hair. She'll also talk to you about the maintenance required for each option, an important deciding factor. (If your color needs a touch-up every few weeks and you're not the disciplined type, you won't be happy with the results.)

There are definite advantages to having your hair colored at a salon. The quality of the color itself is better, and you obviously have the benefit of an experienced professional with a practiced eye to do the job. The colorist will custom-mix your color, achieving a much more subtle result than you can get at home. But let's be real: you don't always have the time or money available; sometimes 2 A.M. is the only moment you have left in the day to color your hair. Okay, go ahead, but don't try anything complicated (especially not at 2 A.M.!). At-home hair color is best left for safe—not sorry—processes: touch-ups, henna, and covering gray. Anything more complicated than that should be entrusted to a talented professional at a good salon.

There are several different types of hair color. Some simply lay color on top of the hair strand like paint on a canvas; others require a chemical reaction that takes place inside the hair shaft. The amount of time the color lasts—how strongly it cleaves to the hair—depends on the complexity of the coloring process and the firepower behind the chemicals used. Whatever your reasons for wanting to color your hair, carefully consider the choices

> *There is no such thing as natural hair color, darling," a veritable institution in the salon industry once admonished me. "Coloring your hair is not natural. All the more reason to do it, I say."*

below—and discuss them with your colorist—because if you use permanent color or henna and you don't like it, you could be stuck with the results until your hair grows out or you pay a colorist a pile of money to correct it.

Permanent Color

Permanent hair color is the most popular choice (making up roughly 50 percent of the hair-coloring business), because it lasts the longest and gives the most dramatic change of tone. Permanent color can take you instantly from light to dark or dark to light. If your hair is more than 30 percent gray and you want to conceal it, permanent or demipermanent color is necessary (see below). But there are several reasons why it's smart to look for alternatives, if possible: (1) permanent color is the most damaging to your hair; (2) you can end up with flat, one-dimensional, unnatural-looking color; and (3) even though it lasts a long time, you still have to deal with the roots every six weeks or so.

Although hair-color companies have managed to lower the percentages, peroxide and ammonia are still necessary to achieve a "permanent" result—and these chemicals are harsh on hair. In a single process (one-step), the ammonia and peroxide (the developer) combine to "lift" your hair's natural pigment. (This combination oxidizes the melanin in your hair, causing it to lose its natural color.) The ammonia also opens up the hair cuticle, while the peroxide activates the new color and it is taken into your hair. "The more permanent the hair color," says Mark Garrison, of the Mark Garrison

MUY LINDA

Linda Evangelista's capricious color changes—from natural brunette to honey blond, platinum, and redhead—are a sign of the times. A while back, women had to rely on wigs and hairpieces to have any fun. But the nineties were, without a doubt, the "coming out" decade for hair color. Developments in technology have made women trust color products more. The baby boomers are going gray—and fighting it. And perhaps the biggest shift is psychological: it's become trendy for young people to treat hair color as a cosmetic. The availability of temporary color has made it almost as much of a fashion item as lipstick, especially among thirteen- to twenty-four-year-olds—who try on a new hair shade as often as they take on a new identity. And if you feel red, black, or even blue, why not switch shades—especially since you can shampoo it right out?

salon in New York City, "the deeper it takes the color into the hair shaft." Permanent color will last until you cut your hair and/or your roots grow out.

It's difficult to remove permanent color from the hair. Today, many salons rely on Modulat, a citric-acid-and-sulfur-based stain remover from

Schwarzkopf, which you may or may not be able to find at a beauty supply store—but it's worth a try.

Here's the catch: ammonia dries out the hair and causes it to frizz—and that's the number one reason women limit their use of permanent color. Some brands may have a harsher effect because they contain more ammonia and are less buffered than others. Some salons use low-ammonia, low-peroxide salon formulations, but these are hard to find in at-home products. For at-home use, try Nutrisse by Laboratoires Garnier, which is applied as a hair mask, then rinsed off in the shower. New Basics, a Boston company, created brush-in color that is placed in the handle of a special "ColorIn" brush: it goes onto the bristles when you brush it through your hair.

Demipermanent Color

This technique, known as "deposit-only" or "tone-on-tone," is gentler than permanent color because it doesn't contain ammonia. It's good for enhancing or brightening natural color and can camouflage up to 75 percent of the gray. But because it only deposits color and doesn't lift it, it won't lighten your hair. (It does contain enough peroxide to make the color penetrate somewhat into the hair shaft.) Benefits include the low level of peroxide, the

absence of ammonia, and the lack of obvious roots (because you haven't altered your hair's natural pigment, you've just added pigment to it). The downside is that it lasts only around six weeks before it fades. Suggestions: L'Oréal Casting Tone-on-Tone, Revlon Shadings, Clairol Second Nature.

Semipermanent Color

These products penetrate the hair shaft and stain the cuticle layer, but the color fades with each shampoo. There is no peroxide or ammonia; coverage of the gray is not as dense as with permanent color, the new growth is less obvious, and, as it fades, it's less obvious that you need to do it again. Semipermanent color can be used on permed hair, while demipermanent or permanent may be too strong, and the combination of color and the perm process can

---

COLOR PATCH TEST

If you have a sensitive scalp, have the colorist apply a one-inch round of hair color on your upper arm or behind your ear before she applies any color to your head. Leave it on for 20 to 30 minutes, while you wait. If there's no rash or irritation, it's safe to go ahead. If you're coloring your hair at home, leave the patch on for 24 hours to be really sure.

damage the hair. Depending on the strength of the product, it lasts either 6 to 8 weeks or 10 to 20 (ask your colorist). Semipermanent color is applied in the form of a liquid, gel, or aerosol foam. Suggestions: Clairol Natural Instincts, L'Oréal Avvantage, L'Oréal Casting ColorSpa, Wella Soft Color.

Temporary Color

If you don't want to make a full commitment to a color change, temporary color is for you. The options range from color that you brush in for 24 hours and wash out; to "hair mascara," which can be used in a pinch to touch up small sections of your roots or a few stray grays; to the standard temporary colors that can last from six to eight shampoos. Temporary color is benign; it contains no peroxide, ammonia, or harsh chemicals, and you won't have obvious roots. Temporary color is applied in a rinse, gel, mousse, or spray. Suggestions: Revlon RevUp, Clairol Xtreme F/X, Wella Color Mousse, henna, and vegetable or "botanical" color. For edgier colors, look to companies like Paul Mitchell, Tony & Tina, M·A·C, and Hot Head.

Natural Hair Color

When I had my hair colored for the first time, I ended up with good-looking hair and a scalp full of itchy red patches. The second time, I developed welts. Apparently, I am the 1 out of every 100 women who has an allergy to aniline—a colorless liquid obtained from coal tar, from which many hair colors and dyes are derived. At that point, I started to investigate "natural" hair color (aka vegetable or botanical

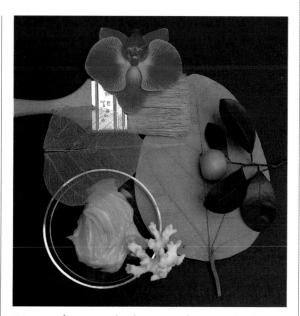

Pigment for natural color comes from tree bark, crushed nut shells, brewed coffee beans, henna, and other fruits, leaves, and flowers.

color), because it has a plant rather than chemical base. And although it can't quite accomplish what chemicals can, it worked for me—but I didn't have much of a choice.

Natural color isn't for everyone. It's especially appealing to women who are pregnant, health-conscious, allergic, or sensitive. But it has its limitations. Natural color (the category includes henna) "stains" rather than "dyes" the hair, because it doesn't oxidize or penetrate into the hair shaft. So it won't do the job if you want

Tip If you love the way your new hair color looks but can't stand the smell, rinse your hair with tomato juice. If you can't stand the way your new vegetable color *looks*, rinse it with a strong detergent shampoo like Prell, Pert, or Breck. Or try a dishwashing liquid (such as Ultra Joy), and it will come right out in the wash.

DID BLONDES ALWAYS HAVE MORE FUN?

With Helen of Troy as their golden-haired standard, the ancient Greeks were the first on record to color their hair blond. They rinsed the hair with a potassium solution and rubbed it with a pomade of pollen and yellow flowers. They also used harsh alkaline bleaching soaps and sat for hours in the sun—which sometimes worked and sometimes didn't. In ancient Rome, blond hair took on a different overtone: prostitutes were required to wear blond wigs to identify their profession. Many centuries later, in the 1660s, women dyed their hair blond with ceruse, a lead compound. Lye or lime was mixed with ceruse and warm water, saffron or turmeric was added for color, and the mix was left on overnight.

to go from dark to blond, blond to dark, or add highlights. And natural color, unfortunately, still doesn't really cover gray (though if you're a brunette, it can give bronze or reddish highlights to a few stray grays).

Right now, only four companies—Schwarzkopf, Aveda, Framesi, Goldwell—sell natural, commercial hair color, although no product is completely natural. (Only pure Egyptian henna is truly organic.) Framesi, an Italian brand whose products are available mostly to haircare professionals, has a 98 percent plant base, with the minimum 2 percent level of ammonia and chemicals that is needed to open the hair cuticle so the color will penetrate. Schwarzkopf, one of the three leading haircare companies in the world, uses a low-ammonia formula buffered with vegetable moisturizers like corn, coconut, or palm oil for its Igora Royal line. The company also makes a powder preparation called Igora Botanic that includes ingredients like bark from the logwood tree in Central America and crushed chestnut and walnut shells. Igora Botanic sits on top of the hair, which is why no strong chemicals are needed to open the cuticle. Aveda Shades of Enlightenment is an essential oil–based color line with 3 percent ammonia. The oils help enhance and accelerate color development, as well as condition and protect the hair.

Henna, the oldest way to color your hair, dates back to Cleopatra. It was also used by the ancients in India, Persia, and Saudi Arabia for decorating the skin. Even now, more than 2,000 years later, henna is still the only 100 percent natural way to color the hair—and it is by far the gentlest.

Henna is made from the leaves of the *Lawsonia inermis* plant, and it colors by coating the hair shaft and staining the cuticle. Neutral henna or red henna without lawsone (the coloring agent) is also an excellent conditioner for the hair. Henna works best as a conditioner for oily hair, and it may also help clear up dandruff. But in terms of color, the exact result is unpredictable, hard to control, and not subtle. And it's permanent: if you don't like it, the only way to get the stain out is to cut your hair off and let your roots grow out. There are three types of henna: red, neutral, and black. The henna can

The owner of Mojo's was a suicide blonde, dyed by her own hand.
—RITA MAE BROWN, *Bingo*

be mixed to color the hair shades of brown and black or by mixing red henna with iron oxide.

Avoid henna if you have a perm or plan to get one. Mineral salts in the henna clash with the chemicals in the perm solution, and you could end up with undulating waves of bright crimson hair. And if you're doing the job yourself, make sure to wear rubber gloves so you don't stain your fingers.

Some salons cook up food-based coloring supplements—like coffee instead of plain old hot water—to enhance the brown shades; concentrated carrot juice, pomegranates, or cherries to bring out the copper in redheads; or chamomile tea for blondes, which can enrich the henna or botanical color. Ask your colorist about these enhancements.

Special Salon Techniques

The techniques below can be beautiful or dramatic or both—as long as they're left to a professional. Even then, they take a talented hand and a skilled eye. At the very least, a colorist can see the back of your head, and you can't!

Highlighting and lowlighting. What was once called frosting is now called *highlighting*. Highlighting brightens the hair by adding light to it. The colorist takes a lighter shade of your natural color (or several shades lighter) and subtly lays it onto strands of the hair. It looks best when you use shades of gold, amber, and red. Even when the highlighting color doesn't contrast sharply with the natural or base color, it

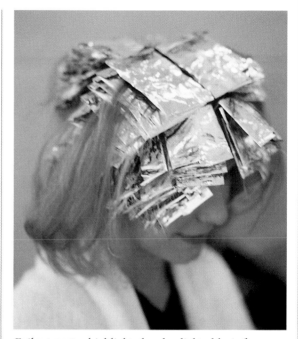

Foil separates highlighted or lowlighted hair from the rest of the crop and protects the scalp from potentially irritating chemical dyes.

still lightens or brightens the overall effect. The process is subtle and time-consuming; it takes about an hour and a half.

Lowlighting is the same technique, with the introduction of darker tones instead of light, which add depth to the hair, especially if it's been lightened too much. Highlighting and lowlighting also help camouflage gray, and, because the color is intentionally uneven, you won't need to be as fussy about regular touch-ups.

Some salons still use bleach to highlight, but I highly recommend that you look for a salon that uses tints instead. Not only is bleach harder on the hair and more limited in its applications, but it continues to lift color until you stop the process. If your colorist happens to get distracted with another client while your hair is bleaching, your hair will go totally white. Then she'll have to add another step to the process and put color back in again. Tints lift and deposit color in one step, which means less potential damage to your hair, less risk of a color disaster, and more control over the end result.

The reason colorists stud women's heads with foil is to keep the highlighted hair away from the rest of the hair on the head and to keep the chemicals away from the scalp during the process. The colorist first places fine sections of hair onto foil, paints on the color or lightener,

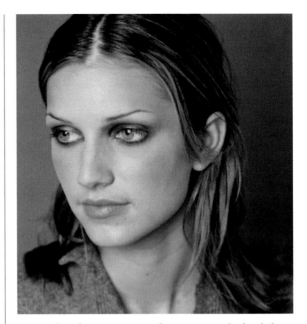

A trendy take on striping: the roots are dark while the ends (and random hanks) are dipped in high-voltage blonde.

and folds the foil to keep it in place. Foiling enables you to get really close to the root without touching the scalp.

Bailiage. Color is hand-painted onto random strands. It can be a great look for curly or wavy hair, and it's a great technique to cover a few random strands of gray.

Chunking (aka striping). This technique is generally credited to celebrity colorist Brad Johns, who first became famous for "chunking" Christy Turlington's hair in 1990. Chunking is similar to highlighting, but the look is much more obvious. The colorist grabs a few random hanks of hair and paints them in high contrast to the hair's natural color. Sometimes both the base color and the chunks are colored. The effect is highly stylized, flagrantly fake, and, for some women, lots of fun.

"GRAY" MARKET

Trade Secret

Unfortunately, the gentlest salon brands—Swarzkopf, Aveda, Goldwell, and Framesi—don't sell directly to the consumer, which enables them to keep the prices high and make the products seem more exclusive. There is a vast "gray" market in the haircare business, however, and some of these products do end up "diverted" to beauty-supply stores, where you can sometimes find them if you're lucky—especially in Los Angeles. Try Number One Beauty Supply, Larchmont Beauty Supply, Wilshire Beauty Supply, or Changes on Melrose. In New York City, try Ray's or Ricky's. Some stores get their hands on restricted salon products by setting up "phantom salons." In other words, they set up a chair in the back of their shop and staff it with a part-time stylist. This makes them, technically, a salon, which means that suppliers will supply them with professional hair-color products, which they can then sell.

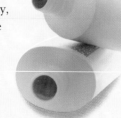

Double processing. Invented in the 1930s, when everyone wanted to look like Jean Harlow, double processing is most often used to go blond. It involves two steps. First, the hair is stripped of its natural pigment with a combination of peroxide and ammonia. Then, a toner that deposits the desired color onto the hair is applied. "The lighter, more ethereal shade of blond you go," says colorist Michael Brimhall, "the more you need heavy artillery."

Double processing is hard on the hair, because when you go from dark to light you need more peroxide to "lift" or remove the color; therefore you must leave it on longer than if you were darkening your hair. If you double-process your hair, make sure to condition and shampoo with special products for color-treated hair (see page 223).

Glazing or glossing. To add shine to the hair, a transparent gloss is layered on top of already colored hair like a polish. Because most glosses are silicone-based, they add incredible shine to the surface of colored or highlighted hair. They can be applied in between color treatments or at the end of your coloring appointment. If your hair is dull, glazing or glossing is an inexpensive way to make it glisten.

Do-It-Yourself: At-Home Color

Most over-the-counter permanent hair color is stronger than professional salon color, which is usually not available to the public. It works more quickly, which makes you feel as if you're getting more bang for your buck, but

The question of whether or not chemical hair color may cause cancer has been hotly debated in recent years. The FDA ruled in 1993 that occasional use of most hair colors probably won't hurt you. Yet studies conducted by the National Cancer Institute as far back as 1978 showed that certain coal tars in permanent hair dyes caused cancer in lab rats. Nonetheless, a loophole in the Federal Food, Drug and Cosmetic Act (FD&C Act) exempts manufacturers from some of the act's provisions and allows some dyes that have been linked to cancer to remain in hair-coloring products as long as there's a disclaimer on the package.

For your health's sake, *absolutely avoid:*

■ Any product containing phenylenediamine. This ingredient has been banned in European hair dyes because it has been linked to cancer.

■ Temporary dyes and rinses containing Acid Blue 168, Acid Violet 73, Acid Orange 87, Solvent Brown 44.

■ Products with this disclaimer on the label: "Caution: This product contains ingredients which may cause skin irritation on certain individuals and a preliminary test according to accompanying directions should first be made. This product must not be used for dyeing the eyelashes or eyebrows; to do so may cause blindness."

it usually contains more ammonia, which means it is harsher on hair. Salon color not only works more slowly but also becomes more diluted when the colorist mixes it to create just the right tone for you. At-home color is premixed and geared to cover a more generic range of shades. Salon color also tends to be better buffered

TOOLS FOR COLOR-TREATING YOUR HAIR

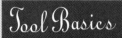

■ A nonreactive bowl—glass or plastic—for mixing color. (Metal interacts with the chemicals in hair color, and you may end up with a surprising result.)

■ Plastic gloves, which come with most hair-coloring products, to protect your hands from irritation. (Salon colorists who tough it out barehanded end up with some of the roughest, driest hands this side of Alligator Creek.)

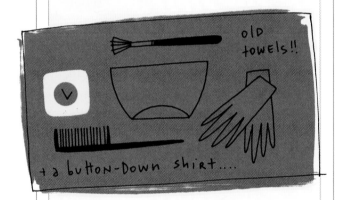

old towels!!

+ a button-down shirt....

■ A small brush from a beauty-supply shop or art store to touch up roots.

■ An alarm clock or kitchen timer to make sure you leave the color on for exactly the time required.

■ A rat-tail comb to lift and separate the hair and large hair clips to hold up some sections while you're working on others.

■ A button-down shirt, which will be easier to peel off than anything that goes over your head.

■ An old, dark towel to wipe off excess color.

with silicones or emulsion bases, which make it gentler on hair.

If you're going to use permanent color, always look for products labeled "low-ammonia, low-peroxide," because they're better for your hair. When it comes to at-home hair color, L'Oréal is one of the best. Also look for hair-color kits with cream formulas that contain conditioning botanicals and polymers that bind to the hair shaft to condition it. Semipermanent color coats the hair shaft, which makes it thicker, and opens up the cuticle, which gives the hair body. A good product can also add shine, which gives an optical illusion of thickness.

You may not want to drag yourself into the salon every few weeks for touch-ups. Once you've become friendly with your colorist (after a few visits), ask if she will mix up a bottle of the color—or color-enhancing shampoo—she uses and sell it to you for in-between touch-ups. Or ask her to recommend the commercially available product and color that would work best for you in between visits to the salon.

1. Choose it. A bad color match can turn your $5 box of hair color into a $100 trip to the salon for color correction. If you're new at coloring your hair, my advice is to start with a temporary hair color, because if you screw it up, it's easier to wash out right away— or in the worst case, it will wash out in six to eight shampoos.

Next, narrow your choice down to the color category you want—black, brown, red, blond. Then zero in on that section of the drugstore shelf. Look at the back of each box, where most kits show "before" (natural) hair colors next to "after" hair colors. Ignore the lustrously shaded locks of the model on the box; she probably didn't start out with your color, and you won't end up with hers. Instead, consider your skin tone. Hold the box up next to your face, look in the store mirror, and see how the color looks against your skin. (It isn't easy under fluorescent lighting, which is why I strongly recommend asking your hairstylist for guidance, if you can.)

If you're trying for a match to cover gray, be honest with yourself. "Look at your natural color and stay within one or two shades of color," says Wendy Bond, co-owner of the Oscar Bond Salon in New York City. The most important thing to know in choosing color is that most companies make their shades too dark. Choose one that's one or two shades lighter than your natural color.

If your natural colors are "warm"—in beauty-speak, that means your makeup palette has yellowish undertones (rusts, bronzes, greens, apricots)—look for warm hair-color shades with golden undertones. (It's easier for women with "warm" skin to go blond, because they already have warm skin tones to complement the warm blond tones.) If you're "cool" and look better in blue-reds, look for cool,

> **Tip** At-home cream hair color is usually buffered better than the liquid versions, and the pH (acid level) is generally lower and more hospitable to the hair.

LEAVE NO TRACE

Before you apply color, apply Vaseline around the hairline to prevent the color from staining your skin. If you do stain your hands or hairline while coloring your hair, use an alcohol-based toner or astringent to remove it. If that doesn't work, a product called Clean Touch Color Remover definitely will.

Trade Secret

ashen shades. For a refresher in determining "what color you are," see pages 106–107.

Next, consider the color of your eyes. If your eyes are brown and your skin has yellow undertones, look for colors with a touch of gold (golden blond, chestnut, orange-reds). If your eyes are blue, green, or gray and your skin has blue undertones, choose from the burgundy-browns, ash blonds, or red-violets. If your skin has red undertones, be careful. The more red you put in your hair, the redder your skin will look. When in doubt, start subtly. Remember, you can always pump up the intensity later on.

2. Test it. Before you dive in and color your entire head, do a test strand first to see how the color really looks on your hair. Take a half-inch-wide section of hair from the nape or bottom, where you can see it but no one else can, and color it from roots to ends. Leave the color in for the right amount of time, rinse it, dry it, and check to make sure that it's the color you want.

3. Color it. Coloring works best when the hair is dry and not freshly washed or brushed. Put on an old button-down shirt and sling an old towel around your shoulders. Mix the formula, and apply it in sections starting with the top, then sides, then back, according to the instructions on the box. (Have you ever seen a woman with spotty color on the back of her head and wondered what happened? To avoid the same fate, get someone to help you apply the color to those areas you can't see or reach too well.)

Make sure to saturate your hair evenly as you go along, and clip each section to the top of your head as you finish it. Do your best to avoid applying the solution directly onto the scalp: you don't want hair color on your skin, and a small percentage of the chemicals can be absorbed by the scalp into the bloodstream. At the end, comb the color through your hair a couple of times to make sure that it's distributed evenly.

4. Wash it. Follow the directions on the box, and use a timer to track the time carefully. Make sure not to leave the color on your head longer than necessary and rinse thoroughly. Then condition and rinse again.

Coloring Tips

- Color your hair when it's dirty to protect the scalp. (Oil from dirty hair will block penetration into the large pores on the scalp.)

- Every time you shampoo color-treated hair you fade the color. Wash hair less frequently, and use cool water. Sometimes just rinsing it is enough.

- If your color doesn't turn out well, your water may be at fault. According to National Geological Survey studies, 85 percent of U.S. households have hard water, which often contains chlorine and lime. When minerals build up on the hair, color and perm treatments don't penetrate as well. If you have this problem, try a special shampoo—Aveda Detoxifying Shampoo or Bain de Terre Hydrogel Purifying Crystals—a couple of days before coloring to prepare your hair for color.

- Never mix different hair-color products, because you can induce potentially harmful chemical reactions—not to mention disastrous color.

- Never use hair color to dye your lashes. The FDA prohibits even salons from doing this, because if it spills into the eyes, it can seriously damage eyesight.

- Avoid chlorine, try to stay out of the sun, and cover your head when you go out of doors. The sun oxidizes and fades color and turns ash blond into red.

- Remove contact lenses before coloring your hair. Contact lenses are gas-permeable, and the eyes get irritated when the ammonia permeates the lenses.

Beauty Bloopers

Too many chemicals will overprocess the hair and make it look fried. If your hair is already permed or relaxed, avoid permanent color and see if you can get the effect you want with semi- or demipermanent. When you use ammonia- and peroxide-based permanent color, you're giving your hair a double dose of harsh chemicals, and that can really damage it. The road to recovery? Deep-conditioning treatments (see page 224).

If your hair looks too flat and dark, you've chosen the wrong color. For example, if you add dark brown to dark brown, it will come out close to black, and the color won't lighten up until you go to a salon to get it corrected or cut your hair off.

You may end up with roots lighter than the rest of your hair if you color already colored hair, says Lissette Martinez of the Rutherford/Lissette salon in Manhattan. "Remember, you don't know how much pigment is in your hair naturally, so it's hard to know what you'll end up with when you recolor." If you want to change your color, you should have the old color removed first.

Touch-ups

Permanent hair color will last until you cut your hair, but the roots will start showing in four to six weeks. When you touch up your own roots, don't recolor your entire head, because there's no need to risk damage to your hair with an unneccessary round of chemicals. Stick to the new growth and, if you can, use demi- or

The art of color: A wide range of shades create a perfect palette for touch-ups. If you only have a few strands to cover, hard-pressed Q-tips are precise enough to work hair by hair, and they won't leave a trail of cotton bits behind.

semipermanent color on it. If your overall color is fading, use a color-enhancing shampoo or conditioner to perk it up. And if your colorist cancels at the last minute because he had to squeeze in Catherine Deneuve or Courtney Love, you can touch up your roots with these quick fixes: 'Tween Time (Cosmetics Plus), Aveda Mask-Hair-A, or any waterproof mascara.

Don't even think about highlighting your own hair. Dark hair can turn orange, especially since you don't know how much red is already in your hair. Besides, how can you possibly know which strands to grab on the back of your head? Most at-home highlight kits are bleach-based, whereas good salons use tints, which are more subtle and easier to control. P.S. If you try to color highlighted sections back to their natural shade, you may end up with a lovely shade of aubergine.

Did You Know?

In the 19th century, "mascaro" was used by both sexes as a touch-up for graying hair. By the 21st century, hair mascara is back, thanks to baby boomers who want to cover up a few stray grays, and Christian Dior's Mascara Flash for Hair has become a best-seller.

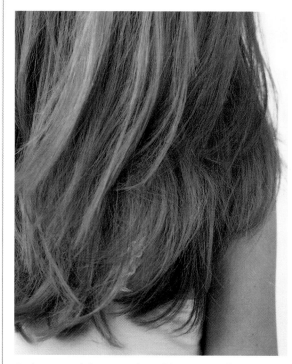

Red is one of the most desirable—and difficult— shades to hold onto.

Go, Red

It's easy to transform yourself into a redhead—especially if you're brunette—but it's a difficult color to maintain, because red is one of the more unstable pigments. Use of a color-enhancing shampoo can really help hold on to the red. A gloss treatment at the salon will also help protect your color, since red oxidizes more quickly than any other color—even blond.

However, choosing the right shade of red (and matching it to your skin tone) can be difficult. "If you do it yourself, chances are it won't be subtle," says Wendy Bond. "Most brunettes have natural red tones in their hair. When a brunette goes to a lighter shade of red, the red she has will be emphasized." The easiest and most obvious way to go red is, of course, with henna (see page 212), but that's about as unsubtle as it gets. Unless you really know what you're doing or don't mind neon, go to a salon—at least the first time.

Shades of Gray

My grandmother, a former millinery model, has had her hair cut short at the barbershop for over 60 years. She slicks it back from her deep-dip widow's peak with some emerald-green goop that must have been one of the first hair gels in history. Grandma saw her first gray hairs at age 77, but most women see their first strands in their mid- to late 30s. (African Americans tend to go gray later, in their mid-40s.)

Gray hair can come as a shock. Psychologically, few women are ready when their hair signals passage into middle age, which is why so many color their hair. But those strands of silvery gray not only can be beautiful, they can be sexy, too, especially when you do something

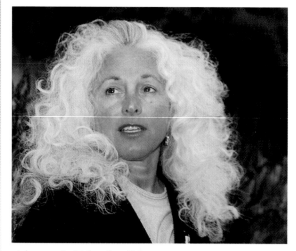

A heavenly halo of stylish gray.

with them. When my cousin Leslie's hair turned gray, she not only let it grow below her shoulders, she got a perm and wears it loose around her head like a crown (see facing page). Her hair has evolved into a mark of her personal style. And everywhere she goes, someone compliments her on her gorgeous hair.

Whether you color your hair or keep it natural, you'll still have to care for graying hair differently. It's not only the color that changes; the texture does, too.

Gray hair can turn yellow due to the effects of pollution, sun, mineral deposits, or product buildup. Shampoos with blue or indigo tints can balance out the yellow, and they do work, but don't use them every day or you'll turn into a "blue-hair." Simply use the shampoo until your yellow is gone, then alternate with your regular shampoo. The following shampoos get the yellow out: Kiehl's Chamomile Shampoo, Sterling Solutions Shampoo and Conditioner (a true find!), Matrix So Silver, Nexxus Simply Silver Toning Shampoo, Phyto Therathrie Phytargent Shampoo. Conditioning is also important, because gray hair can be both coarse and dry. Because of this, most gray hair can handle conditioning without getting weighed down. It keeps the gray shiny and will also beat back frizz.

Gray or white hair can be gorgeous, but if you want to put off the moment of truth and cover your few strands,

HAIR DRESSING

Colored (or permed) hair needs extra moisture, especially in the summer. Before you go out in the sun, comb a dime-sized dab of conditioner through color-treated hair. Then, of course, cover with a hat.

use vegetable color or semipermanent color. It will turn your grays a reddish or golden hue (depending on the shade you choose and how much red you have naturally in your hair), and they'll look like mini highlights.

Lots of women (even former brunettes) decide to go blond when their hair starts to gray. It makes sense, because gray is the shade visually closest to blond, and that makes maintenance easier. But it's not always a great idea, especially if you have fair, ashen skin, because the gray-blond can make you look really washed out. Of course, a dark color can look unnatural and harsh. There's a natural, aesthetic reason we turn gray at a certain point—it's softer and complements our changes of skin tone and our new wrinkles better than a dark color around the face. A smart choice for brunettes is to highlight (or lowlight) their hair when it starts to gray. If you create a deeper base color and

The fashion model Carmen grows even more attractive as her hair gets grayer over the years.

highlight against that, you'll get more depth, and it will balance out your skin tone. Plus, highlights soften the lines of demarcation as your roots start to show, and you won't need touch-ups as frequently.

Loss of pigment can make your hair's texture wirier, frizzier, and coarser. "Gray hair can be extremely resistant to color," says Arlene Bradley, a colorist at Manhattan's Kim Lepine Salon, "and the coarser it is, the harder it is to cover." Sometimes, even permanent color won't cover gray. In that case, you can try a one-two punch: demipermanent color and lowlights.

If you have only a few gray strands, ask the colorist if she can hand-paint them without applying color to the entire head. If you are a dark brunette with less than 30 percent gray, consider semipermanent color that's a shade lighter than your natural color; you'll cover the gray without darkening your own color. (But if you go too light, the gray will stay gray.) On the other hand, color that's too dark can wash out your skin tone.

"Most women don't want a flat, one-dimensional color," says Lissette Martinez, "or to be tied into maintenance every three weeks." The solution? If you've got a lot of gray but you want to imitate the hair you were born with, she suggests putting in 50 percent permanent color (brown), leaving some gray, and foiling in some highlights. Or let's say you're 30 percent gray in one area and 10 percent gray in another. "You need to use permanent color on the gray streak and something softer [like semipermanent color] on the rest of the head. Why go for permanent color all over and lock yourself into heavy maintenance and flat color?" Why, indeed?

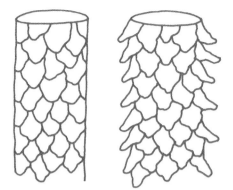

The cuticle (outer) layer of healthy hair lies flat and fits together like shingles on a rooftop. An unhealthy, overprocessed cuticle (right) will tangle and break because it sticks straight out like the top of a telephone pole.

Caring for Colored Hair

Color-treated hair needs special care. "Coloring weakens the hair, breaks down the disulfide bonds in the hair shaft, and gradually breaks down elasticity," says Philip Kingsley, a trichologist and owner of salons in Manhattan and London.

The best thing you can do to keep color-treated hair healthy and shiny is not to color it too often—although a lot depends on the type of color and the chemicals used. Always choose the gentlest treatments that will accomplish your

Her locks had been so frequently and drastically brightened and curled that to caress them, one felt, would be rather like running one's fingers through julienne potatoes.

—DOROTHY PARKER

FOR COLOR-TREATED HAIR

Whether your hair is colored, processed, damaged, or simply dry, it needs special care. Shampoos that target these problems are emollient and contain more conditioners than other shampoos. Use a shampoo designed for any of these conditions, and your color will last longer and look better. Avoid shampoos with Castile soaps, Castile oils, and glycerine, because they will fade the color (or loosen the perm) with each shampoo. Clarifying shampoos can also strip color, so use them in moderation.

★Best Products

Shampoos. Thermasilk Heat Activated Shampoo Revitalizing Formula, ABBA Crème Moist, La Coupe Color Safe Moisture-Rich Shampoo, Aveda Pure-Fumé Brilliant Shampoo, Revlon Colorstay Shampoo, Rio Vista Equine Shampoo, Vidal Sassoon Shampoo for Permed or Color-Treated Hair, Artec Kiwi Shampoo.

For blond hair, try Frédéric Fekkai Baby Blonde, Aveda Blue Malva Shampoo, Emerald Bay UV Activated Hair Lightener, Aveda Chamomile Shampoo, Kiehl's Chamomile Shampoo.

Color-enhancing shampoo. Artec Colorist Collection Shampoo, Goldwell Colorance Color n' Care, L'Oréal ColorVive, Redken Shades EQ Color Enhancing Shampoo. (Don't use a color enhancer each time you shampoo. Alternate with a regular color-safe shampoo or you may find your color overly enhanced.)

Conditioners. Aveda Damage Control Leave-In Conditioner, Nexxus Humectant, Aussie 3-Minute Miracle, Klorane Oil of Safflower Conditioner, Artec Kiwi Conditioner, Thermasilk Heat Activated Revitalizing Conditioner, L'Oréal ColorVive Crème Conditioner, Artec Colorist Collection Conditioner, TIGI Moisture Maniac Conditioner, Paul Mitchell Awapuhi Moisture Mist.

Deep conditioners. Philip B. Botanical Deep-Conditioning Crème Rinse, Ouidad Deep Treatment (for curly hair; fixes frizz), Goldwell Kera-Fix Deep Conditioner, Peter Hans Nourishing Conditioner, Mastey Basic Superpac Protein Complex Reconstructor.

goal. For example, if you can use semipermanent instead of permanent color, do it.

In the first week after a color treatment, your hair may be especially dry or frizzy, and the lighter the color, the more frizziness. Don't freak out about dryness; simply use a conditioner for color-treated hair, specific to your hair type, and it will help smooth down the cuticle.

If your individual strands are very fine, they're probably also dry and fragile. If you relax or process fine hair, it becomes even drier and more fragile. Because this type of hair has a thin cuticle layer to begin with, it can't take much abuse. Besides, it tends to react to color very quickly, which is why it's advisable to use mild products.

If you both color and process your hair, leave at least two weeks in between—and never do both on the same day. Stick to semi-permanent or vegetable color to keep hair in good condition. Some hair just can't take both, and you may have to make a choice.

Long term, you'll need to use a low-pH shampoo for color-treated hair. Conditioning with a conditioner for color-treated hair will moisturize your hair, keep it looking and feeling healthier, and give it more shine. "Hair is dead," says Philip B., a stylist and owner of Philip B. Botanical Haircare. "It has a grain like wood. You want to go with the grain and smooth the cuticle layer with a conditioner."

Deep Conditioning

Deep-condition your hair regularly. If you've gone blond and double-processed or high-lighted your hair, you should use a deep conditioner once a week. Otherwise, once every two to four weeks will do it. If your hair lacks moisture, use a moisturizing conditioner. If it lacks strength, use a protein-based conditioner.

When Hollywood clients come to Philip B. with hair that's been working overtime, he recommends a four-step oil-based treatment. "When you color hair, you burn away natural oil with caustics. For soft, healthy hair, try to balance out the damage by adding oil to the hair." Philip uses Philip B. Rejuvenator for Dry to Damaged Hair, a special essential-oil blend, along with other custom-blended oils in his salon treatments, which is also available for home use. Or try "Oil or Nothing."

LOOSE ENDS

Take a moment to read the ingredients label when you're shopping for products. A little more or less of this or that can really improve the quality of life for processed hair.

For colored hair. Avoid products containing mineral oil or silicone at the top of the ingredients list—these can strip color.

For permed hair. Look for ammonium —rather than sodium—cleansers and for shampoos with keratin or wheat amino acids, which strengthen the hair fiber. Silicones and dimethicone will make combing easier. Avoid polyquaternium or resin listed in the first few ingredients. These can weigh down your hair.

For brittle, heat-damaged hair. Look for shampoos with added moisturizers like glycerine; butylene glycol; extracts of kukui, chamomile, or jojoba; and betaine-based cleansers.

OIL OR NOTHING

¼–¾ cup olive or almond oil (depending on the length of your hair) A few drops of lavender oil

1. Shampoo your hair.
2. Heat the olive or almond oil until it's warm to the touch. Add the lavender oil.
3. Gently massage the oil into your scalp and hair, from top to tips.
4. Heat with a blow-dryer (using a diffuser attachment) at low speed until dry. (The heat opens the cuticle and helps the oil absorb better.) Then shampoo again.

Here are two more home remedies—one moisturizing and one protein-based—that I've adapted from my salon travels.

SOUTH OF SHANGHAI MOISTURIZING TREATMENT

In Chinese medicine, ginseng is believed to cure impotence. It can also rejuvenate dry, colored hair and scalp.

½ avocado
2 pinches of ginseng powder
1 egg yolk

1. Mash the avocado and mix in the ginseng powder and egg yolk.
2. Massage the mask into your scalp, wrap a thin towel around your head, and leave on for 10 minutes.
3. Rinse, then shampoo.

TUSCAN PROTEIN PACK

Egg is rich in protein, and the oil will moisturize your hair. After applying, wrap your head, go into the backyard, and imagine yourself sitting outdoors on a terrazzo in Tuscany.

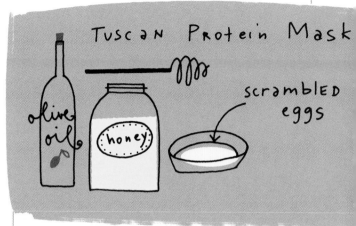

½ cup honey
¼ cup olive oil
1 egg

1. Mix the honey and olive oil.
2. Scramble the egg and mix it in.
3. Massage into the hair, and let it sit for 20 minutes.
4. Shampoo out. Rinse.

Now that your hair is soft and shiny, and you've chosen a shade that makes your skin glow, it's time to talk cut and style. Read on.

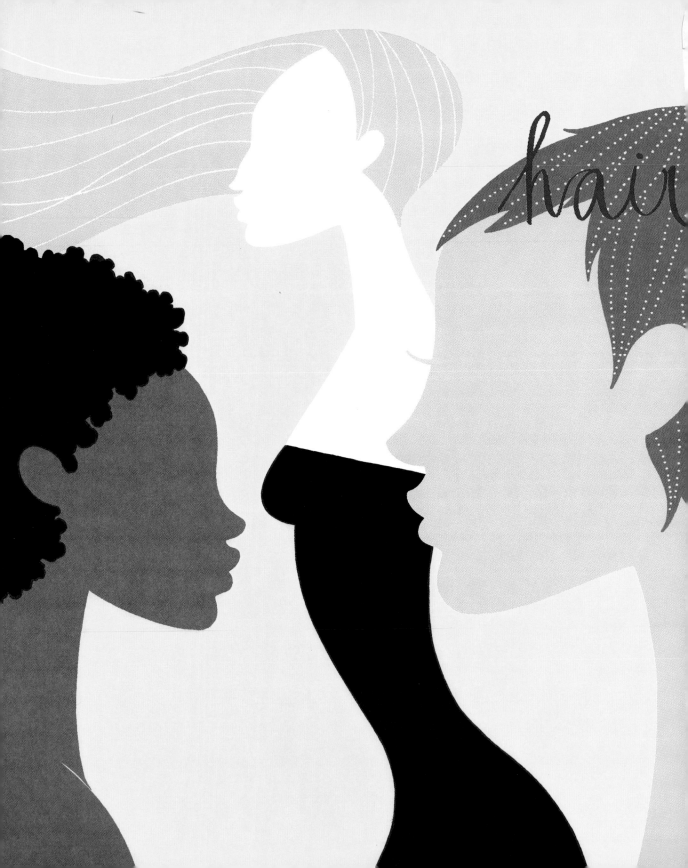

cuts & styles

*To Crystal, hair was the most important thing
on earth. She would never get married because
you couldn't wear curlers in bed then.*

—EDNA O'BRIEN

No matter how chaotic life was in my childhood, there was one thing we could always count on: Mom's weekly trip to the "beauty parlor." My mother was totally dependent on those appointments, and it always amazed me how she—and most women of her generation—seemed to be incapable of combing or even washing their own hair. By the end of the week, she would enter the salon with hair that was droopy, if not totally deflated. When she came out, her hair was pumped back up, and so were her spirits. For her, the hair salon was a haven—as it should be. A lot of things have changed since then, but one thing has not: many women are still dependent—to some extent—on their stylist to look good.

Today, most women still want a haven—a soothing place where they can feel relaxed, pampered, and secure. After all, trying a new haircut is risky enough. You don't need an intimidating salon setting to make you feel even more insecure about your looks. If only all stylists could take Vidal Sassoon's credo to heart: "Haircutting is a very kind art form," he told me. "You're only there to make people feel better."

A good haircut moves beautifully, it's easy to style, it's soft and tactile, and it looks good from any angle—even when it's a tousled mess. It can give you a huge boost, make you look fabulous, and fit you like a second skin. "A good cut becomes your style," salon owner John Sahag once said. And your style becomes you. Of course, the more you take control of the process from the beginning, the greater chance you have of getting the look you want in the first place.

Finding the right style for you is key, and to do that you need the help of a good stylist. This chapter will help you figure out the cut that's best for you and your hair, and how to find a stylist who can deliver.

Finding the Right Style

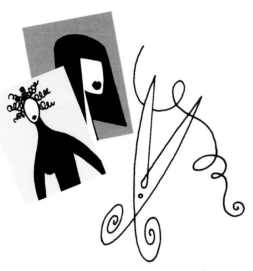

W hether your hair is blunt cut or layered, coaxed into finger waves, braided into cornrows, or simply set loose, it decorates your body and expresses who you are. That's why it's so important to find a style that suits the real you—not only your hair type, face shape, and body type, but your personality and lifestyle as well.

Before you experiment with a new cut, ask yourself how much time you want to devote to your hair each day: 5 minutes to wash and walk out the door in the morning, or 20 minutes to blow it out? If a bob is the look you want but you have curly hair, consider this: either you'll have to blow it straight with gels and round brushes every time you wash it, or you'll need to relax your hair. Are you really up for that?

Trends in hairstyles can be fun and will update your look, but first you need to figure out the basic cut that's right for you. Getting a haircut is not a good time to be impulsive. Plan ahead—do you want a big change or a small one? If you're making a major change—a dramatic cut or new style—before a big event, do it a week or two ahead so that you have time to play around and get comfortable with your new look. It's crushing when you have your heart set on a chic bob and you leave the salon looking like Prince Valiant.

The importance of a good haircut can hardly be overstated. Whether or not you choose to color, curl, or otherwise treat your hair is a matter of personal preference. But no one, no matter how beautiful, can look her best with a bad haircut. Here are the main things to consider before taking that big step.

Face Shape

A good stylist will obviously want to accentuate your most beautiful features—high cheekbones, strong jaw, swanlike neck—and play down the less beautiful ones. The shape of the face is underplayed by many stylists these days, but it's a good way to establish general guidelines for a cut.

If you don't know the shape of your face, tie your hair back, stand up close to your bathroom mirror, and trace your reflection with a lip pencil. Then step back and see which shape it most resembles: round, square, oval, or heart. Here are some styles that are most flattering to each.

Round. Cheeks are as wide as your jaw and forehead; wide, full chin, no visible jawline.

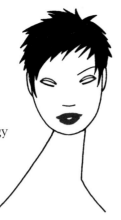

STYLE: A side part will make your face appear longer. So will a short, fringy cut brushed toward the face, a short cut that tapers in above the ears and has lots of layers at the crown for height, or a long style that's layered around the face. Extra width or curl at the sides will make your face look even fuller—unfortunately, there's no Louise Brooks bob in your future.

Square. Prominent, squared-off jaw, wide forehead with squared-off hairline, may have strong cheekbones.

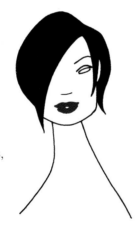

STYLE: To soften the angular shape, avoid blunt-edged jaw-length cuts and straight bangs. Hair length is best above or below the jawline. Fringy, tapered bangs, side parts, off-center layers, and curling the ends of your hair under will all soften the line of your jaw. Adding height at the crown will elongate your face and make it look less square.

Oval. Somewhere between round and square. High forehead, prominent jawline, long and narrow chin.

Tip If your neck is thick, bring some hair forward from the sides of the neck or cut your hair in longish layers to distract from the thickness. A short, boyish cut or hair worn up and away from your face will only call attention to it.

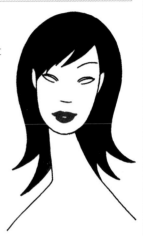

STYLE: To widen a narrow face, go for short or chin-length hair that's subtly layered at the bottom or full at the sides (not on top) and tapered in. Soft, side-dipping bangs are a good bet, as are face-framing layers in front; they de-emphasize the length of an oval face. Long straight hair with a center part is not for you. Asymmetrical parts or cuts add width to a narrow face.

Heart. High cheekbones, delicate, pointy chin, and wide forehead.

STYLE: Avoid super-short cuts or styles with center parts. Hair tucked behind the ears, soft bangs, curly or wavy styles, short layers on top, hair that's long on the neck and wispy at the bottom, flippy ends, and tousled layers will all nicely emphasize your bone structure and soften the effect of a pointy chin.

Hair Texture and Type

Is your hair curly, straight, fine, coarse, wavy, thin, or thick? Even if you're willing to put a lot of effort into retooling your hair, the best cuts work with your hair's natural texture instead of fighting it. The hair falls better that way.

Fine Hair

There are countless styling tricks to make fine hair look more voluminous, involving Velcro rollers, volumizing sprays, and blow-dryers, but the best way to build in volume is with a good cut. A slightly graduated or layered cut can make fine hair look thicker and give it more volume. "To give body to flat hair, get a cut with soft layering in the top of the hair," says Kim Lepine of the Kim Lepine salon in Manhattan. Feathery layers add body, and tapering the ends with a razor can also make it look fuller. "Angling takes weight off the hair so it can lift up," Lepine adds.

Trade Secret

I f your hair is *long*," says Mark Garrison, owner of the Mark Garrison Salon in Manhattan, "brush the hair upside down with a flat brush. Then put volumizer on the roots, and either add a bit of heat at the roots or wait a few seconds and brush the tips of the hair without brushing the roots. This gives you a cushion of air around the roots, which gives bounce." If your hair is short and flat on top, brush it in the opposite direction from the way it lies, and change back and forth. Brush upside down throughout the day to add air. But don't add more product—it will weigh the hair down.

Here are three surefire styles for fine hair:

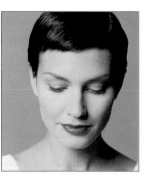

Super-short. If you have delicate features, your hair will take beautifully to a wispy, boyish, Mia Farrow fringe that's short on the sides and razored on top. Just run a little cream or gel through the roots, and tousle with your fingers as you blow- or air-dry.

Longer. Still lightly layered at the crown and around the face; longer layers at sides and back. Keep the layering short on top—anything longer than three inches on top will start to weigh it down.

Round bob. Cut above the jaw with baby-bang fringe, ever so slightly beveled (cut on the slant) at the ends, to add body.

Curly Hair

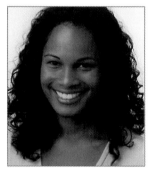

See if you can find a stylist who specializes in curly hair—it's a special skill, and not everyone has it. "It's important to cut curly hair when it's wet, so that you can see its natural shape," says Kao, co-owner of Salon AKS in Manhattan. "I like to cut into it and create some layers, but not fuss with it or fight with it too much. Curly hair is all about movement and a little messiness."

A cut that's layered just right will work well with your hair's natural shape. A bit of layering around the face and at the ends will give curly or wavy hair—both thick or thin—a nice shape. But if the layers are too short, it will spiral off into the stratosphere and pouf.

Layered around the face. If your curly hair is also coarse, a little extra length is a good idea, because the length will weigh it down, which helps control it. But beware of the blunt cut, which

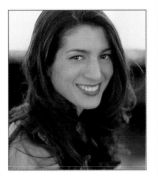

doesn't really work for curly hair. It looks like a wedge, because curly hair tends to levitate when it's short and cut all one length.

All one length. Tightly textured curls look good long, because the length makes the curls look well defined; just make sure the ends are nicely groomed.

Super-short. A close-cropped Afro lets your hair go its own way naturally—but barely.

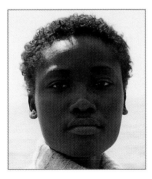

Wavy Hair

Like curly hair, wavy hair needs enough length to fall into its natural pattern: think Andie MacDowell. Cut it in long enough layers so that it's shaped where the natural wave falls; if you cut it too short, you'll lose the wave, or it can devolve into frizz.

RAZOR CUTS

Trade Secret When a stylist uses a razor to cut hair, it creates a tousled, messy, rock-'n'-roll type of cut. When he uses a razor-scissor combination, it can look wispy rather than choppy. Razoring the ends, or tapering them a bit with scissors, will take weight off the hair and allow it to fall in soft angles. "A razor cut is good for straight, thick hair or Asian hair because it creates texture," says Kao of Salon AKS. "Never use a razor on curly hair because it makes it frizzy. Curly hair already has so much texture, you don't want to add more."

Underlayering. This technique (formerly known as "thinning") is used on wavy or straight hair to reduce excess bulk and beat back frizz. Because the surface layers are relatively long, the

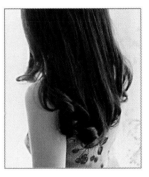

hair keeps its natural shape, as the top pieces fall over the sheared ones.

Thick, Straight Hair

Because thick, straight hair is naturally voluminous, it's perfect for blunt cuts like pageboys and bobs, which emphasize volume. This is the type of hair that Vidal Sassoon's blunt, geometric cuts or slightly layered bobs were made for. "When the geometrics happened in the sixties," says Sassoon, "that was the change from hairdressing to haircutting."

STRAIGHT TALK

Asian hair is the same color—dark—and it's always straight," says Younghee, owner of the Younghee Salon in Manhattan. "But there's a big difference in textures: it's either silky and fine or coarse with lots of body." Ideally, you want to condition it well so that it looks lustrous and get a good cut for it to move beautifully. For conditioning, Younghee says that cream products are preferable to oily products, which tend to look oily on Asian hair. Use a hairstyling cream, or try her styling trick: "After you put

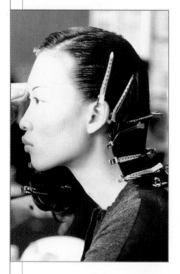

on body lotion or hand cream, use whatever's left over on the ends of your hair," she says. "It's especially good for fine, short, or medium-length hair, because it makes the hair look more lustrous, less perfect, and more textured."

When it comes to shape, a blunt cut can be beautiful, but it's definitely a traditional look. If you want something more modern, "try layering or texturizing cuts," she says, "for example, short cuts with fringe around the forehead or long hair with long layers from the top down." She uses a combination of scissors and a razor because a razor alone can be too blunt. "What I like," she says, "is weightless layering. If you want to take out weight, you start from the top. If you want to build weight, you start from the bottom." Sounds like a plan.

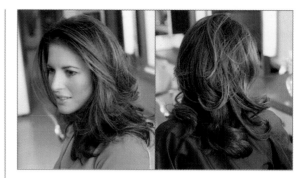

Long shag. The challenge with thick hair is to make it move—it prefers to just hang—and long layers cut into the sides make the ends flip or turn under. A cut with layers starting at ear level is a simple, interesting look. You can also pin it up and let pieces hang down.

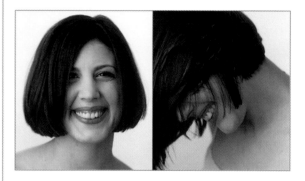

Blunt bob. Everyone with straight hair wants a bob—but not everyone can have the classic version with bangs because bangs don't suit everyone. But it's easy to wear a fairly traditional bob parted slightly off center. For an edgier version, think blunt, fringy bangs, sides tapered into points, and a slightly graduated back. A beveled bottom—cut vertically or on a slant—gives it some swing. A bob is an easy, low-maintenance style that looks good tousled or tame.

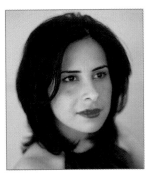

Short cut. Strong features can handle more hair. A short or medium cut with shorter layers around the face will attract attention to your eyes and the middle of your face. If you prefer an edgier, shorter style, a razor cut with tapered sideburns, longish spikes, and short layers should satisfy the latent rock star within.

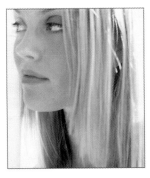

Stick straight. Hair that's thick and straight as a stick can be silky and beautiful but tends to just hang there because it's so heavy. To make the most of your hair's natural volume and give it some movement at the same time, you can razor feathery layers throughout the crown or have the ends cut vertically and taper it at the back for a softer shape. (To give the layers some lift, you'll need a paddle brush for styling.) If you prefer a longer length, blunt cut the ends, and taper layers throughout the sides for a curvier shape, like Mariah Carey's.

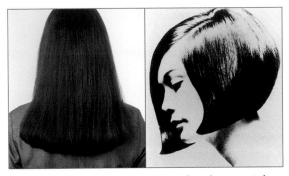

In the 1960s, Vidal Sassoon streamlined women's lives with "wash-and-wear haircuts," like the "geometric" cut on actress Nancy Kwan (above right).

Body Type

A good haircut not only takes into consideration your hair texture and quality but also needs to work in proportion to the rest of your body. So it's important to factor in your head shape and body type. A close-cropped cut that frames the face with bangs or a bit of fringe will look terrific on a slim, tall, fine-featured woman. If you are short, a short or medium-length cut with a little layering on top can create the illusion of height. Longer hair makes people look shorter.

In general, a short haircut will emphasize your weight. If you have a small head on a big body, you won't want to cut your hair too short. When it comes to the length of your hair, factor in your head shape: Is your head round, flat, or oval? Super-short hair is more flattering on a perfectly shaped head.

Finding a Stylist

If you see a woman with hair that is similar to yours who has a great cut, ask her where she got it. Don't be embarrassed—she'll be flattered. If you like a cut in a magazine, read the styling credits to find out who styled the hair in the photo and the name of his or her salon. Once you collect a few names, book a consultation. In fact, book a few. They're free.

The consultation. The most important part of any haircut, the consultation is your opportunity to discuss your ideas with the stylist—and listen

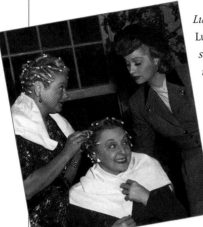

Lucille Ball, of I Love Lucy *fame, kept a salon in the back room of her house, where she gave egg shampoos and perms to friends. "It's where I gab with the girls while I give them beauty treatments," she said. As far as I'm concerned, it's just another reason to love Lucy.*

to hers. If you can, book the last appointment of the day. It's easier to talk things through in a leisurely way if no one else is waiting for her turn. Even so, you'll get only about 10 minutes of a stylist's time, so be organized.

1. Go to the salon with hair that's clean and as product-free as possible, so the stylist can see it in its natural state. Talk to her about the health and condition of your hair. She should have good, helpful suggestions that may need to be factored into your cut.

2. Flip through women's magazines ahead of time, including the cheesy-looking hair magazines like *Sophisticate's Hairstyle Guide* and *Hairdo*. They're jammed with both classic and trendy style ideas. Tear out photos of cuts you like—even if it includes Shawn Colvin's cut and you're more of a Mary-Chapin Carpenter

Tip The expected tip for a stylist is 15 to 20 percent of the cost of your cut and $5 for the assistant who does your shampoo.

type. Bring the clips to the salon to show what kinds of looks you like so that you have a point of reference.

A picture is worth a thousand words, because words like "sophisticated," "simple," even "layered" may mean one thing to you and something quite different to the stylist. Include a few pictures of yourself—or your mother or sister—when you think your hair looked good. Tell the stylist what you like—and dislike—about your hair.

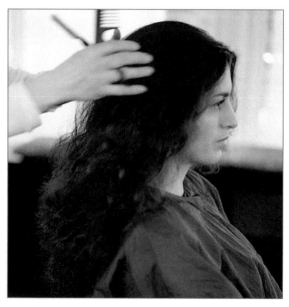

Trendy or traditional? Soft or spiky? It's smart to know what you want before you sit down in the stylist's chair.

3. Ask questions. Let's say you've brought a picture of Winona Ryder. Discuss whether Ryder's pixie cut would work for you. If not, ask why not and if there's any way to adapt the look so that it would. What style would be best for your face shape and hair texture?

To get out of a hair rut, ask the stylist to suggest ways to assimilate current trends into a style that works for you. Beware of stylists who get stuck in a single look and crank out the same trendy cut for everyone who walks through their door. "My biggest complaint about haircuts," says Susanna Romano, co-owner of Salon AKS, "is when you have the most gorgeous, stylish haircut, but it does nothing for the woman who's wearing it."

4. Talk about your lifestyle, your time constraints, your business, your wardrobe, your personality. Let the stylist know who you are—and what you need from your hair. Do you want your haircut to whisper or scream? She needs to find some way to get a sense of who you really are and the type of look you're after.

5. Finally, assess whether or not the stylist (and salon) makes you feel comfortable. Stylists don't need attitude to have aptitude. Beware of stylists who trash your current haircut. Remember, the salon industry is a service industry, just like the hotel or restaurant business. It's a stylist's job to make you relax and

feel good. Some women prefer a dishy stylist who will keep them up to date on gossip; others prefer a quiet cut. It's up to you to choose.

The Cut

Make sure the stylist assesses your hair before it's shampooed, so that she can really analyze its texture. Pay attention while she's cutting, and if you start to feel panicky, about the direction she's going, stop and discuss it while she can still do something about it.

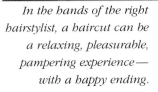

In the hands of the right hairstylist, a haircut can be a relaxing, pleasurable, pampering experience— with a happy ending.

Ask your stylist to give you two or three easy styling ideas that will work with your cut. If you're happy with your cut, book your next appointment before you leave. You can always cancel later, but at least you're down in her book. It's almost as important to maintain a good cut as it is to get one in the first place.

Just like the most disastrous experiments in color, even the worst cuts can be corrected. But you have to get right back in there the next day and try again. Or if your hair has been snipped really short, experiment with clips, headbands, or even extensions to create new styles until it grows out.

Super-short cuts need a trim every four weeks, short to medium cuts every six weeks, and long hair can go for eight weeks. Hair grows more slowly in winter and faster in the summer, so schedule your cuts accordingly.

Top salons have a bargain night once a week, when you can go and get your hair cut by a junior stylist and feel secure because she will be supervised by the owner the entire time. (See appendix E, page 375.) It's usually easiest to score an appointment in a busy salon on a Tuesday or Wednesday. Midweek is also the best time to get a discount. Obviously, Fridays and Saturdays are the busiest days. Or find a young trainee at a high-end salon, someone whose level of training is high but whose price is not.

Mass vs. Class

What's the difference between a $15 "super-cut" and a $150 cut at a top salon? Obviously, a more expensive cut is not necessarily better. But there are substantial differences in salon training procedures that you should know about.

Most reputable salons hire licensed stylists who've trained for six months to a year in beauty school. But what they do next with

Tip To save money, you might want to go to a high-end salon for your initial consultation and cut. Then go to a cheaper place to maintain it.

their novice stylists is where the difference lies. Budget salons or chains—Regis, MasterCuts, SuperCuts—will typically train their stylists with a video of the salon's top four to six cuts. After a couple of weeks, the stylists are out on the salon floor getting the rest of their training by practicing—on you.

At a budget salon, the menu is strictly à la carte. If a $15 haircut is advertised, that's all you get—a haircut. A shampoo or blow-dry costs extra. You can expect quick service, no frills, and a more generic cut. So if your needs are simple—for example, you have straight hair and want a blunt cut or a bob—a budget salon is cheaper, probably can do no damage, and you can get in and out on your lunch hour.

At a high-priced salon, everything is included—the shampoo, blow-dry, and amenities like fruit, coffee, and tea. In addition to the cut, you're obviously paying for pampering, location, maybe even a trendy CD collection and robes. There, the novice stylist trains from the bottom up: shampooing, fetching tools for the head divas, blow-drying, sweeping up, and, most important, observing the masters. She learns which cuts flatter which faces and types of hair and how to finesse an intricate cut by watching it done over and over. Eventually, the novice is ready to begin her own heavily supervised work with the clipping shears and continues to attend training workshops until she becomes a senior stylist, a process that can take up to five years.

Styling Your Hair

When I was a child, my best friend, Rosita, and I used to play with a doll named Tressy. The gimmick was Tressy's hair, which would "grow" if you pushed a button somewhere on her hard plastic body and "retract" if you pushed the same button twice. Tressy taught me how hair offers almost immediate gratification, with just a few basic tools. If you want loose, loopy Jerry Hall curls, you can just put in heat rollers for a few minutes. If your hair is curly, you can blow it straight. If you want ringlets, pick up a curling iron. It doesn't have to take a lot of time to make a major change. It just takes the right apparatus and an intrepid attitude. Besides, you can always undo your 'do by washing it out—unlike poor Tressy, who lost it all when I gave her a buzz cut!

The best way to learn to style your hair is from your stylist. She's actually studied this stuff and practiced it, over and over, on people like you. Take advantage of her expertise and watch and ask questions as she styles your hair. Have her show you what to do when you leave the salon: how to hold the blow-dryer, how to use the brush, and how to use styling products to get the look you want.

Tip Unless your hair is super-fine, I recommend using gel instead of mousse. Both will style and hold the hair, but mousses tend to be drying. If you prefer mousse, look for one that's alcohol-free. Comb it through with a brush or comb to distribute it evenly through your hair; the stickier it is, the more alcohol it contains.

How To: trim your own bangs

Bangs will emphasize your eyes and camouflage an irregular hairline or a high forehead. There are endless ways to style bangs, from a wedgelike Louise Brooks fringe to wispy Amy Irving–style tendrils.

Bangs usually need trimming every four weeks. Most salons will offer to trim your bangs gratis between cuts. But if you don't have time to go, and decide to do it yourself, always trim your bangs dry. If you do it when they're wet, they'll just shrink up as your hair dries.

First, twist your bangs together in one piece and cut the ends in a slight zigzag.

Next, release the hair, and cut the longer pieces until they're even with the shorter ones.

How to Apply Styling Products

Styling products are one of the great technological advances of the 20th century. Well, almost. But when it comes to hair goop, a little goes a long way—a dime- or quarter-sized dab will do. If your hair is fine and you use too much or too many products, you'll weigh it down. If your hair is curly and you glop it on, you'll look like there's an oil slick on your head.

Here's what to do: place a small dab in your palm and rub your palms together. Scrunch it into the roots if your hair is straight or wavy and

The Toolbox

Styling your hair at home can be easy and rewarding, as long as you've got the right tools.

The range of styling equipment to be found at the salon, the beauty supply shop, or even the drugstore can be absolutely mind-boggling. The trick is to pare your tool kit down to the basics and learn to use the few that you live with in your daily life wisely and well.

The Essentials

Paddle brush. *A wide, square-shaped natural-bristle brush is best for long or fine hair because the spaced-out bristles put air into the hair, which adds body. Boar's bristles are gentle but not too soft. The crown prince is the Mason Pearson brush, but it costs almost as much as a small pony; the nylon-natural hybrid works about as well.*

Round brush. *A round brush gives a*

smooth, polished look; it curls the ends under and adds volume while blow-drying. Round brushes are great for styling straight hair with a blow-dryer, but get the right size: big enough to wrap your hair under once, but no more, or you increase your chances of tangling.

a. A narrow-width round brush is best for styling bangs and short hair. It gives it more "bend" and adds volume.

b. A midsized brush is best for shoulder-length or shorter hair, for blowing hair straight, curling ends under, and adding "bounce."

c. A large round brush is best for shoulder-length or longer hair. The diameter makes it easier to smooth and straighten longer hair without tangling.

Hairpins, metal clips. *Useful for sectioning off your hair when you're styling.*

Blow-dryer with diffuser. *If your hair is wavy or curly, you need a diffuser because it dries hair less forcefully and won't blow away your curl. Any inexpensive drugstore diffuser*

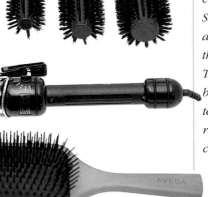

(or "sock") should attach to the end of your blow-dryer (check the size)—you don't need anything fancy.

Curling iron. *To touch up a curl here or there, or create a cloud of ringlets. For ringlets, you'll need a half-inch iron; for looser curls, an inch-and-a-half iron*

will do the job. Make sure it has more than one heat setting and fits comfortably in your hand.

Flat iron. *For straightening; with the proper attachments, it can also crimp hair.*

Rollers. *Heat rollers are heated on a platform base. As they cool, they "set" the hair. Steam rollers set the hair as steam pumps through the soft sponge rollers. They're best for dry hair but not for hair that tends to frizz. Steam rollers and velvet-covered heat rollers are the gentlest, because the fabrics insulate*

the hair from the heat and prevent it from tangling, but Velcro rollers are great for styling.

Hot sticks. *These long, squishy pieces of bendable plastic are heated before you wrap your hair around them. I love them because the ends fasten together without extra prongs or clips. They're easy to use and great for a quick curl or for smoothing out frizz.*

Tail comb. *The rat-tail handle will lift, separate, and part your hair in a nanosecond, and the comb will help with styling.*

BAD BUYS

Plastic-bristle brushes. They're cheap, but they're unyielding and snag the hair. They're not porous, so they don't carry moisturizing oils down to coat the ends of the hair. If you must, use one with nubs on the bristles, which are gentler on the scalp.

Metal-bristle brushes. These should be reserved for cats and dogs— not humans. They actually increase static, scratch the scalp, and the metal will heat up with a blow-dryer and fry your hair.

Wide-toothed comb. *Use a wide-toothed comb on curly hair. It's also the best way to spread conditioner and comb out wet, curly hair without pulling. Stick with wood or rubber: plastic snags and encourages flyaways; metal tears the hair.*

Fork comb or pick. *These separate tight curls and let the air into tightly curled hair.*

How To: clean your brushes

Hairbrushes collect oils from your hair and scalp, as well as the residue from styling products, so you must clean them regularly (at least once a month). First, remove excess hair with your comb. Then dip natural-bristle brushes several times in a basin of warm water and mild liquid soap. Do not soak the brush, or the bristles can separate from the handle, and a wooden handle can warp. Let it air-dry. Wash synthetic styling brushes the same way, but you don't need to be as careful.

LESS IS MORE

The gel that defines your curl and the spray that holds your style can cause flaking, especially if you hold your hairspray too close to your head; keep it at least six inches back. To control flakes, alternate a gentle, "frequent-use" shampoo with a clarifying shampoo.

you want a fuller look with more body, or into the middle of the hair down to the ends if your hair is curly and you want to define and hold your curl.

Apply styling products—gels, creams, thickeners, volumizers, mousses, pomades—to hair that is damp, not wet. (They stiffen wet hair and weigh it down.) When the hair is merely damp, it retains its elasticity and ability to bend. If your hair is straight, wait until it's almost dry before you use a styling product. If your hair is curly, don't brush the product through, or you'll brush out the curl. Scrunch it on with your fingers, or spray it on. For straight or wavy hair, comb or brush it through to distribute it evenly.

The stickier a gel feels in your palm, the heavier it will be on your hair. If you want a soft hold and your gel feels really sticky, mix it with a dab of cream or conditioner to dilute it. If you do want a stiff, slicked-back look, use a spritz gel, or try La Coupe Hair Gelée, Kiehl's Extra Strength Styling Gel, or Joico's Ice Spiker.

How to Defrizz

For curly or wavy hair, if you want a strong hold, mix two-thirds gel with one-third texturizing balm or pomade. For a softer hold, mix half

SOFT AND SPRINGY

African American hair tends to be dry, so you need to moisturize it to keep it from becoming brittle. Layering grease, waxes, or pomades on your hair may help make it less dry and easier to manage—temporarily—but over the long run, it will clog your scalp and the products will build up on your hair. Massage your scalp regularly to stimulate your own natural oils (see page 198). Avoid products with a high alcohol content, which will really dry the hair. And no matter what texture your hair is, lighter products are better than heavier ones.

According to Ademole Mandella, founder and creative director of Locks 'n' Chops, a natural hair salon in Manhattan, "Everything has to be lighter than the hair." Avoid ingredients like mineral oil and lanolin, which build up and weigh down the hair. Use sweet almond oil instead, suggests Mandella. If your hair is coarse, a light oil will also make it easier to comb.

And if it's oily at the scalp and dry at the ends, apply oils and conditioners from the middle of the hair shaft on down to the ends.

gel with half texturizing balm or pomade. For the softest hold, mix half gel with half finishing cream. Scrunch through the ends of your towel-dried hair. (Stay away from the roots, or you'll flatten the curl.) Let dry naturally, or blow-dry with a diffuser set on cool or a low setting.

Let's say you're not washing your hair today, but you want to resuscitate your curls. Dampen your hair (with a little water from a spray bottle) and work a light cream or gel from midstrand down. Remember: the less you handle your hair, the better it will look.

Heat styling. If you use heat regularly or your hair is dry, fine, or fragile, use a thermal styling product when you style it to protect it from dryness. Many thermal products contain heat-activated moisturizers and conditioners that buffer the heat. If you use heat irregularly, be sure to condition your hair when you do; the conditioners that coat the hair will also protect it from heat damage.

★ Best Products

A little dab will flatten the frizz: Artec Textureline Smoothing Serum, Ouidad Climate Control Heat & Humidity Gel, Bumble and bumble Defrizz, Revlon Texture and Volume Silky Pomade, Phyto Therathrie Phytodefrisant Gel, Phytoplage Gel, Kiehl's Silk Groom, Wella Liquid Hair Reconstructor.

Best Hairstylists' Lines

Vidal Sassoon started his own highly successful haircare line in 1973, but few stylists followed his lead until almost 20 years later. Now salon lines are so much in demand that many are sold—and sometimes bootlegged—in cosmetics discount emporiums and beauty supply stores around the country. Others retain an aura of exclusivity with limited distribution and upscale pricing. Some stylists, like Philip B. and Ouidad, actually work in the lab to help formulate their products, but many have a more distant relationship with the goods, and they're unique in name only. In any case, these lines are some of the best.

■ AVEDA

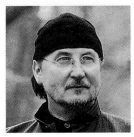

FOUNDER: Horst Rechelbacher; the company is now owned by Estée Lauder

THE IMAGE: Eco-Chic; one of the first beauty companies to incorporate a message of environmental conservation in the manufacture and development of their products

SPECIALTIES: Phytomollient Volumizer; color conditioners; brushes; chamomile, clove, blue malva shampoos; hair detoxifier; Pure-Fume Brilliant Retexturizing Gel; Self-Control Hair-Styling Stick

QUOTE: *What's healthy is what's beautiful. We strive to set an example for environmental leadership and responsibility, not just in the world of beauty, but around the world.*

BUMBLE AND BUMBLE

FOUNDER: Michael Gordon

THE IMAGE: Runway Style for Real Women

SPECIALTIES: Thickening spray, styling cream, brilliantine polish

QUOTE: *We strive to make looks that are wearable and suitable, to make women look modern and feel comfortable.*

DEVACHAN

CO-FOUNDER: Lorraine Massey

THE IMAGE: Hair Herbologist and Curly Hair Specialist

SPECIALTIES: Lavender-based Herbal Hair Cleanser

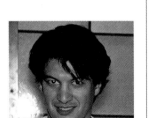

QUOTE: *Keep your haircare as simple and pure as possible. I believe in maximizing your natural growth pattern. Let your hair be for a while, and see what else it can do. Work with what you've got.*

FRÉDÉRIC FEKKAI

FOUNDER: Frédéric Fekkai

THE IMAGE: High-End Haircare with a French Twist

SPECIALTIES: Crème Hydrante, Apple Cider Clarifying Rinse

QUOTE: *The most simple and natural is the most beautiful.*

KIEHL'S

FOUNDER: John Kiehl, 1851; owned by Jami Morse Heidegger's (right) family for three generations. Though not a stylist herself, Jami's line is a universal favorite among stylists—for good reason. The company is now owned by L'Oréal.

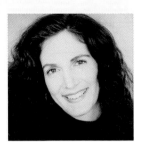

THE IMAGE: Old World Apothecary Integrity

SPECIALTIES: Silk Groom, Styling Creme, Thickening Spray

QUOTE: *We look toward the longevity of hair and skin, and we do that by being gentle and using gentle ingredients.*

NEXXUS

FOUNDER: Jheri Redding

THE IMAGE: Mass Market, Mass Appeal

SPECIALTIES: Volumizer/Infusium 23, styling gel Regular Hold, Vita Tress Hair Volumizer

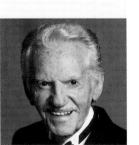

QUOTE: *Nexxus is short for nature and earth united with science.*

OUIDAD

FOUNDER: Ouidad

THE IMAGE: Queen of Curl and Frizz-Buster Extraordinaire

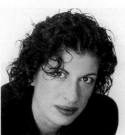

SPECIALTIES: Ouidad Deep Treatment, Climate-Control Hair Gel, Botanical Boost Spray

QUOTE: *Ninety percent of curly hair is fine hair. You don't want to weigh it down with waxes and silicones. It needs light, breathable products that feed it from the inside. You have to eat to survive, and so does your hair.*

PHILIP B.

FOUNDER: Philip Berkowitz

THE IMAGE: Top-of-the-Line Essential-Oil Guy

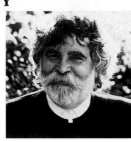

SPECIALTIES: Deep-conditioning essential-oil treatment, antiflake dandruff shampoo, botanical detangler, deep-conditioning cream rinse with shea butter

QUOTE: *If you start at the root—the skin of the scalp—you can extend the life of your hair.*

PHYTOTHERAPY

FOUNDER: Patrick Ales

THE IMAGE: Godfather of Chic Botanicals

SPECIALTIES: Phyto 9 and Phyto 7 moisturizing shampoos

QUOTE: *When I began, over 30 years ago, everyone said I was crazy. Now they realize that nature—and natural haircare—is not a fad. It's the future.*

SEBASTIAN

FOUNDER: Geri Cusenza; the company is now owned by Wella

THE IMAGE: Trendy, mass-market salon line

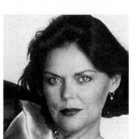

SPECIALTIES: Potion 7, Potion 9, the laminates, shaper hairspray

QUOTE: *Hair was once tough and tacky with spray, but now it's tactile and touchable with glosses and gels.*

Blow-Dry Basics

The best thing for your hair is to let it dry naturally. But of course, that's not realistic—especially for women with fine hair, most of whom are addicted to the master-blaster, with good reason: it's the ultimate volumizer. "If you do blow-dry all the time," says Jami Morse Heidegger of Kiehl's, "at least take a break on the weekend, when you can condition your hair and give it special care."

To do as little damage as possible, follow these ground rules. If your hair is curly, use a diffuser, which not only helps hold the curl but also diffuses the heat. Also, keep the blower at a low, cool setting as much as possible, and hold it four to six inches from your head. A 1,200- to 1,500-watt dryer is powerful enough for most women; if your hair is thick or coarse, you may need 1,700 watts.

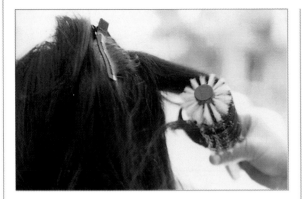

1. Section it off, with clips or a scrunchy, and dry it one section at a time on the lowest setting possible. Keep the dryer moving, so it won't burn your hair.

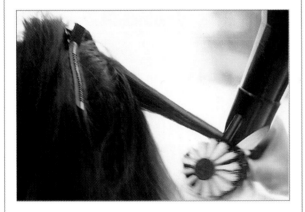

2. Dry the bottom layers first. Start at the back and dry the underlayers first. For straight hair, always direct the blow-dryer down toward the floor: this smooths the hair and prevents frizz. Lean over and blow-dry at the roots to give your hair volume. To add height or volume to the top of your hair, lift the hair from the roots with your fingers (or use your round vent brush or paddle brush) and blow-dry at the roots. For wavy or curly hair, hold the diffuser into the hair (with your head straight up) and work your way around your head, from bottom to top (do not use a brush).

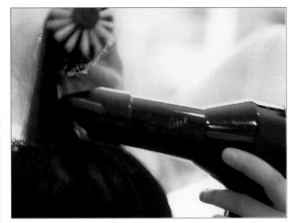

3. Smooth the top. When the underlayers are dry, use your brush to shape the top layer. Put the bristles against your scalp, turn and lift back small sections of hair, and curl them under until dry.

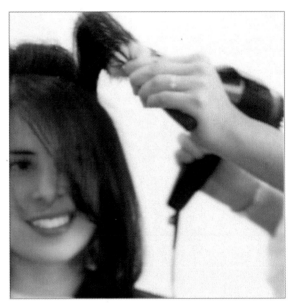

4. Curl the ends. Take your brush and curl the ends under. Brush through and follow with the blow-dryer directed toward your hair. Finish styling with a shot of cold air, which "sets" the style and makes hair shinier.

TAKING A SHINE TO YOUR HAIR

Products that contain silicones coat the hair and reflect light—just as they do in a car polish. Silicone styling products smooth the hair cuticle, making it lie flatter, and give hair a high-gloss shine. But they tend to be sticky and can weigh the hair down, and regular use can dehydrate your hair. Use two or three drops, max, and don't use them all the time. Suggestions: Wella Insta-Seal Recovery Treatment, Jheri Redding Replenishing Hair Shiner, Redken's Glass Smoothing Complex, Citré Shine's Shine Miracle Hair Polisher, Phyto Therathrie Brilliantissime Spray, Sebastian Laminates, Bumble and bumble Brilliantine.

★*Best Products*

Ready to Roll?

They're called rollers instead of curlers because they're no longer used only to "curl" the hair; rollers add body, height, wave, or smoothness as well. The great thing about rolling is that it gives you so many options. When you're in a hurry, you can give a quick roll to your bangs, the top of your head, or wherever you need a lift.

Rollers are an easy way to add lift to fine, straight hair. After your hair is dry (spray lightly with a heat-styling product or volumizer), put heat rollers in for a few minutes. Take the rollers out, tousle your hair, and, if you're lucky, it'll end up looking like Meg Ryan's.

If you prefer big hair with loose curls—think Farrah Fawcett or Cindy Crawford—you'll need Velcro rollers and thickening lotion. Velcro rollers are great for coarse, thick hair, and, because of

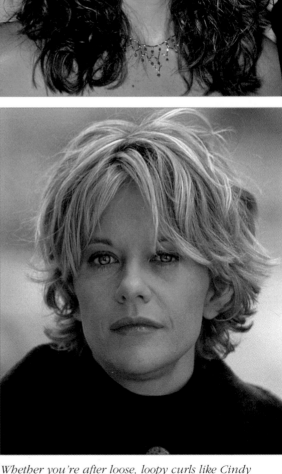

Whether you're after loose, loopy curls like Cindy Crawford's (top) or tousled "bed-head" hair like Meg Ryan's, rollers are the way to go.

their "grab," they really hold. They also give the hair a lot of body. Here's how to get that look.

1. Apply volumizer or thickening lotion to the roots. Blow your hair with a round, vented brush or a paddle brush until it's almost dry.

2. Roll big sections of hair around seven or eight rollers. Roll downward toward your scalp, but make sure to keep your hair smooth on the roller. (The danger with Velcro is that if you don't roll smoothly and carefully, you can tangle and then break the hair.) Leave rollers in for 10 to 20 minutes, until your hair is dry.

3. Unroll the same way you rolled, taking care to release hair in a smooth movement. Don't get impatient and try to slide it out, or it'll snag. Shake your head, finger-comb it (use a brush or comb if it looks clumpy), and go!

Ironing

There are three types of irons: curling, flat, and crimping. Curling irons roll the hair on an electrically heated rod whose size depends on the size of curl you're after. Flat irons and crimping irons press the hair flat between the jaws of two hot metal pieces. They are all fun to use occasionally, but if you use them often, get a perm or use a relaxer instead. It's much better for your hair in the long run.

Never use an iron on wet hair: not only will it fry, it'll frizz, too. Apply straightening balm to dry hair, position your hair between the clamps (not too close to your scalp), and flat-iron or crimp it. (Flat ironing adds an inch or two to the length.) Crimping irons create a tight wave. If you're using a curling iron, wrap the hair around the rod, hold for a couple of seconds, and release.

> **Tip** Instead of an iron, you can use a brush with nylon bristles and a metal shaft to curl your hair, along with a blow-dryer. The blow-dryer heats up the metal shaft, and it acts almost like a curling iron. There's less risk of overheating your hair, and the brush is easier to control than an iron.

Try to keep the heat of your curling iron at the lowest setting that will enable you to achieve the result you want, especially if you have fine or medium hair. You'll need to turn up the heat for coarse or thick hair in order for it to curl. Don't use an iron too near the roots or scalp. It's not necessary, and you can burn yourself. Start toward the top of the hair, and turn the iron as you work down toward the ends.

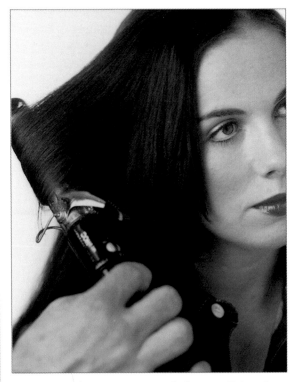

To use a curling iron, start with dry, conditioned hair, and roll the ends down and around the iron.

Putting It All Together:
FIVE
EASY STYLES

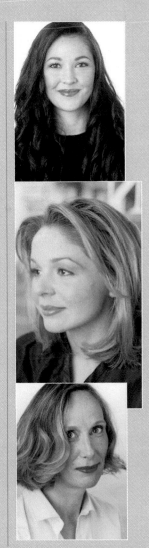

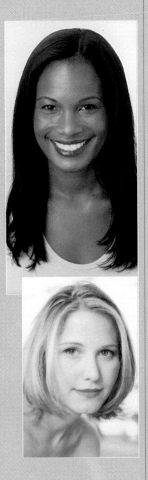

Everyone needs a change. A new hairstyle is the easiest way to reinvent yourself, and, unlike a new cut or color, there's no risk involved. Blowing your curly hair straight, giving fine, limp hair a lift, or making straight hair curly does involve an investment of time, but it's time well spent if you like the result. Besides, it feels good to pamper yourself once in a while.

Here are five simple styles, along with the tools, products, techniques, and expert advice you'll need to achieve them on your own. Once you hit on a look you love, it will become second nature to achieve after a little practice. And if you're not happy with your new look, hey, just wash it out.

LIFTOFF
or BIG HAIR:
from flat to voluminous

Leah's hair has a good texture—not too fine, not too coarse. Although it's basically straight, it has enough of a natural wave that it's easy to work with. She wanted to learn a few tricks that would give her hair more body, especially on top.

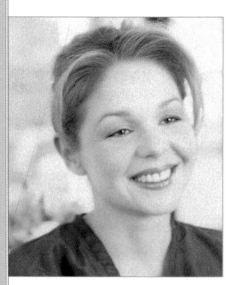

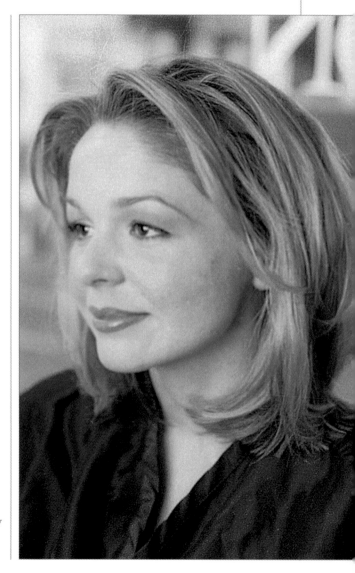

Tools. A blow-dryer, a round brush, big metal clips.

Products. A volumizer or thickening spray. Good ones: Redken's Fat Cat Body Booster, Bumble and bumble Thickening Spray, Aveda Phomollient, Hair Putty by Fudge, Sebastian Perfection Volumizer, L'Oréal Body Vive Add-In Body,

Phyto Volume Actif, Pantene Pro-V Essentials Body Enhancer, Kiehl's Thickening Spray.

Techniques. Leah's hair was cut into long layers. "When you cut the weight off the top, it gives the hair more movement," says Kao, co-owner of the AKS salon in Manhattan. He starts the layers around the chin, though, because short layers on long hair can look choppy.

To style, first apply volumizer to the roots, especially around the crown and hairline. Then, lift the hair up with your fingers and give the roots a short blast with the blow-dryer (no diffuser). Then, clip your hair up on top of your head, and take hair down section by section, starting at the nape. Wrap each section around a round brush and blow it dry. (Blow-drying against the direction in which the hair grows will give you more volume.) Let it cool on the brush for a few seconds. Finally, spray

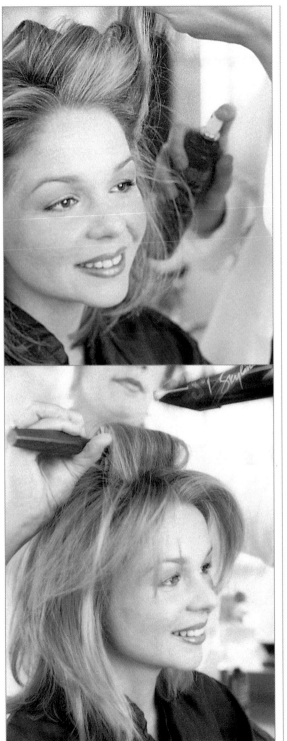

a light-hold hairspray such as Phyto Silk Protein Hairspray or Aveda Flaxseed Spray at the roots and lightly brush it back along the hairline at the crown and the sides.

FOR A QUICK LIFT

Spray dry hair with volumizer, and place a few large Velcro rollers strategically around the head. Heat with a blow-dryer for about 5 minutes, then leave the rollers in for about 10 minutes more, until they cool. Take them out, style with comb, brush, or fingers, and go.

Easy Style 2 SUPERSLEEK:
from curly to silky straight

Robinne's hair is on the dry side, so she doesn't blow her hair straight very often and tries to minimize her dependence on the blow-dryer. To make this simple style hold, she relies on pomade.

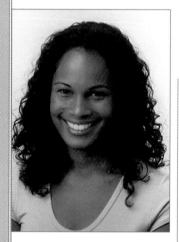

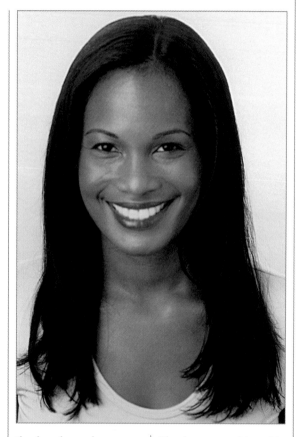

Sebastian Performance Active Texturizer, Palmer's Coconut Oil Formula, Kiehl's Silk Groom, Bumble and bumble Sumo Wax, Redken Water Wax, Aveda Purefume Brilliant Anti-Humectant Pomade, Modern Organic Products (MOP) D-Curl.

Tools. Wide-toothed comb, large silver clips, blow-dryer with diffuser, big round brush.

Products. Good straightening balms or pomades: Citré Shine Styler Straightening Balm, Phytotherathrie Phytodefrisant Straightening Balm,

Technique. Shampoo and condition the hair. Towel it dry.

Clip your hair to the top of your head with large clips. Take a small section down from the bottom, starting close to the nape. Roll hair around the brush, and move the brush and dryer downward to the ends, which smooths the cuticle. When you reach the ends, hold the hair down with the brush or your hand until it cools, or it will curl up again.

The key to making this style work is the heat. "It's not about how many times you go through the hair with the brush," says New York hairstylist Brett Strange, "it's about the hair getting enough heat to shape it."

MAKING WAVES:
from straight to curly

Brenna likes a change every once in a while, and her hair curls easily because it's so thick. But since there's so much of it, it takes patience—and a whole lot of goop.

Tools. Heat rollers, Velcro rollers, or curling iron; paddle brush.

Products. Cream or gel. Good ones: ABBA Ultimate Styling Cream, Phytodefrisant Gel, Bumble and bumble Styling Crème, Ouidad Climate Control Gel. *Optional:* a curl rejuvenator, like L'Oréal Pumping Curls or Ouidad Botanical Booster.

Technique. Heat rollers are the quickest way to curl straight hair—but if your hair is really silky, you may need a curling iron (top right). Remember, the smaller the roller, the tighter the curl.

Start with dry hair. If your hair is fine, spray with a volumizing heat-styling spray before and after you put in the rollers. If your hair is coarse, use a leave-in conditioner. Roll hair starting at forehead and working back. On the sides and back, work from the bottom up. Let the rollers cool (about five to ten minutes), then remove. Flip your head upside down, and, if your curls are small, lightly scrunch a dime-sized dab of gel on the ends all around your head. If your

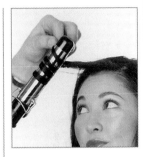

curls are large and soft, use a flat, paddle-shaped brush to brush your hair. Then smooth a sculpting lotion or gel through the hair.

To use VELCRO ROLLERS, wrap towel-dried hair around rollers and blow-dry on low to medium setting. Dab the ends with pomade, and spray with water-based hairspray.

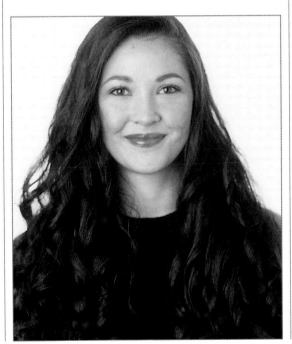

FINE SHINE:
from baby fine to full and wavy

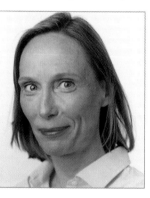

Susan has limp, lackluster hair, but she was ready to polish up her look and give her hair some shine, fullness, and style. If you have this type of hair, here are several simple ways to go from flat head to flowy, fluid waves.

Tools. Curling iron, clips, hairbrush.

Products. A shine product and a spray gel. Good ones: Phyto Brilliantissime Spray, Bumble and bumble Brilliantine, Redken Glass Smoothing Complex, John Frieda Frizz Ease Spray Gel, ABBA Instant Recall Spray Gel, Wella Liquid Hairspray Gel, L'Oréal's Tee Ni Pli Spray Thermal Fixant Sculpting Lotion.

Technique. Start with dry hair. Spray with a light gel. Take the hair in sections, from the nape area, and wrap it around a curling iron. Remove the curling iron, and clip each curl in place. When you've gone around the entire head with the iron, spray with a shine product. Unclip the curls, starting at the nape. Run your fingers through the hair to loosen the waves, and brush hair lightly into place.

Cool Waves

Here are a few ways to get a wave or curl going without heat or a blow-dryer.

Braid it. Braid damp hair at night, and you'll wake up with crimped hair in the morning. Or rag it for a soft curl: Divide damp hair into sections, apply gel, and roll each section around a piece of rag. Tie the ends of the rag together and let the hair dry.

Twist it. Apply gel. Divide damp hair into sections (the larger the sections, the looser the curl). Keep twisting until it curls into a knot. Pin. Repeat until

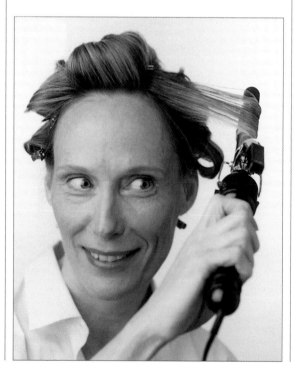

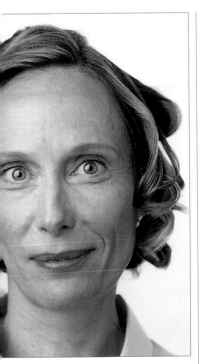

Pin it. Spray some gel in your damp hair. Separate your hair into one-inch sections, twist it, wrap it around your finger, clip it.

Go through your entire head or just the ends this way. Leave until dry, then take it down and you'll have perfect little curls.

Or brush it out (lightly) and it will wave.

you've curled and pinned each section. (Don't do more than three or four clips at the crown if you want it to be relatively smooth on the top of your head.) Dry with a diffuser and take out the pins. You'll have a soft wave.

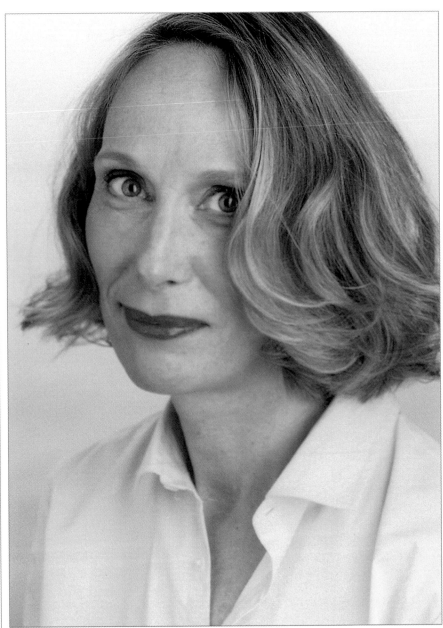

Easy Style 5 LIGHT 'N' LAYERED:

from girlish to grownup

Andra thought she looked too young. "In a work environment, if your overall look is young, your clients don't take you seriously. My hair was my biggest problem." Granted, looking

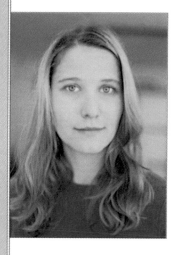

young is not a problem most women complain about, but it can put a crimp in your professional style. When Andra consulted Angelique Flynn, a stylist at the AKS salon in Manhattan, they came up with a shorter, softer, layered cut. "I worried about layered cuts looking too trendy, but this cut is sophisticated and it makes me feel confident," says Andra. "Looking too young is something I don't have to worry about any longer."

Tools. Round brush, blow-dryer.

Products. Heat-activated volumizer spray. Some volumizers are designed to work with heat, and these work extremely well with fine hair: Phyto Actif Volumizer, Joico Thermal I.C.E. Heat-Activated Volumizer, Infusium 23. The heat stimulates the polymers or resins in the product to bind to the hair. Avoid waxes or pomades—they're too heavy for fine hair.

Technique. Andra's hair was highlighted, cut, and styled. She knew that she wanted to cut her hair above her shoulders, but not above her jaw. And no bangs—too young. "With such fine,

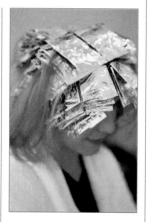

straight hair you can't cut too many layers or it looks choppy," says Flynn. So she angled it around the face, for more definition, and at the ends, so that it would move nicely.

To create this style, start with slightly damp hair. Lift hair with fingers, and spray volumizer on the roots. Don't use too much product, or you'll weigh down the hair. Section by section, put the round brush up under the roots and blow the hair with the blow-dryer on the warm setting. Keep the hair on the brush, and switch the setting to cool to "set" the hair. Do the same to the ends, cooling and setting. Take care not to use too much heat, or your hair will fall flat like a soufflé. When it comes to fine hair, less is more.

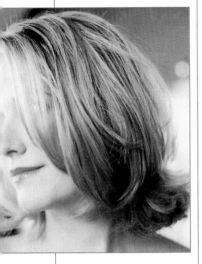

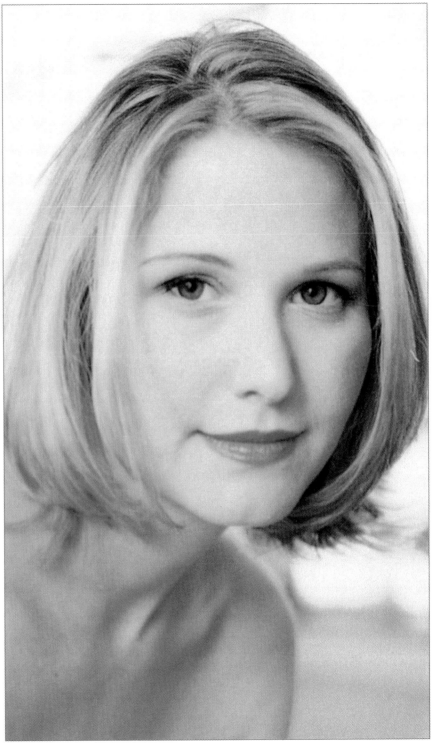

Head Trips: Perming and Relaxing

Growing up with a long, tangled mass of corkscrew curls, I would have done anything for the stick-straight styles so many of the other girls had. They, of course, coveted my curls. Why do we always want what we don't have? Never mind, that's what salons are for.

If you yearn to change your hair texture, try not to make it too drastic. The greater the difference, the more obvious it will be when it grows out, which puts you into the high-maintenance zone. If you retexturize your hair, you'll need to be diligent about touching up the roots and take more time to condition and care for it.

Perming and relaxing both rely on chemical processes to break the bonds in the hair's structure and reestablish them in the shape of a curl (permed) or straight (relaxed). But if you're already using blow-dryers, curling irons, heat rollers, and flat irons to retexturize your hair on a daily basis, you're already damaging your hair. So you may as well get the look you want, avoid the daily wear and tear on your hair, and save yourself some time and trouble. Besides, there are new products and methods available (especially in the salon) that are not as harsh and damaging as they used to be.

Permanent Waves

Perms have come a long way since they were first developed in 1902, when quicksilver, nitric acid, and heat were used to wave the hair. The wet hair was wrapped in treated papers, dried, and greased. The perm lasted for around three weeks.

Today, stylists can control not only which part of the hair they want to perm (such as a "root perm" to add body to fine, limp hair) but also the softness of the curl. Show your stylist a picture of the type of curl you want so she can choose the right-sized rods. Almost any type of hair can take a perm, but some hair types take more skill. If you are an Asian American woman with thick, heavy hair, for example, or an African American with fine hair, it may be hard to get your hair to take the perm. You will need to find a stylist who is experienced enough with your kind of hair to know how to wrap it. "When you're creating an artificial curl," says Younghee, owner of the Younghee Salon in Manhattan, "you have to work with the weight of the hair and see what the density of the hair will handle."

The stylist will apply one chemical solution to break the bonds in the hair and another, a "neutralizer," to re-form the bonds and change its texture. The tightness of the curl depends on the size of the rods used. If you want a tighter curl, your hair will be rolled around smaller rods while it "processes." For a softer, looser curl, the rods are bigger. A perm takes 48 hours to settle; you won't have the full style impact until then.

There is no such thing as a chemical-free perm. (Don't be misled by "botanical perms"— these contain added plant extracts, but they also contain chemicals!) Traditional perm solutions contain ammonia or the sulfur-based chemical thioglycolate. Not only do they smell bad, they can wreck your hair. The gentlest, top-quality perm solutions—Zotos Distinctly Different, Helene Curtis Insite, Senscience Inner Strength Waving Lock, Système Biolage Style Support Wave—can be found only in salons, which is where I recommend you perm your hair anyway. At-home treatments take longer to process, the technique is difficult to master, and misuse of the chemicals can result in frizzy, fried hair.

But if you want to do it yourself, look for "thio-free" solutions, which contain conditioner to soften hair, and don't roll the hair too tightly. If you want a loose curl, forgo the curling rods altogether. Divide the hair into sections, wrap each section around a piece of cloth, tie the ends together, and apply solution. For a really subtle look, divide your hair into four or six even sections, twist the hair into Princess Leia buns, clip to the head, and apply solution.

Prepping for a perm. If you make sure your hair is healthy before you perm, you'll avoid broken, brittle hair afterward. In the weeks before, use a protein conditioning treatment, as well as a moisturizing conditioner after you shampoo. But do not deep-condition your hair for at least 24 hours before the process—it may interfere with how well your perm takes hold. And do not shampoo for at least 48 hours afterward to give the process time to "set."

After your perm, shampoo with ammonium- rather than sodium-based shampoos with keratin or wheat amino acids, which strengthen the hair fiber. Matrix Perm Fresh and Nexxus Rejuv-A-Perm are a couple of good choices. Products with silicones and dimethicone make combing easier. Avoid polyquaternium or resin listed in the first few ingredients because they weigh down the hair.

Relaxing

Almost all hair types can be relaxed (straightened), but the process is most popular among African American women, because their hair tends to be the most naturally curly. With a relaxer, you can make your hair straight as a stick or simply soften your curls without really straightening them. Whichever way, relaxing your hair will make it more manageable.

Relaxing loosens the curl and cuts back frizz. But because the chemicals in the process are so strong, it's important to protect your scalp. Your stylist will first apply a cream or oil to your scalp. Then she'll work the chemicals into your dry hair, one section at a time. As with perming, the hair will "process" until it is as straight as you want it. Then a neutralizer is applied to stop the process. There are different strengths for different types of hair: strong for coarse hair, regular for normal hair, mild for fine hair. Some contain lye; others don't. No-lye relaxers are milder and less irritating to the scalp, but they can make the hair a little drier.

If you're thinking of relaxing your hair, remember two things. First, it can be extremely damaging to hair that has permanent color in it. Some people need to choose between color and other chemical processes, because their hair can't withstand both. (Ask your stylist first, but it should be okay to use semipermanent color.) Second, once you relax your hair, touch up *only the new growth* every six weeks. Don't repeat the process on your entire head, or you could end up with hair like straw.

Styling Solutions

We all have days when our hair won't look right, we're too lazy to bother, or we simply want a change. Sometimes the solution can be as easy as studding your hair with clips, sticks, or other glittery bits, which are a great way to camouflage loose ends while your hair is growing out or spiff up a less-than-stellar hair day. "There's a drama about putting your hair up with sticks and then taking it down," says hair accessories designer Colette Malouf. "Learning to be good with sticks is like learning to be good with makeup. It creates options, which everybody needs."

You can slick your hair back in a headband or ponytail or twist it into a chignon. You may also want to consider a more long-term styling solution like dreads, braids, or extensions. Here are a few ideas.

HOLD THAT SPRAY!

Nonalcohol, nonaerosol hairsprays are the least drying. They dry soft, not stiff like traditional sprays, and they are much more eco-friendly. The trade-off: they don't hold as well. Try Vidal Sassoon with Formesilk Flexible Hold Hair Spray, Wella Liquid Hair Brilliant Spray Gel, Aerogel from the Institute of Trichology, PhytoSilk Protein Hairspray, Aveda Flaxseed Spray.

The Ponytail

There are dozens of variations on this chic classic. Pulled high on the crown like Wilma Flintstone's or clipped low on the nape like Audrey Hepburn's, the only caveat is not to pull your hair back too tightly over an extended period of time, because it can break and, over time, you can lose your hair (see page 201).

(Go for 100 percent elastic—without metal clasps. That tiny metal bit may seem harmless enough, but it really snags the hair.)

Brush your hair back or part it on the side. (If your hair is curly, separate out a piece from the front, set it on a Caruso curler or heat curler for a few minutes, and let it hang smooth and loose.) Slick the top back with gel or pomade, and fasten with a banana clip, a ribbon, or a scrunchy—or, if your hair is really long, use several bands, spaced out every few inches. You can also smooth the hair back, bind it with elastic, then separate a section of hair and wrap it around the elastic—or let it hang loose.

French Twist

Brush your hair back with a bit of gel or pomade, or part it on the side. Gather hair at the nape of the neck, twist, and pull upward, tucking it in and securing with hairpins as you go—or wrap in a bun. Spray for extra hold.

If your hair is super-silky, you may need help with your twist. Try a hair rat. (Couldn't someone have come up with a less unfortunate name for these things?) Rats became popular in the 1930s and 1940s when upsweeps, French twists, and chignons were the locks du jour on screen pinups like Betty Grable. These soft, mesh buns, available in drugstores, come in different sizes and shapes and enable you to take your medium-length hair and transform it without a hairpiece.

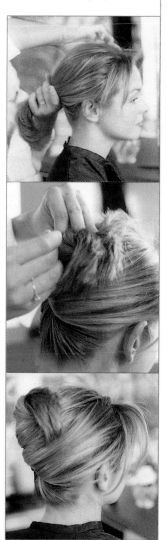

Hold the rat where you want to place the style, twist or roll your hair around it, and pin it in place with bobby pins or hairpins, then spray, since you'll want extra hold.

Chignon

A chignon (soft bun) is an easy, elegant style for everyday or special occasions like a black-tie wedding or cocktail. For a chignon, you can start with a side part or a flamenco-style center part. According to Liell Hilligoss, resident chignon expert and stylist at the Avon Centre Spa and Salon in New York City, "The classic chignon looks sleek and beautifully groomed, but if you want it to look younger, fresher, and less formal, let the ends stick out a bit."

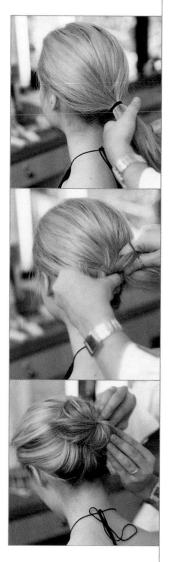

The traditional French chignon is an elaborately sculpted bow-shape at the base of the neck. For a simpler, more manageable version, gather the hair in a ponytail at the base of the neck, twist, and wrap around the elastic. Use hairpins to hold it in place. Thick hair may need a thin net or snood on top to hold it in shape. A slick of gel should coax any loose hair into submission.

How to French Braid

Whether your hair is thick and sleek or a tendrily pouf, a soft braid can be fun as well as fetching. Divide your hair into three equal sections at the crown. Start braiding your hair at the top, and pick up a piece of hair with each of the three sections as you braid down. At the end, all of your hair should be woven in. Fasten with an elastic or a ribbon.

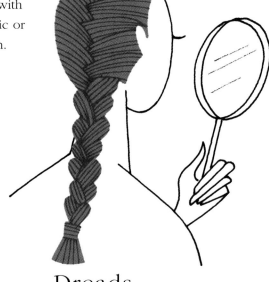

Dreads

Whether you call them "dreads," "locks," or "dreadlocks," the natural style once exclusive to Rastafarians in Jamaica has become more mainstream over recent years. "Dreads are now what the Afro was to the sixties," says Dael Orlandersmith, an Obie award–winning actor and playwright, pictured (see facing page), with braids. "It's a way of saying, 'This is our hair, we don't have to look like Cheryl Tiegs or Cindy Crawford.' This is our standard of beauty, and we're proud of this hair."

The style is achieved by twisting sections of hair together with the hands, starting about an inch from the scalp, until the hair "locks" in place. The only styling tool required is the hands. The twist is most vulnerable closest to the scalp, but once the hair locks, there is no way to unlock dreads unless you cut them off. You can keep dreads short or grow them long, but they do require a minimum of care: you need to twist them with almond oil or beeswax every week, otherwise they can get matted. When you wash dreads, use a gentle shampoo and, if possible, allow the hair to air dry.

Extensions

Extensions can really simplify your styling regimen, make your hair look thicker, and add a lot of style. If you want extensions that look natural, go for the texture and color that match your own hair. If not, anything goes!

Extensions are synthetic or real hair that you can have braided, woven, sewn, or "bonded" into your own hair with something like glue. They work for women with all hair types, especially African American women who want to extend their natural braids or any woman with thin hair. Extensions can be expensive—if you go to Lisa Mitchell, New York City's celebrity extender, you can pay up to $1,000—but they don't have to be. Smooth extensions can be left in until they fall out or you cut them off, but when they're braided in, they can pull on the hair and need to be redone after three to four weeks.

Braids. Braids can be sectioned off into "cornrows," soft-sculpted into thicker "dooky braids," or double-braided and twisted around your head. If you get your hair braided, be careful that the braids aren't too tight. (One friend says hers give her an "automatic face-lift"!) But if your braids pull too much, they will not only feel uncomfortable and give you headaches but also break your hair. Over time, the hair loss can be permanent. Of course, the looser the braids are, the more often you'll need to have them redone, but considering the alternative, it's worth it. Wash your hair and scalp once a week with braids in. It's important to keep your scalp clean. Don't leave them in too long, or they'll be hard to take out and you can break your hair trying.

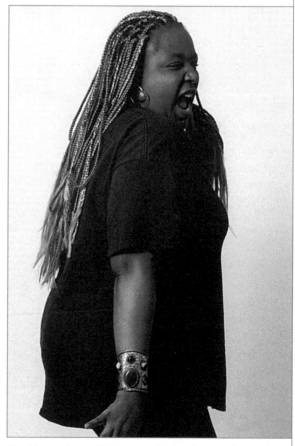

Braids are beautiful, especially on playwright Dael Orlandersmith, who has made them her signature style.

hair time line

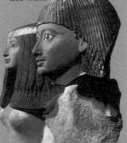

4000 B.C. Egyptians use dried fish backbones as combs.

2000 B.C. Egyptians mix water and citrus juice to make shampoo and mix animal fats and plant oils to create hair conditioner.

1800 B.C. Babylonian men powder their hair with gold dust.

1500 B.C. Assyrian slaves curl the hair of kings and other nobles with heated iron bars.

1370–1352 B.C. The heavy wigs that adorn Egyptian nobility are made from intricately braided human hair, to which horsehair and lamb's wool are sometimes added. The wigs both decorate the head and protect it from the sun.

500 B.C. In western Africa, sticks and clay are early versions of curlers and setting gel. The end result resembles dreadlocks.

35 B.C. Cleopatra adorns hair with jewel-studded ivory pins.

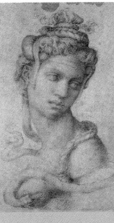

First century A.D. Although Romans believe that washing hair disturbs the spirit guarding the head, Plutarch recommends doing it once a year.

First century A.D. Dark hair is fashionable among Romans, who create a dye from boiled walnuts and leeks.

40. Roman prostitutes are required by law to dye their hair blond.

100. Saxon men color their hair and beards green, blue, or orange—presumably to terrify their opponents on the battlefield.

200. In Rome, sculptors affix detachable marble wigs to their sculptures so they can update them to reflect rapidly changing hairstyles.

300. Hair nets and snoods become fashionable in the Roman Empire.

1300s. European women condition their hair with dead lizards boiled in olive oil. The fashion is to shave the hairline to emphasize a high forehead and to pile hair high on the head to show off a long neck.

1500s. In Italy, married women are expected to cover or braid their hair in the interest of modesty.

1500s. Frenchwomen frizz their hair with heat, then sculpt it to towering heights.

1500s. Queen Elizabeth I makes red hair—and wigs—fashionable in England.

1550. "Blonding" peaks in popularity. One recipe for lightening hair calls for a mixture of honey, celandine roots, olive madder, white wine, cumin seed oil, box shavings, and saffron. This concoction was left on the hair for 24 hours, then washed off with lye and ashes.

17th and 18th centuries. In France, aristocratic hairstyles become intricate tableaux, bedecked with flowers, jewels, even birdcages.

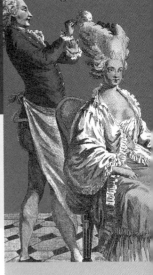

1740s. The rise of the "pompadour." Named after Madame de Pompadour, the style is combed high, frizzed above the forehead, and held in place with paste and glue.

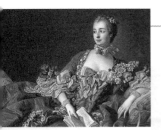

1780s. In France, long before the advent of punk, hair is powdered in blue, violet, white, pink, and yellow pastels.

1790s. The French Revolution occasions a brief period of shorter, less elaborate styles.

Early 1800s. In keeping with the general interest in classicism, short Greco-Roman hairstyles come into vogue.

1820s and 1830s. Hats, hoods, and headdresses are the rage in France.

1840s and 1850s. Plain and plaited hair, like the Brontë sisters', prevails in England.

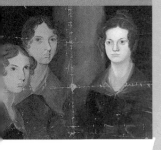

1860s. Clip-on hairpieces come into fashion. In England, big hair creeps back.

1870s. The first beauty parlors open in the United States. The styles of the day are chignons and dainty little bunches of curls.

1880s. Hair is worn all the way down the back, sometimes even to the ankles.

EDWARDS' HARLENE FOR THE HAIR

1902. "Gibson Girl" hair is the ideal—wavy, poufy, feminine, piled loosely on the head—as in this photo of Edith Wharton.

1905. Charles Nestle creates the first permanent wave machine.

1906. Madame C. J. Walker (below) begins selling haircare products for African Americans, which becomes a multi-million-dollar beauty business. (She later becomes the first female African American millionaire and a prominent figure in the Harlem Renaissance.)

1907. Josephine Baker's sleek style and the marcel wave become fashionable in the United States *and* Europe.

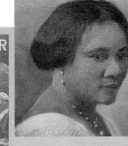

1907. French chemist Eugène Schueller creates Auréole, one of the first commercial hair colors; a year later, he changes his company's name to L'Oréal.

1917. Louise Brooks starts the hair trend that dominates the 1920s—the bob.

1920s. The double-process blonding technique is invented.

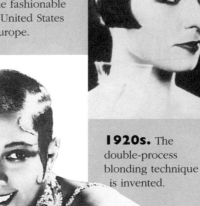

1920s. Brightly colored wigs— red, green, orange, purple—are inspired by the Cubist art movement.

1920. The first hair-dryer is invented, inspired by the vacuum-cleaner hose.

1925. There are now 25,000 beauty parlors in the United States.

1930s. Pin curl styles are first created for couture houses Mainbocher and Madeleine Vionnet.

1930s. John Breck becomes a haircare entrepreneur when he develops hair and scalp products to thwart his encroaching baldness.

hair time line

1930s. Listerine is widely used—and fails—as a "cure" for dandruff.

1930. Shirley Temple inspires little girls to wear bouncy curls.

1931. Jean Harlow stars in Frank Capra's film *Platinum Blonde* and kicks off a haircolor craze.

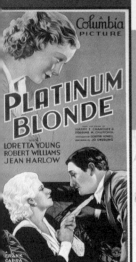

1934. "Dry cleaning" becomes a popular, time-saving alternative to shampooing. The two best-known "dry cleaners" on the market are found to be highly flammable and toxic; one woman becomes disfigured when her "dry" shampoo explodes.

1939. In Angola and other parts of southwest Africa, styling aids include fruit seeds and sinew, along with cowrie shells and beads.

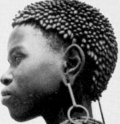

1940. Rita Hayworth popularizes sultry side-parted finger waves.

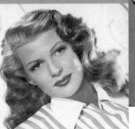

1940. Veronica Lake's cascading blond waterfall makes her a 1940s glamour girl.

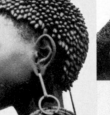

1941. Rosie the Riveter dons the snood for factory work in WWII.

We Can Do It!

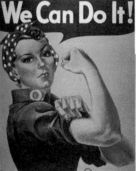

Late 1940s. In postwar Paris, sisters Maria and Rosy Carita (above) open up a beauty shop—becoming the first women to break into the predominantly male hairstyling profession.

1950s. The first commercial conditioner is conceived when chemists discover that ingredients used in fabric softeners can also soften the hair.

1950s. Highlighting becomes popular.

1950s. Lucille Ball makes red the rage.

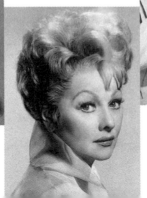

1952. Doris Day's helmet hair enslaves her—and women who tried to emulate her—to the beauty parlor.

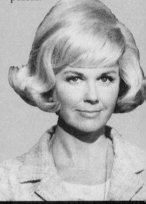

1953. The modern pixie cut is born when Audrey Hepburn gets one in this memorable scene from *Roman Holiday*.

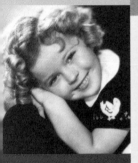

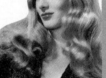

1954. Gina Lollobrigida popularizes the short, curly "poodle cut."

1960s. Women wear Dynel wigs and flippy falls or up 'dos like the Supremes.

1970s. Grace Jones's natural box cut brings in the disco look.

1967. Angela Davis's Afro becomes a symbol of black pride.

1963. Vidal Sassoon initiates the first simple "wash 'n' dry" cuts.

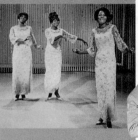

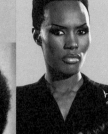

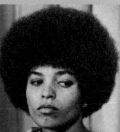

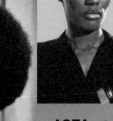

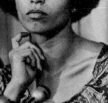

1960s. Redken popularizes pH-balanced and protein-enriched shampoos.

1967. Long, natural hair symbolizes freedom for countercultural men and women.

1971. The first handheld blow-dryer makes a new range of "blow-and-go" styles possible.

1955. Clairol's provocative "Does She . . . or Doesn't She?" ad campaign makes it more acceptable—and appealing—for women to color their hair.

1960. Hairspray gives rise to the age of beehives and bouffants. Most spray jobs last a week, until the next beauty-parlor appointment.

1972. Geri Cusenza invents the crimping iron.

1973. Gloria Steinem's signature center-parted straight hair is an antistyle statement.

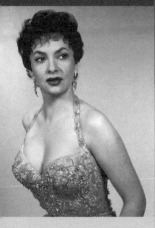

1960s. Twiggy's boyish, no-maintenance crew cut indicates an end to the tyranny of the 1950s.

1974. The feathered hair of Charlie's Angels becomes the decade's most iconic 'do.

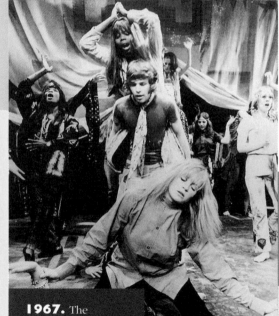

Does she... or doesn't she?

Hair color so natural only her hairdresser knows for sure!

MISS CLAIROL HAIR COLOR BATH

1956. The aerosol spray can is invented.

1967. The musical *Hair* opens, epitomizing the rebellious, let-it-all-hang-loose 1960s ethos—from hair to politics.

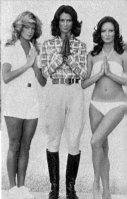

hair time line

1975. Endless variations on Afrocentric braids (formerly known as cornrows) are widely embraced and considered beautiful.

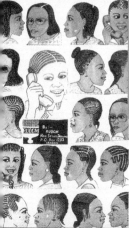

1976. Punk rock brings purple, green, blue, and orange to the hair landscape, along with Mohawks and other spiky styles.

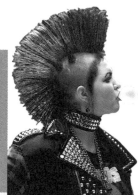

1977. Suave sells its billionth bottle, becoming the best-selling shampoo in the United States.

1976. Dorothy Hamill wins a gold medal at the Olympics; her short, layered wedge cut becomes almost as famous as her double axel.

1979. A crossover craze for cornrows is sparked when Bo Derek wears them in the movie *10*.

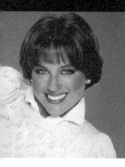

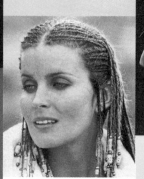

1980. Melanie Griffiths's hair in *Working Girl*—from big hair to a sleek Manhattan hairdo—parallels her career rise.

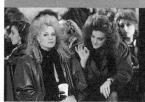

1981. After Lady Diana's wedding, thousands adopt her short, softly layered hairstyle.

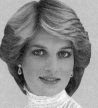

1988. Sinéad O'Connor's shaved head starts a trend among rebellious young women.

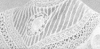

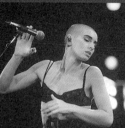

1990s. Courtney Love ushers in the dark-rooted platinum look.

1994. Jennifer Aniston's layered shag becomes the most emulated—and ridiculed—style of the decade.

1995. The Montreal Protocol on Substances that Deplete the Ozone Layer, an international agreement to eliminate the production of chlorofluorocarbons, takes effect.

Late 1990s. Long, straight, pale blond hair, parted in the middle, is made fashionable by the late Carolyn Bessette Kennedy and Gwyneth Paltrow.

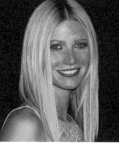

1998. Lauryn Hill makes dreadlocks glamorous.

1999. Halle Berry is stunning in a short, natural style.

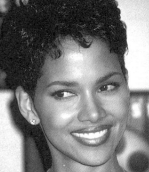

2000. Traditional Tanzanian-style combs carved of wood or woven from basket fibers are all the rage.

2000. The return of the "Curly Girl," à la Sarah Jessica Parker. Locks that have been blow-dried straight for decades find their natural inner curl. The straight heads get perms to be "in."

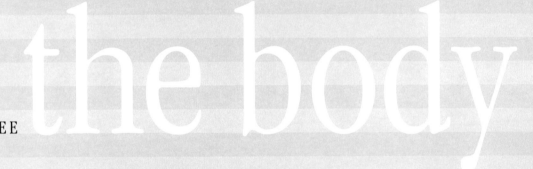

PART THREE the body

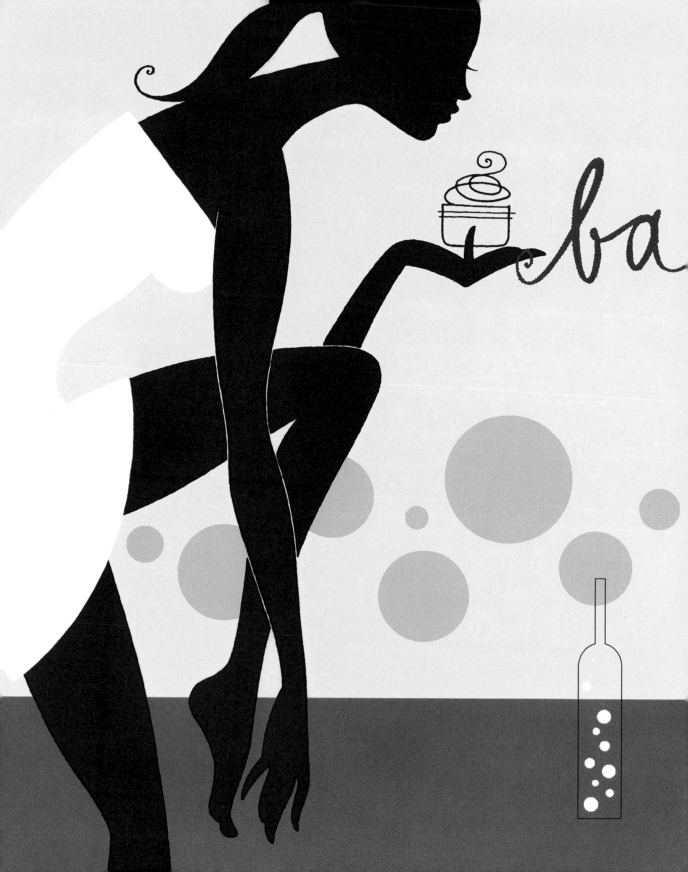

th & body

I believe that the physical is the geography of the being.

—LOUISE NEVELSON

The physical cues we express with our bodies—the way we touch, move, stand, adorn, and care for ourselves—reveal the way we feel about ourselves deep inside. If we feel good in our skin, we look good, too. It's as simple as that.

Unfortunately, when it comes to our bodies, most women obsess about one thing only: weight. The American standard of beauty, though slowly changing, is still the fashion model ideal—size 6, five feet seven inches, 110 pounds—an ideal that only 1 percent of the population has in their genes. (Standard size-6 or size-8 models are very tall, very thin, and very rare—which is why they make so very much money.)

But no matter how much you weigh, you'll look beautiful if you feel comfortable with your body. Like a dancer who expresses who she is through movement, a woman's physical ease expresses her ease with herself. As soon as you start to like, respect, and take care of your body (whether you're 5 pounds under- or 30 pounds overweight), you'll feel better, and your confidence will come across.

One way to start feeling good in your skin is to take long, languorous soaks in the tub. The bath has become the designated decompressing zone in our high-stress modern lives—a safe, sweet-smelling haven. Since the bath-and-body market is today a $1.1-billion-a-year business, it seems we're beginning to understand what bathing cultures like Japan have known for centuries: R & R—relaxation and renewal—is as much a part of the bath as cleansing.

The bath is a wonderful place to relax, but it also serves a more basic function. It's the place to establish a skincare regimen for the rest of your body. While most women are on intimate terms with just about every pore and freckle on their face, skincare from the neck down is often given short shrift.

Though the skin on the body is thicker and hardier than facial skin, it, too, demands attention. There are three main elements to healthy skincare for the body: cleansing, exfoliating, and moisturizing—basically, the same regimen I recommend for the face. *Now here's my little skin secret: if you exfoliate regularly—especially if you give your body a dry-brush treatment a couple of times a week—you will not need to moisturize!* Of course, you may want to moisturize occasionally, because it feels good and smells good—especially on extra-dry areas like the décolleté, elbows, and knees, and at the change of seasons. But take my word for it: dry-brushing is the secret of healthy, supple, hydrated skin.

Cleansing

So many skin problems (such as flaking and itching) that people blame on everything from diet to weather to indoor heating come down to the soap they use. If your skin is always dry, it's probably the fault of your cleansing bar. To counter the dryness, you probably overmoisturize and find yourself in a cycle that will never really correct the problem, especially if you use a mineral oil– or petroleum-based moisturizer.

Now that many of us are going to the gym, working up a sweat, and taking two or more showers a day, dryness has become even more of a problem. We don't have to bathe or shower every day, especially during the winter months, and doing so is one reason we suffer from lizardlike skin. But if you do shower often, a simple change like switching to a vegetable-based soap will make your skin feel hydrated and smooth.

A good soap should leave your skin feeling and smelling fresh. It should not leave a greasy film, it should not clog your pores, and it should not dry the skin. Like good foundation and face powder, a good soap is a necessary splurge, and *the very best* is a milled vegetable-based soap. I love the heft and tactile quality of a sweet-smelling almond, lavender, rosemary, or sandalwood bar. Milled vegetable soap is gentle on the skin, it's long lasting, it's a pleasure to use because it smells so irresistible—and it leaves you smelling that way as well. These soaps contain extra oil, which tempers their stripping action and seals moisture into the skin.

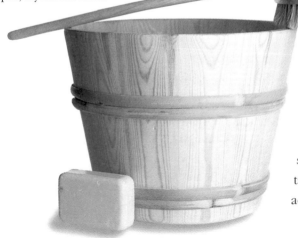

THE DISH ON SOAP: WHAT TO AVOID

Amazingly, in spite of huge technological advances in the beauty industry, the mass-market soap available today has not changed much since Procter & Gamble, Colgate, and Lever Bros. first set up shop in the early 19th century. Most supermarket soaps are still made from lard (sodium tallowate) and lye (sodium hydroxide), and you don't need a Ph.D. in chemistry to guess that there are gentler ways to clean your skin.

Deodorant soaps. Avoid them. Period. Deodorant soaps contain chemicals that kill odor-causing bacteria. But any soap will kill these bacteria without the harsh additives that dry and irritate skin.

Antibacterial soaps (liquid). Doctors have scrubbed with antibacterial soaps containing triclosan for years, but in our present germ-phobic culture, they're catching on for household use. But unless you have a good reason to use anti-bacterial soaps—for example, your family has very young children and recurrent strep infections—I would avoid them.

Medicated soaps. Medicinal substances (sulfur, tar, resorcin) are added to the soap to aid in treating skin conditions like acne. Sulfur is an antiseptic and dries up acne, but so does tea tree oil, and it's not as harsh. Try tea tree oil soap instead.

Body washes and shower gels are actually shampoo, and like shampoo they contain the drying ingredient sodium laureth sulfate. They may feel slinky on your skin because they contain silicone, a common (because it's cheap) lubricant in many beauty products. Silicone sits on top of the skin; it doesn't penetrate (the molecule is too big). So, in spite of the hype, body washes and gels do not moisturize nearly as well as a super-fatted shea butter, milk, or milled vegetable soap.

Exfoliating

Soaps and cleansers scrub away everyday dirt, but exfoliation actually improves the health of the body's skin. It stimulates blood flow to the skin, helps the circulatory and lymphatic systems release waste, and gets rid of built-up skin scales that can clog pores and lead to ingrown hairs. Exfoliating softens and smooths the skin, makes it easier to absorb moisturizer, gets rid of flakiness, relieves itchiness, and, over time, results in healthier-looking skin.

For all these reasons, it's a good idea to exfoliate the entire body (except for the face) at least once or twice a week. Washcloths, loofahs, sea sponges, silk mitts, exfoliating soaps, dry brushes, bath salts, or body scrubs will all help you get the job done. In a pinch, you can even use a gauze square or some cheesecloth.

Nothing feels more luxurious than an all-over rubdown with a big, floppy sea sponge and a simple bar of sweet-smelling soap. Sea sponges exfoliate without harshness, because they're soft and extremely absorbent. Moisten the sponge, soap it up, and rub it gently, in circular motions, beginning at the bottoms of your feet and heading north toward your knees and elbows, stopping at the neck. The only problem

The Soapbox

A necessary luxury

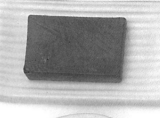

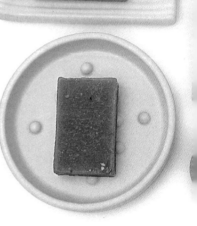

Milled vegetable soaps cost more than the supermarket variety, but at anywhere from $4 to $12 each, a bar is certainly an attainable luxury. It also lasts much longer than a drugstore brand because of the compacting process—so you come out about even in the end. Back in the Middle Ages, Marseilles became a soap-making center, and it still is. (Many high-quality French soaps brought into the United States are stamped "savon de Marseilles.") The French, not surprisingly, were the first to add fragrance to soap.

The Essentials

MOISTURIZING SOAPS

French-milled or hand-milled is soap that has been shredded, remelted, and mixed with essential oils or perfume to give it a sweet scent. It tends to be gentler than most other soaps, and a bar lasts a long time.

Triple-milled is a really dense and long-lasting soap that's pressed three times to get rid of any air. The bar is hard, lathers well, and is moisturizing.

Castile is an extremely gentle soap composed of olive oil and water. It has a whitish green color and virtually no trace of a scent. Rich, soft, and slightly greasy, Castile soap is best for very dry skin. (Although Castile originated in the Castile region of Spain, the most readily available, authentic Castile soaps today are imports from Greece or Italy.)

Glycerine or translucent soaps are made from oil and the emollient glycerine. Because they are extremely mild, soft, and gentle, they are good for babies, children, and adults with normal, dry, or sensitive skin. (In France, where these soaps are wildly popular, it's a custom to present newborns with their first translucent honey-colored bar.)

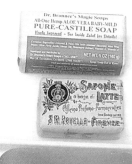

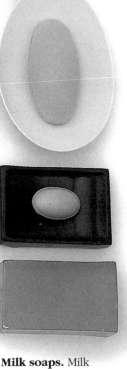

Tip **D**on't leave your soap in a puddle of water, or you are literally throwing money down the drain. Leave it in a soap dish on a draining rack, and it will last a lot longer. Another thrifty trick: cut a soap bar in halves or thirds, wrap the extra pieces, and use as needed.

Seaweed soaps and gels, also called "kelp" or "sea vegetable," are rich in iodine and minerals and very slippery. Some claim that seaweed soap, in tandem with massage, can help break down cellulite and improve circulation. In any case, these soaps are nice and gentle, though some, unfortunately, have a faintly fishy smell.

EXFOLIATING SOAPS

These are gritty bars that work as a combination cleanser–body scrub. They get rid of dry, flaky skin on the body, and they're especially good if your skin is oily or prone to blackheads or ingrown hairs.

Almond meal soap is an abrasive made from ground almonds. Because it absorbs excess oil, it is good for oily skin.

Oatmeal soothes sensitive or irritated skin and soaks up oil. An excellent exfoliant, it works particularly well on rough patches like elbows, knees, feet.

Pumice or lava soaps actually contain pulverized volcanic rock that's added to soap as an abrasive. But it can be rough stuff. So restrict the use of pumice soap to the bottoms of your feet.

Clay soaps (aka French clay) draw out and absorb oils from the skin, which makes them best for oily skin.

Milk soaps. Milk moisturizes, softens, and soothes itchy dry skin. They are good for dry, normal, or sensitive skin.

Shea butter. Indigenous to Africa, shea butter comes from a nut grown on the karite tree. This rich emollient makes a lovely, creamy, soft soap, good for normal to dry skin.

Super-fatted. Extra oils or emollients (olive oil, cocoa butter, even milk or cream) are added to make super-fatted soaps even creamier and more moisturizing, especially for dry or sensitive skin. They don't lather well, but this isn't necessarily bad.

𝒣𝑜𝓌 𝒯𝑜: dry-brush

Use a good, natural-fiber bath brush (available at drugstores, bath and body shops, and health food stores) that's about the size of your hand with a handle long enough to allow you to reach down your back.

With your skin dry—not wet—begin with the toes of your left foot and brush toward the heel. Work up your leg, with 6 to 12 long, quick strokes. Brush your knee in a circular movement, and then move up your thigh, using circular motions on your hips and glutes. Repeat on the right leg.

Then brush each arm, moving up toward your heart. (You always want to stimulate the flow of blood toward the heart.) Keep the pressure light but firm, as you do when shaving, and brush until your skin lightly tingles. Don't forget your back, especially if you're prone to blackheads or clogged pores. If you're lucky, your mate or a good friend might scrub your back for you while you're in the tub—it's nurturing, and it feels really good. The skin on your breasts and neck is more sensitive, so be very gentle on those areas or skip them entirely.

WARNING: Don't dry-brush at night, because it stimulates the circulatory system, and you'll get yourself all revved up. And *never* dry-brush your face because facial skin is too tender for this treatment.

with sponges is that you can't sterilize them. Because soap residue and dead skin remain in the sponge, it's important to wash and dry a sponge well after each use and replace it every couple of months.

While sponges may be the most sensuous skincare treatment, dry-brushing is the most effective. Dry-brushing is actually an ancient beauty ritual 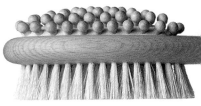 that has fallen out of favor in our fast-paced modern times. But it takes only a couple of minutes to dry-brush your entire body, and the benefits are more than worth it.

Dry-brush your skin with a natural-fiber brush before a bath or shower once or twice a week, and your skin will be so naturally soft and healthy, *you won't need a moisturizer.* "Dry-brushing eliminates the need for remoisturizing because it stimulates the circulatory system and keeps bringing fresh nourishment to the skin through the blood," says Deborah Evans of the PGA National Resort and Spa. "Exfoliating also allows the body's oils to surface and moisturize the skin naturally."

If you prefer, you can exfoliate with a loofah (or sisal) instead of a dry brush. (Sisal is

> **Tip** **I**f your skin is sensitive, oily, or prone to breakouts, use a raw silk mitt—the texture is closest to a washcloth, but far more delicate—and rub gently. Once you begin to exfoliate regularly, however, you'll find that your skin will adapt to an increasingly vigorous exfoliation.

rougher, but effective if you're prone to ingrown hairs.) Loofahs work especially well on elbows, knees, and heels to remove rough, scaly dead skin cells—they're usually too harsh for other parts of the body, but not if you've got tough skin. Unlike the dry brush, the loofah should be used wet. Stand in the tub (or move out from under the nozzle if you're in the shower). Apply a soap or shower gel (if you prefer it) to the wet loofah, and rub the loofah over your body in gentle circular motions.

After you exfoliate, make sure to rinse, rinse, rinse to wash all those bits of dry skin away. First wash with a warm shower, then rinse with cool water.

Elbows and Knees

According to folklore, the true way to tell a woman's age is to look at her knees or elbows. Whether plump and dimpled or dry as the bones in a Georgia O'Keeffe landscape, these areas are a dead giveaway. The skin on the elbows and knees is some of the thickest and most neglected on the body, which, in most cases, means the dead skin just keeps piling up until it resembles your pet lizard's hide. The first line of attack is to exfoliate them with a dry brush. If they need extra help, use a body scrub, kosher salt, or dry oatmeal and a loofah.

If your elbows and knees have attained true lizard status, use an AHA body lotion. AHA moisturizers work beautifully to exfoliate calluses and get those areas up to speed, especially in the spring when you're ready to bare them after a winter of being covered up. The best

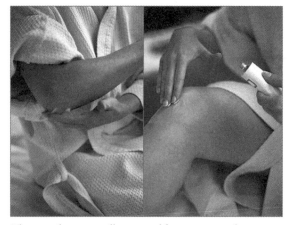

The rough spots—elbows and knees—can always use a little extra dollop of moisturizer.

way to *keep* elbows and knees looking smooth is with balm, which is just a prettier name for ointment or salve. A balm soothes and softens even the body's roughest terrain, despite the fact that its thick, waxy texture—a blend of semisolid wax and sweetly scented oils—bears an uncanny resemblance to Crisco. Balms don't contain water, so they don't need preservatives—a plus for those with sensitive skin. Most have a moisturizing blend of sweet almond, lavender, jojoba, neroli, and rose oils. The following are some of the best "elbow grease" products I've found: Bag Balm, Decleor Baume Aromatique Harmonie for Sensitive Skin

LEMON AID

Nestle your elbows, knees, and heels in a lemon half for a few minutes every couple of weeks. Sit for two minutes, then wash off with soap and water. Or mix the juice of a lemon with a couple of teaspoons of sugar or salt, and rub lightly onto the scaly area.

BEAUTY Rx

(African shea butter, neroli, and sweet almond oil), Guerlain Lipbalm (almond oil), Elizabeth Arden Eight-Hour Cream, Origins Rough Skin Soother, L'Occitane 100% Shea Butter, Natura-Bisse Glyco-Skin Exfoliator Lotion (AHA), Common Sense Chamomile and Primrose Balm.

Shaving

Many people don't realize it, but shaving is a form of exfoliation, too. Shaving the legs first became popular for women around World War II, when a shortage of nylon stockings kicked off a bare-legged trend. Today, shaving is still the easiest, cheapest, and most convenient way to get rid of unwanted hair—under the arms, on the legs, and around the bikini line. The downsides are stubbly regrowth in two to three days and cuts and irritation. These are some reasons that make waxing a better choice for hair removal (see page 97). But here are some tricks to smooth shaving and ways to cut down on irritation.

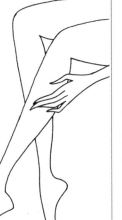

The trick to a close, smooth shave is to wet the area first, and wait a couple of minutes until the moisture soaks in. Then apply shaving

> **Tip** The absolute best razor is the nondisposable Gillette SensorExcel for Women (along with Gillette Satin Care Shave Gel). I know, I've tried them all. Electric shavers don't even come close.

gel, liquid body cleanser, or shower gel. (A squirt of shampoo will do in a pinch, but don't use soap if you want a close shave, and forget about dry shaving—bits of loose skin will clog up the razor.) Since your leg hair grows in one direction (down), start at the ankle and shave in an upward direction *against* the hair growth. Since underarm hair grows every which way, shave it in every direction as well. When you shave the bikini line, pull the skin taut to get a smooth surface. If you need to go back over an area, apply more gel first. Rinse the area when finished, pat dry, and apply oil or moisturizer.

Shaving No-nos

To avoid irritation, do not shave . . .

▨ Before jumping into a chlorinated pool or before a massage, salt rub, or any other exfoliating treatment.

▨ Sunburned skin.

▨ Dry skin. You're more likely to cut yourself.

▨ Immediately before a long bike ride, spinning class, hike—because you can chafe.

Also:

▨ Do not apply an AHA product or sunblock immediately after shaving.

▨ Do not share a razor, especially not with the man in your life. His hair is coarser than yours, so the blade blunts more quickly and is apt to nick you.

Body Smoothers: Salts, Scrubs, and Masks

When the seasons change and your skin is shedding like a snake's, a body scrub—salt glow, herbal wrap, or mud mask—is an alternative way to exfoliate and pamper yourself at the same time.

For an at-home salt rub, run a warm bath ankle-high—or stand in the shower, away from the water. Wet your body. Take a palmful of bath salts, moisten your palm, and massage the salts, gently, in circular movements, directly onto your skin with your fingers. Start at your feet and work your way up, always working inward, from your extremities toward your torso. Finally, scrub your torso. (Never apply to your neck, face, or broken skin, and avoid your décolleté.) Rinse with warm water.

When you're done, empty and refill the tub, throw in a small scoop of bath salts, and take a muscle-relaxing soak. At home, I always keep a big glass jar of bath salts on my shelf, with a flat seashell inside the jar. I use the shell to scoop up the salts, and toss a couple of shellfuls into the bath. Contrary to what you might think, bath salts do not dry out the skin—too much water does. Rinse with cool water.

You can easily make your own bath salts by spiking sea salt with a few drops of essential oil (your choice). Bath salts mixed with essential oils pack a three-fisted punch: the salt exfoliates

THINGS THAT GO BUMP ON THE SKIN

Ingrown hairs curl back under the skin and can cause red bumps, also known as "razor bumps" or folliculitis—an inflammation of the hair follicle. Folliculitis usually plagues the bikini zone, legs, or underarms where the skin has been irritated by shaving or waxing. If you're ingrown-hair prone, exfoliate the area daily with a loofah or scrub to help hairs grow in the right direction. If you've got a chronic case, try Tend Skin, which works like a charm. Apply twice a day—in the morning and at night—and they'll disappear within a day or two.

To keep ingrown hairs away, use a glycolic acid body lotion (Aqualglycolic, Avon's Renew, Lac-Hydrin, Lacticare) or a hydrogen peroxide product (Karin Herzog's Oxygen Body Lotion)—but not on days when you wax or shave. And if your bumps become infected, use a topical antibiotic ointment (Bactroban or Bacitracin).

Exfoliating will also help remove those hard bumps, known as KP (keratosis pilaris). KP looks like a vast swath of bumps or pimples, without the redness or irritation. They most often appear on the back of the upper arms, buttocks, and outer thighs. The bumps are actually plugged hair follicles, and though they can be controlled, they can't be cured. The best way to control KP is to keep the affected areas very clean and exfoliate regularly with a body scrub on a sea sponge—but do not rub. After a bath or shower, apply an alpha-hydroxy or beta-hydroxy gel or lotion such as Oil of Olay's Age-Defying Lotion. If your bumps are particularly stubborn, see a dermatologist, who may prescribe Retin-A, Renova, or a series of glycolic peels.

Did You Know? The actress Sarah Bernhardt was renowned for her flawless skin, which she claimed she owed to a beauty bath concoction that included six pounds of bran and two pounds of barley. It's a little too heavy on the fiber for my taste, but it's interesting to see what beauty sometimes boils down to.

the skin, the aromatherapeutic oils soothe the spirit, and a mineral-rich soak afterward can relax tired muscles.

There's a reason why bath-and-body shops are almost as ubiquitous as Starbucks: some of the store-bought bath salts are irresistible, and they last forever because a little goes a long way. Read the labels, and you'll usually find three main ingredients: sea salt, sodium bicarbonate (baking soda), and essential oils. Remember: this is a case where less is more. Lists that go on with endless ingredients are loaded with dyes, fragrances, and preservatives. These products contain just the good stuff: Bliss Hot Salt Scrub (Dead Sea salt with rosemary oil), Burt's Bees Dead Sea Salts, Ahava Dead Sea Bath Salts, Elizabeth Arden Green Tea Tub Rub, Essentiel Elements Essentiel Oil Bath Salts, Fresh Brown Sugar Body Polish (a pricey splurge!), Origins True Grit Fruit-Sloughing Body Gel (apricot pits and peppermint).

Here are a couple of body scrub recipes for all skin types. You can use your fingers, a sponge, or a washcloth to apply a body mask or scrub. Avoid a loofah or brush, because the combination is overly abrasive.

BIRDBATH SCRUB

1 cup oatmeal, wheat germ, cornmeal, or ground sunflower seeds
4 tablespoons water
2 sprigs peppermint, rosemary, or sage leaves

1. Mix the oatmeal and water to make a thick, smooth paste. (Add more water if necessary.)
2. Smash the leaves with a mortar and pestle. Mix into the paste.
3. Massage the paste gently into the skin, rinse with warm water, pat dry, and moisturize.

MUD BATH FOR BLEMISH-PRONE SKIN

If you are prone to breakouts on your back or chest, a nonabrasive mud (clay) mask is the best choice for your skin. All of the following ingredients are available at health food stores.

1 cup powdered clay
¾ cup powdered kelp
1 cup aloe vera gel
½ cup water mixed with a pinch of sea salt

1. Mix the ingredients together to form a paste.
2. In a dry bathtub, brush or spread the paste on your body.
3. Relax and allow to dry for 10 minutes. Rinse off with warm water.

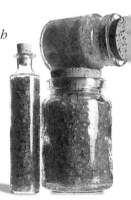

Here are a few down-and-dirty mud masks to play with at home: Ahava Dead Sea Body Mud, The Body Shop Africa Spa Hair & Body Honey Mud, Erno Laszlo Sea Mud Body Skin Polisher.

Moisturizing

A soak in a tub for about 15 minutes will rehydrate your skin, but add a good bath oil and you'll soften and moisturize the skin like you can't believe. The oil, which smells nice and floats in shimmery little slicks on the water, actually clings to the body as you leave the tub—instantly sealing in the moisture the skin has soaked up from the bath.

Wait until after you've run a warm bath, then sprinkle in five or six drops of bath oil. Salts can be added as the bath runs, but if you add the oil under running water, the vapors will dissipate by the time you get in, and you'll lose much of their olfactory benefit.

Remember, if you dry-brush your skin a couple of times a week before your bath or shower, you won't need a moisturizer after a bath. But if you enjoy the way it smells or feels, go ahead and tantalize your senses—especially on dry or sensitive areas like the elbows, knees, and décolleté. When you use scented moisturizers, you will smell good without using perfume. The ideal time to moisturize is directly after a bath or shower, when the skin is wet and most receptive to moisture.

If your skin is oily, stick to lotions rather than creams. Lotions are lighter because they contain less oil and more water. Avoid products that contain olive oil and mineral oil–based lotions and creams, which can clog the skin. Look for lotions with silicones (ingredients ending in "-one"), because they won't clog the pores.

DAIRY DIP

Poppaea, wife of the Roman emperor Nero, used to literally bathe in milk—asses' milk, in her case—because she claimed it softened her skin. It probably did, because milk is a source of lactic acid, one of the alpha-hydroxy acids. Milk helps exfoliate the skin, which is why your skin feels softer after a dip in dairy products. Poppaea was such a lacto-lover, she was said to have led a caravan of 50 asses with her when she traveled, in order to make sure she'd have enough milk for her daily baths.

But today, few of us lead caravans of asses around (or, at least, we don't admit to it), and aside from it being highly impractical, the aesthetic of bathing in dairy products has somehow lost its cachet over the centuries. The benefits of bathing in substances that make the bath *milky,* however, are another story. Milk, oatmeal, and baking soda will all soothe dry, itchy skin and gently exfoliate flaky patches. Starting with Aveeno baths recommended for young children, rice starch, oatmeal, or almond meal can be incredibly soothing in a bath for dry or itchy skin, especially in winter. They also loosen flaky skin, just like milk. Or try The Body Shop's Powdered Milk Bath with Avocado Oil and Oat Flour.

It pays to be picky and avoid petroleum- or mineral oil–based moisturizers. Mass-market cosmetics manufacturers almost always use petroleum and mineral oil in their moisturizers because they are vastly cheaper than alternatives like beeswax, jojoba, vegetable squalene, and shea butter. Okay—it won't harm you to use these occasionally, and it won't harm some people at all. But it doesn't help much, either. Unlike plant and certain animal oils (kalaya), mineral oil won't absorb into even the top layer of skin. It just sits there, greasing up and smothering the skin, which means that if your skin is oily, it can lead to breakouts. If your skin is dry, it can actually make it drier—like some soft drinks that make you more thirsty—by mopping up your skin's natural oils.

Stretch Marks

Stretch marks can occur with pregnancy, yo-yo weight loss and gain, bodybuilding, or anytime the skin is required to make a significant and abrupt stretch. Stretch marks are most commonly found around the belly, hips, upper thighs, and breasts, and behind the knees; some people get stretch marks on their upper arms, too. The best thing to do, obviously, is to stop them before they start, and the best mode of prevention is to keep your weight from fluctuating wildly. If your weight goes up and down, using a body moisturizer on the problem areas after the bath or shower may help.

If you are pregnant, apply a rich body cream every day, but check with your doctor first to make sure there aren't any potentially harmful ingredients in the cream (although the chances are minuscule, you'll want to make sure). I'm convinced that the reason I got through my pregnancy stretch-mark-free is because I slathered on truckloads of Kiehl's Creme de Corps daily.

White stretch marks that you've had for a while are quite resistant to treatment. But if you notice red ones (the beginning stage) and they bother you, see a doctor soon. There are two approaches to treating early-stage stretch marks. The first is Retin-A or Renova, the prescription medications used to reduce wrinkles and treat acne. In a study done at the University of Michigan several years ago, women who applied Retin-A to stretch marks for two months significantly decreased their length and width, although it's too soon to know if the results will be permanent.

The second treatment is laser therapy. The pulse-dye laser is the type generally used to eliminate scars, and it is the one used on stretch marks. Temporary side effects can include itching, irritation, and discoloration, but in terms of overall effectiveness, studies look promising.

THE BEE'S KNEES

Roxanne Quimby was a medicine woman before she became a millionaire. Thirteen years ago, Quimby was a "back-to-the-lander," an herbalist and organic gardener eking out a subsistence on a few cheap acres in Guilford, Maine. When her marriage broke up, she supported herself and her children by selling herbs and homemade candles at craft fairs and flea markets.

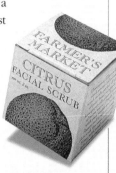

Everything changed one day when she met Burt Shavitz, a local beekeeper who sold his honey by the side of the road. "I told him he could get more for it," says Quimby. Besides, she wanted to use Shavitz's discarded beeswax to make candles. "He cut me in," she says, "and I kind of took over the business."

The two partners molded candles and bottled honey together, and they started to look for other uses for beeswax. Quimby knew that beeswax had long been used as an emulsifier. It also acts as an occlusive and seals moisture into the skin. "So we sort of stumbled on skincare," says Quimby. And Burt's Bees, an earth-friendly, natural skincare product company, was born.

Despite its success—Burt's Bees brings in over $4 million a year and can be found in 3,000 stores around the United States—Quimby and Shavitz have held on to the eco-friendly ethics of their business, using beeswax rather than petroleum, which can be toxic to the environment. That and the fact that their products contain 97 to 100 percent natural ingredients really set Burt's Bees apart. "We're trying to reestablish meaning to the word *natural*—because in this industry, it doesn't really mean anything," says Quimby.

Cellulite

Known colloquially as "mattress," or "orange peel," because of its unfortunate resemblance to both, cellulite plagues 80 to 90 percent of women. It's a myth that cellulite is an affliction of overweight women. It makes no difference if you're heavy or lean—you're either genetically predisposed to cellulite or you're not. Women, unlike men, are prone to cellulite because of the way our connective fibers are arranged in our bodies. Men's connective tissue is set at an angle, but women's is arranged vertically. Female hormones help make our hips, thighs, and buttocks home to a large and thriving population of fat cells, which makes them especially susceptible to cellulite.

Cellulite forms when the fat cells within the connective tissue enlarge, which restricts blood and lymph circulation. Waste matter then accumulates, and fluids build around the waste, which swells the connective tissue and bloats the fat cells. The fibers exert a downward pull on the swollen fat, like the buttons on a Chesterfield couch. Voila! Cellulite.

You can make cellulite look a little bit better—but it takes persistence bordering on obsession. No one-shot "cellulite recontouring massage" at the day spa or salon will do it. No miraculous cellulite product on its own will beat cellulite. All cellulite creams are expensive and their application is time-consuming. But if you apply them to the area with regular, vigorous, circular massage (a small brush will help), you may see some improvement after two to three weeks. But it's the massage action, not the cream, that is making the difference.

So my advice is to follow the same rules you would follow as part of a general good-health regimen—avoid fatty and junk foods, get plenty of exercise—and, if you want, massage the areas you want to keep cellulite-free. But most important, try to cultivate a healthier attitude toward those dimpled spots on your thighs. After all, if 80 to 90 percent of all women have it, doesn't it make it normal? We may not like it, but we don't have to beat ourselves up about it either.

Create a Home Spa

After my daughter was born, it seemed the only time I had five minutes' peace was in the bath. Needless to say, the tub became my sanctuary, and a soak a much-needed luxury. Even today, whenever I'm really stressed, I retreat to the tub with a sea sponge in hand to smooth out the rough spots. I turn the bath into a bouillabaisse spiked with aromatic mineral salts, drizzled with glistening bath oils, and infused with herbs and flowers. An aromatic candle fills the room with scent, and its relaxing effects take hold of my psyche like the soothing oil on my skin. Immersed in warm

water, solitude, and delicious smells, I am weightless. All burdens lift. By the time I step out on the mat, my cares have slipped down the drain and I'm ready to go another round.

You'll be amazed at how much mileage you can get out of a simple soak, surrounded by a bit of sweet-smelling soap or some scented bath oil. The ritual of soaking and cleansing not only strips the body bare but also clears the mind and lifts the spirit.

You don't need much to create your own home spa—a bathtub, some imagination, a few plants or a vase of cut flowers does a lot to make the atmosphere fresh and renewing. Ask your local florist if he has any leftover rose petals and strew them in the water. Buy an aromatic candle (or several small candles) and use it as your only light. The lingering scent and warm glow are instant relaxers. A loofah or brush, some salts, oils, and a sweet-smelling soap, and you're ready to float. Many appealing bath and body products are available at body shops and health food stores as well as through mail-order catalogs, spas, and Internet Websites (see appendix B, page 355).

If you really want to relax, the most important thing is to block out some time for yourself. Allow anywhere from 20 to 30 minutes to luxuriate in your home spa. Even if you don't have that much time to make the transition between work and an evening out, you can still benefit from a soak. (And remember, if you're in the state where you think you're too stressed out to take a bath, *that's* when you need it most.) Unplug the phone. Let your family, roommate, or partner know not to disturb you. (In your best Greta Garbo imitation, announce, "I vant to be alone!")

Equipment

Set up everything for your soak in advance so that once you enter your sanctum, you can totally relax and clear your mind. For the ultimate sybaritic soak, you'll want to have the following:

- *Soft cotton terrycloth robe and slippers*
- *Milled vegetable soap*
- *Sea sponge*
- *Long-handled, natural-bristle bath brush*
- *Bath crystals and/or aromatherapy bath oil*
- *Body scrub*
- *Bath pillow*
- *Seashell*
- *Scented candles*
- *Two large, fluffy bath towels*
- *Body moisturizer or oil*
- *Thick cotton bath mat*
- *Water with a slice of lemon or herbal tea*
- *Herbal eye pillow*
- *OPTIONAL: Favorite music, face mask, hair oil*

Beauty Culture

In Japan, cleansing begins before you actually enter the tub. The Japanese either shower quickly before their baths or sit on a little stool in a tiled bathroom and meticulously scrub every inch of their bodies with a brush, soap, and a bucket of hot water. This is done however many times is necessary until one is clean enough to step into a tub. To the Japanese, the idea of washing off dirt and then soaking in the same water is disgusting. If you share this sensibility, take a modified Japanese bath: cleanse yourself in the bath first, then drain and refill the tub, and pick up at step 4 (see page 287).

A Bath of One's Own

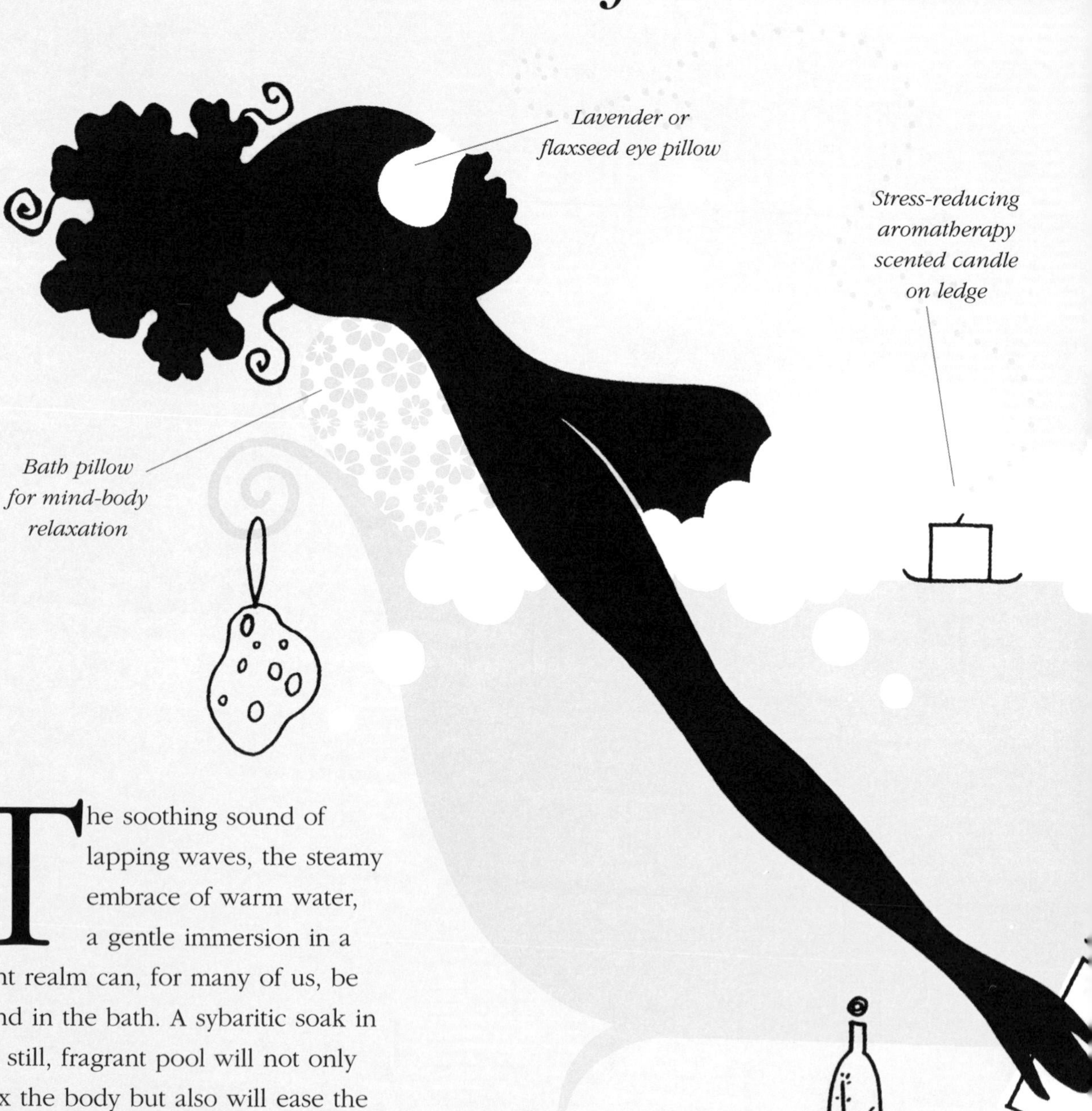

*Lavender or
flaxseed eye pillow*

*Stress-reducing
aromatherapy
scented candle
on ledge*

*Bath pillow
for mind-body
relaxation*

soap

The soothing sound of lapping waves, the steamy embrace of warm water, a gentle immersion in a silent realm can, for many of us, be found in the bath. A sybaritic soak in that still, fragrant pool will not only relax the body but also will ease the mind. Shut your eyes, and a whiff of sandalwood can transport you to exotic realms.

I have had a good many more uplifting thoughts,
creative and expansive visions—while soaking in
comfortable baths . . . in well-equipped American bathrooms
than I have ever had in any cathedral.

—EDMUND WILSON

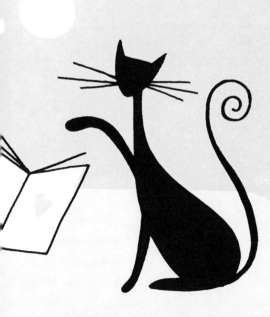

Fill tub with
bath salts and
fragrant oils

A SHORT SOCIAL HISTORY OF BATHING

Throughout history societal attitudes toward bathing have revealed a lot more than just skin. For the ancient Romans, communal bathing was a social—and business—obligation that eventually developed into a decadent national pastime. In Islamic cultures, bathing was a way to remove the stains of sin. The early Christians believed the opposite: the bath was a temptation of the flesh and must be resisted. It was preferable to live with stains on the body than a stain on the soul. St. Francis of Assisi considered an unwashed body a sign of purity.

In Europe, up until the 19th century, washing and bathing were denounced as decadent, sensual pastimes, even among the upper classes—certainly a bit of hypocrisy since they were intimately acquainted with other forms of sensual indulgence. Water was thought to weaken the body as well as the spirit, making it soft and vulnerable to disease, and washing was limited to the hands and, rarely, the face. Lotions and creams were the preferred means of cleansing, along with rubs, perfumes, and floral-scented toilet waters. Not surprisingly, stench was a way of life.

In 18th-century America, Puritans considered bathing impure, and laws in certain states banned or limited its practice.

Soap was subject to prohibitively high taxes—similar to those on cigarettes today—which discouraged common folk from using it for anything but laundry. When cheap tropical oils were first imported from Britain's colonies, soap became available to the masses.

By the late 19th century "taking the waters" became a medical prescription or curative, and people began to realize, once again, how therapeutic bathing could be. The personal-care giants—Colgate & Company, Procter & Gamble, and Johnson & Johnson—all set up shop around

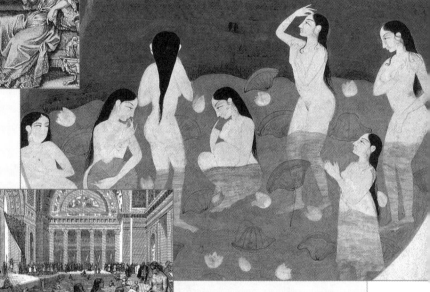

this time and made their fortunes on soap.

Today, the popularity of bathing has reached an all-time high. According to a recent study, about 47 percent of American women relax by taking a bath. As a nation, we're so obsessed with cleansing and deodorizing, it's not unusual to shower twice a day.

1. Put on your robe and slippers, and make yourself a cup of herbal tea. Bring it into the bathroom, turn down the lights, and light some scented candles. Sit, sip, and relax for a couple of minutes.

2. Draw a warm bath. With a small seashell, scoop out your bath crystals (two or three scoops) and toss under the running water.

3. While the water is running, give yourself a dry-brush treatment by the side of the tub, or gently rub bath crystals over your body.

4. Turn off the water, and swirl in a few drops of bath oil with your hand. Step into the bath slowly, sink down, put a bath pillow behind your head, and place an herbal pillow over your eyes. Take a few slow, deep breaths—in through the nose, out through the mouth—and focus on relaxation. Soak for 10 to 15 minutes (any longer than that, and you'll look like a prune).

5. Remove the eye pillow. Take the soap, rub it on the sponge, and wash slowly and thoroughly.

6. Empty the tub. Rinse yourself off with a handheld shower spray or use a pitcher to pour water from the faucet over your body.

7. Step out of the bath, and pat yourself dry with thick, luxurious towels. Apply moisturizer or body oil (see page 279), especially on the rough patches: elbows and knees. Wrap yourself in the terrycloth robe, and drink a tall glass of water or tea to rehydrate.

8. If you can spare an extra half hour, the best time to give yourself a pedicure (see page 307) is after a bath.

SOAK SUDS ALERT

Bubble baths and foaming washes are not as glamorous as they appear. Unlike bath oils and bath salts, they don't offer any great benefit. On the contrary, **warning** they can be irritating to skin and the mucous membranes, and they've been known to cause vaginal yeast infections. In fact, manufacturers are now required to put a disclaimer on these products telling the consumer that they may cause irritation. Try to avoid products that contain the ingredient sodium lauryl sulfate, which is the most irritating of them all.

As a general rule, the more foam you get from a product—this includes shampoos, soaps, and body washes—the more drying it is to the skin. But since we expect lots of foam from a bubble bath, cosmetics companies give us what they think we want.

P.S. Le plus extra. While the water is running, dampen your face and apply a mask to your face and throat. If your hair is dried out, apply an oil treatment. Leave both on while you soak for 15 minutes, then rinse off under the running faucet.

P.P.S. Little luxuries. Make an herbal sachet from dried or fresh herbs. Take a piece of muslin, gauze, or cheesecloth the size of your palm and place rose petals, a bit of oatmeal, and some chamomile or lavender flowers in the center. Close at the top with ribbon or twine and tie to the faucet while the bathwater is running.

Use a mortar and pestle to crush some fresh rosemary leaves, or open an herbal tea bag (jasmine or chamomile is good) and wrap the herbs in muslin or cheesecloth. Tie to the faucet under warm running water.

Aromatherapy

Smells influence our moods in ways we're just beginning to understand.

Aromatherapy is the therapeutic use of botanical oils that are distilled or cold-pressed from plants and flowers. The oils, which are introduced into the body topically or by inhalation, have been used to soothe the psyche, heal the body, and soften the skin for thousands of years. As far back as the 4th century B.C., Hippocrates wrote, "A perfumed bath and a scented massage every day are the way to good health."

Modern aromatherapy took hold in the United States in the 1980s, when natural healing and mind-body medicine were brought into the mainstream through the work of doctors like Herbert Benson and Dean Ornish. I remember the day when Gabriella Neurath, our flamboyant Hungarian beauty editor with a nose for news, burst into the editorial meeting at *ELLE* magazine with the imperative: "Aromatherapy, dahlinks, it's in the air. I can smell it."

Although aromatherapy is now a multi-million-dollar business, it took a while to catch on. When Aubrey Hampton founded Aubrey Organics in 1968, he was one of the first to market a cosmetics line based on natural plant essences. Horst Rechelbacher, another early proponent of aromatherapy, founded Aveda in 1978, but it took a few years before he could sell the idea that the natural aromas in plant oils could affect the psyche. The mainstream officially caught up with aromatherapy in 1990, when cosmetics giant Estée Lauder launched an aromatherapy-based company, Origins, headed by Lauder's grandson, William Lauder. In 1997, Lauder bought Aveda and aromatherapy officially lost its "alternative" status.

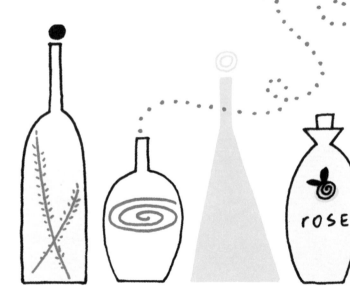

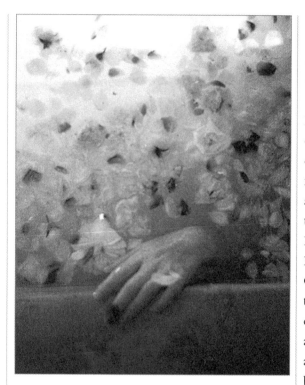

The Nose Knows

Recent scientific research on the olfactory system is beginning to back up some of the anecdotal claims about aromatherapy. The "smell molecules" in essential oils are picked up by exquisitely sensitive nerve receptors in the nose and transmitted directly into the limbic system, which is the emotional center of the brain. It responds by secreting a variety of chemicals that can create different psychological effects: for example, endorphins to reduce pain, serotonin to relax and calm.

In other words, the nose knows. Smells also evoke memories and trigger powerful whiffs of nostalgia. A hint of vanilla can bring up delicious memories of baking cookies with Mom. Mint or eucalyptus may conjure up soothing childhood sickroom rubdowns. Perhaps the smell of pine provides an exhilarating reminder of camping in the Great North Woods.

Studies conducted in Japan and France have also suggested that inhaling different essential oils can shorten or lengthen alpha or beta waves in the brain, resulting in a feeling of calm or of stimulus, depending on the particular oil. Researchers at Yale's Psychophysiology Center are claiming that certain scents can reduce stress and increase alertness. But because our sense of smell is so subjective, proof that plant oils can penetrate deep into the psyche is hard to come by. In the meantime, aromatherapy smells good, it softens our skin, and it makes us feel good. And that's good enough for me.

(continued on next spread)

Tip Look for an "Herbal Comfort Pack," a pillow stuffed with flaxseed, lavender, chamomile, or jasmine. Throw it in the microwave for a few seconds so that the plant oils fully release their scent. Place over your eyes while relaxing on the sofa or in the tub.

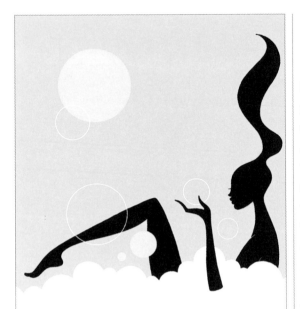

ROSIE'S
GODDESS BATH

My friend Rosie, a poet, has classical taste in literature—and bath soaks. Here's her simple but fabulous recipe for a soak that will leave your skin as supernaturally soft as Aphrodite's.

2 cups dry, nonfat milk
2 cups baking soda
1 cup kosher salt
Drops of your favorite essential oil
   "to taste" (lilac is exceptional)

Mix the ingredients together. Store in an airtight jar. Scoop out and sprinkle in the bath with a seashell—in keeping with the Aphrodite motif—if you like. Keeps up to one year.

Aromatherapy
at Home

For those moments when you feel yourself practically vibrating with stress, an aromatherapy bath can be extremely relaxing. Aromatherapy also works in the shower, where a zippy rosemary- or spearmint-scented soap can provide an invigorating jump start to your day, and it's a pleasurable addition to any massage oil. Although die-hard aromatherapists dabble in 300 essential oils, most of us, for the purposes of bath and body care, can satisfy our needs with products containing the dozen or so listed on facing page.

Because pure essential oils are so strong, commercial products are always diluted with a "carrier" oil. The best carriers are almond, apricot kernel, grapeseed, safflower, and sunflower oils because, unlike olive oil, for example, their scents don't interfere with the scent of the essential oil. If you want to make your own, mix a drop or two of essential oil with a few teaspoons of carrier oil.

Buying Essential Oils. Now that there are so many good essential-oil preparations available commercially, there's no need to mix them yourself. It's easy to buy what you need from a bath-and-body shop, health food store, cosmetics emporium, or quality pharmacy—but there are vast differences in price and quality. For something to provide an aromatherapeutic benefit, it must contain pure essential oils that are derived from plants or pressed from flowers. Products that contain pure essential oils will say so, and this is what you want. Watch out for phrases like "extract of . . . ," "essence of . . . ," or "aromatic oil of . . ."—these are ways companies fudge about exactly what's in a product. Most often, products labeled Oil of Rose, Oil of Geranium, and so on are inexpensive synthetics. Unfortunately, most mass-market drugstore brands are worthless.

It pays to spend a bit more on aromatherapy products, because pure, quality oils contain vitamins, antibiotics, natural hormones, and antiseptics not available in synthetic formulations. Besides, they smell nicer. Here are some companies you can trust: Aromatherapeutics, Baudelaire, Essentiel Elements, Jurlique, Kniepp, L'Occitane, and Aroma Vera.

Pure essential oils are strong and can irritate, even burn, the skin. This is especially true of the spicy ones (clove, cinnamon, oregano). The citrus oils (grapefruit, lime, lemon, orange, tangerine, bergamot, neroli) are photosensitive and if applied directly to the skin can cause hypopigmentation (sun spots).

Red Alert

THE ESSENCE OF AROMATHERAPY

Scents	Effects
Bergamot	Stimulating, energizing
Chamomile	Calming, soothing to skin
Eucalyptus	Strong, invigorating, clears the sinuses
Geranium	Calming, uplifting
Jasmine	Stimulating, uplifting
Lavender	Soothing, relaxing, good for burns (my personal favorite because it evokes delicious memories of the south of France)
Lemongrass	Stimulating, energizing, tired-muscle tonic
Mint	Stimulating, soothes tired muscles
Neroli	From orange blossoms, soothing
Rose	Soothes stress, uplifting
Rosemary	Invigorating, energizing, clears the mind
Sandalwood	Soothing, calming
Ylang-ylang	Soothing, calming

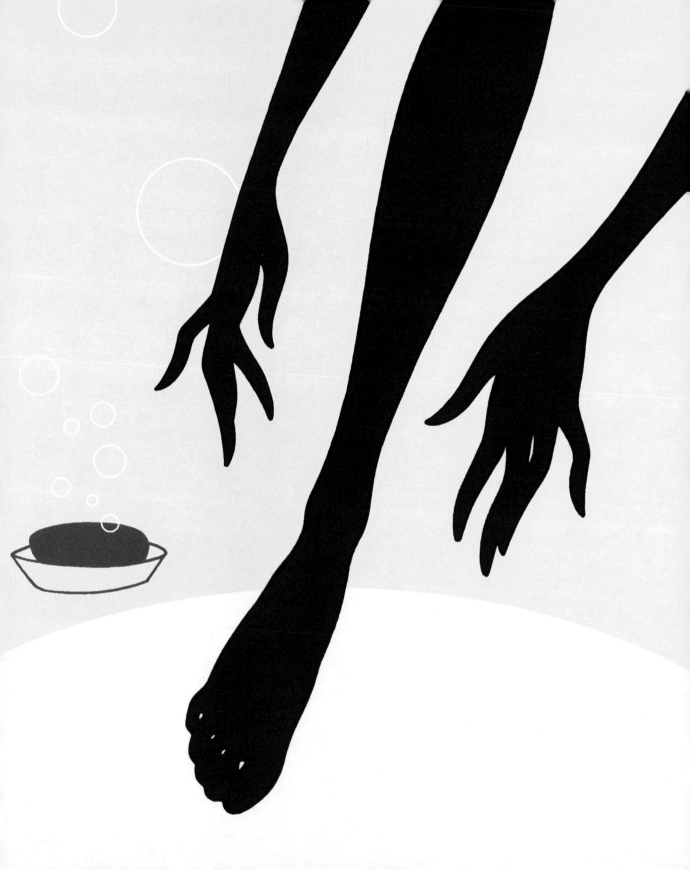

hands & feet

Hands have a history of their own, they have indeed, their own civilization, their special beauty; we concede to them the right to have their own development, their own wishes, feelings, moods, and favorite occupations.

—RAINER MARIA RILKE

Several years ago, I was introduced to Georgette Klinger at a luncheon in New York City. As we shook hands, hers slowly began to stroke mine. Just as I started to wonder what in the world she was doing, she peered out at me from under her wide-brimmed hat and quietly said, "My dear, you need a hand cream. Let's just make sure you get one—and use it, right away."

Ah well, everyone has her weakness, at least one beauty spot that's overlooked and under-cared for. For me, it's my hands. I hate using hand cream, because I can't stand to have my hands rendered useless, not even for a couple of minutes. I am a writer, a knitter, a toucher. My hands need the freedom to move, unencumbered by tacky, greasy cream, at all times.

But the hands need moisture, perhaps more than any other part of our body. It's especially difficult to keep the hands soft and smooth, because they are unprotected by clothing most of the time. The hands flutter around and gesture in the open air; they are exposed to harsh chemicals, dishwater, the sun's rays, and extremes of temperature; they stretch and wrinkle whenever they move, which is almost all the time. Unfortunately, a good hand cream is hard to find—but not impossible. Read on.

Caring for Your Hands

The hand—that appendage Aristotle called the "divine tool"—is masterfully designed, a brilliant feat of engineering efficiency in which tendons, muscles, nerves, veins, and arteries are jam-packed into an impossibly small space and covered with a glove of skin, fat, hair, and sweat glands. Each hand has 27 bones, with 19 muscles to control its movement and drive its power. Rich in touch receptors called "Meissner's corpuscles," the fingertips transmit exquisite sensations of pleasure and pain to the

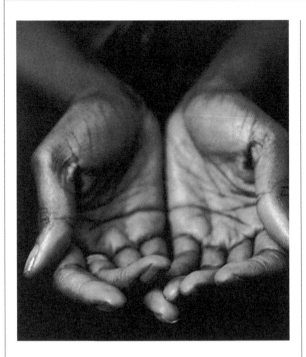

brain. The lubrication provided by sweaty palms and swollen fingertips actually improves our sense of touch. Yet, despite the fact that hands are so essential to human life, they have, apparently, a low biological priority: during winter, the blood flows away from the hands toward the vital organs.

As we age, especially around menopause, the skin on the back of our hands wrinkles and loses elasticity, just as it does on our face. The fatty layer below the epidermis thins, and the skin becomes more flaccid. When it's pinched, it just doesn't snap back as easily as it used to. The sebaceous glands slow down and produce less oil. (The hands have very few oil glands, which is why they get so dry in the first place.) Washing the hands also strips them of oil and dries them out. And American women, on average, wash their hands five times a day. In addition, the cumulative effects of sun exposure eventually yield a brown spot or two.

Hands-On Regimen

Just like the skin on your face or the hair on your head, your hands need a little extra-special attention if you want them to look good. The same basic principles that apply to caring for the rest of your skin apply here, too—but you'll need different products for the extra-dry skin on your hands, along with an occasional manicure.

1. Cleanse and exfoliate. Wash with a gentle glycerine or Castile soap and gently exfoliate, once or twice a week, with an oatmeal- or clay-based soap. If your hands are extremely dry, use a super-fatted soap.

2. Moisturize. Twice a day, and always after doing dishes or washing your hands, apply moisturizer. Hands that are dry, cracked, or chapped are not only uncomfortable but also

OUT, OUT, DAMN SPOT

AHAs can help get rid of brown spots, but the solutions need to be fairly strong—like those in a dermatologist's line, such as M.D. Formulations or Exuviance—and it doesn't happen overnight. Hydroquinone is another ingredient to look for, but you'll have to wait four months or so to see results. In the meantime, try Magic by Prescriptives Brown Neutralizer (a cosmetic concealer that rubs 'em out!). For other options—kojic acid, azelaic acid, Retin-A, and, of course, lasers—you should consult a dermatologist. Some of the best products are: Neutrogena New Hands (AHA and SPF), Esotérica Bleaching Cream, Estée Lauder Revelation Complex for Hands and Chest, Samuel Parr Whiter Skin Cream (hydroquinone).

more susceptible to infection: the skin is a protective covering, and when it's ruptured, bacteria can get through its tiny cracks.

Centuries ago, women wore emollient-saturated gloves to bed in order to keep their hands soft. The modern-day equivalent of this trick is an oil-doused glove, such as Spa Mani Moisture Restoring Gloves by Borghese. The idea works well, especially if your hands have become positively reptilian. Or, you can create your own intensive treatment: if your hands are dry, even to the point of cracking, pick up a balm (see pages 275–276) or a small bottle of sweet almond oil or wheat germ oil at the health food store. Massage it into your hands before you go to bed, and cover your hands with a pair of thin white cotton gloves (inexpensive versions can be found at a garden or art supply shop). The only drawback—and it can be a big one—is that it keeps your hands out of commission overnight.

3. Use sunscreen. Exposure to the sun accelerates aging on the hands as well as the face, which means wrinkling and brown spots (formerly known as "liver spots" or "age spots"). Brown spots most commonly appear on the hands and face. They are concentrations of melanin triggered by too much sun exposure over too long a period of time. Regular use of a good sunscreen—minimum SPF 15—will prevent brown spots over 90 percent of the time. So when you apply sunscreen to your face in the morning, make sure to put some on the backs of your hands, too.

4. Protect your hands. Wear rubber gloves when you clean with harsh detergents or wash

---

HANDS-DOWN BEST HAND CREAMS

★*Best Products*

The following products are good because they moisturize but are not greasy: Aveda Hand Relief, Bloom Care & Repair Hand Cream, Clarins Hand and Nail Treatment, Jurlique Hand Care Cream, Kiehl's Very Unusual Rich But Not Greasy Hand Cream, L'Occitane Hand Cream, Nivea Lotion, Penny Island Body Lotion, Shiseido Essential Energy Hand Cream, Tisserand Hand and Nail Cream, Vital Thymes Hand Care.

For really chapped hands—let's say you're a gardener—take a tip from the farmers. These cult favorites were farmers' friends first, and now you can find them in the drugstore: Bag Balm, Badger Balm, Burt's Bees Farmer's Friend Hand Salve, Cornhusker's Oil, Udder Balm.

---

dishes. Because heavy-duty rubber makes you sweat, which makes the skin dry and pruny, apply a thin layer of moisturizer before you put them on. Or wear latex gloves, which are thinner and easier to manipulate, though not as durable. When outdoors working in the yard, always wear gardening gloves.

Hands at Work

▓ Use armrests to reduce tension in the upper back, neck, forearms, and hands.

▓ Use equipment designed to reduce repetitive-motion injuries: a headset if you're on the phone a lot and wrist rests if you use a computer.

▓ Massage your hands to stimulate circulation (restricted circulation is a cause of carpal tunnel syndrome).

◼ Take one- to two-minute breaks away from the computer every 15 minutes to relieve cramping and tension.

◼ Avoid exposing unprotected hands to extremes of temperature or harsh chemicals for prolonged periods. If you must expose your hands, protect them with gloves.

◼ Keep a moisturizer on your desk and lubricate your hands often during the day.

Caring for Your Nails

Most mammals have claws, and humans are no exception. Our nails are designed to protect the fleshy fingertip and help us manipulate small objects. (But if your nails are three and a half inches long, you'll need a tweezer to remove your bank card from the cash machine!) Incredibly absorbent, nails can take in 20 to 25 percent of their weight in water. When they do, the keratin (the same protein that makes up hair and skin) swells and splits, which can cause the nail to become weak and brittle.

Although nails are actually dead tissue, they grow from a matrix of living flesh beneath what is called the nail bed, or the fold of skin at the base of the nail, at a rate of one-eighth inch per month. A complete nail grows in six months. As the cells push up from the fold, they harden and become keratin.

Nails grow constantly, but if you're right-handed, your nails grow faster on the right hand because the additional activity stimulates circulation. They also grow faster in warm-weather seasons and just before your period. Also, believe it or not, nail-biting actually stimulates nail growth. (Though it's not a good enough reason to do it!) And aging slows down the rate of nail growth.

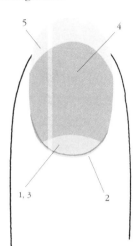

THUMBNAIL SKETCH

1. The matrix lies below the lunule (half-moon) and nourishes new growth.

2. The cuticle is the skin overlapping the nail, which acts as a protective layer against bacteria. It's not a good idea to trim the cuticle, because it can easily become infected. Instead, just push it back with an orangewood stick.

3. The lunule is the white, crescent-shaped area at the base of the nail that is commonly known as a half-moon. It's white because the matrix blocks out the pinkish, capillary-rich nail bed. The larger the half-moon, the faster your nails grow.

4. The nail plate, or fingernail, is a hard layer of keratin that covers the blood vessels and nerves below.

5. The free edge is the white bit that grows beyond the fingertip.

The Classic Manicure

A professional manicure, at $8 to $20, is a small luxury within reach for most of us. If you go often, I highly recommend investing in your own manicure kit and bringing it to each appointment (or have your manicurist keep it for you). It will protect against the risk of infection. Even though most manicurists sterilize

A DECORATIVE TOUCH

In the East, women paint their hands (and feet) with henna—an ancient art that originated in Egypt and spread through the Middle East, India, and Africa thousands of years ago—long before anyone had dreamed up nail polish or nail piercing.

Mehndi, the Indian name for this technique, means different things to different people, says Rabia Islamia, former owner of Allah's Sacred Earth, the company that first commercialized the practice in the United States and opened a string of studios around the country. In India, delicate floral designs are more aesthetic than symbolic. But in Arab and African cultures, certain symbols are said to protect the wearer from evil, symbolize compassion, or increase fertility.

"In America," says the Palestine-born Rabia, "some people want to know about the cultural uses of *mehndi.* But others simply want to feel like Cleopatra for a day." In any case, *mehndi* is trendy—especially after celebrities like Mira Sorvino, Demi Moore, Laurence Fishburne, and Erykah Badu went for it.

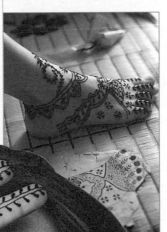

Depending on the intricacy of the design, an application can take 20 minutes or several hours. The stain fades after two to four weeks, but you can take it off sooner by exfoliating.

Henna designs range from simple geometric bands to highly elaborate scrolls, florals, vines, and paisleys. The henna is painted on with a pastry-bag-like cone or an instrument that resembles a toothpick, and the colors include orange, red, brown, khaki, and maroon.

their equipment between clients, it's possible, in a rushed or reckless moment, for that step to be overlooked and for you to fall victim to a pesky infection. Better to travel with your own tools!

At the Salon. The best manicure in New York City is a seat on the balcony at Henri Bendel with Grace Koniecko of the Garren Salon. Grace has perched up in her aerie since the salon opened in 1995. Unfortunately, the best manicure in New York is also one of the most expensive. But even though I don't go back every week, which is what Grace recommends ("the cuticle keeps growing, and you want to keep the nail's shape"), it's

become the standard by which I've measured all manicures since—even the ones I give myself at home (see facing page). It's state-of-the-art.

What is it about this manicure that makes it such a standout? Well, Grace files but doesn't cut the nails. She's an expert shaper. She is a gifted color adviser. She's fastidious, gentle, and methodical. Her table is quiet, sedate, relaxing. You don't feel like you're inhaling the contents of an 11th-grade chemistry lab. ("Those fumes aren't healthy," Grace says, "for you or for me.") And the view onto the heart of Fifth Avenue through Bendel's original Art Nouveau windows can't be beat.

Grace is not a talker; discretion is a good quality if you plan to keep Naomi Campbell and Linda Evangelista on your client roster. Grace's quiet expertise has endowed many fashionable Manhattan women—and cognoscenti—with beautiful hands.

Once I have been given my choice of beverage, Grace pulls out her wide file and gets down to work. After an initial shaping (square or oval), she soaks each hand, one at a time, in a finger bowl filled with warm, soapy water and tea tree oil (a natural disinfectant). In a few minutes, she lifts my hand out of the finger bowl, places it on a tissue, and gently blots it dry. Then she buffs the nails all over with a circular buffer. (A little extra elbow grease is needed on my thumbnails, where horizontal ridges need flattening.)

CUTICLE CURES

These top products keep the cuticles feeling soft and looking as good as possible. They're also a pleasure to use. FACE Stockholm Nail Food (sesame oil, lavender, and myrrh), Creative Nail Design Systems SolarOil (jojoba oil, Vitamin E, almond oil), Decléor Nail Treatment Oil. If you prefer a cream: Nailtiques Hand and Cuticle Cream, Kiehl's Cuticle Cream, Chanel Nail Repair Cream (shea butter), Christian Dior Crème Apricot Cuticle Softener, Burt's Bees Lemon Cuticle Cream, Avon Mira-Cuticle Vanishing Complex (AHA and apricot kernel oil), Barielle Nail Strengthener Cream, Clarins Jeunesse des Mains.

Or rub in a massage oil, the contents of a Vitamin E capsule, or some sweet almond oil around the cuticles.

Best Products

get a manicure

How To: give yourself a manicure

It's easy, of course, to follow the same steps described in the salon treatment at home, but you'll need a bit of practice to get your weaker hand up to speed.

1. Remove any old, leftover polish with cotton—it's the most absorbent fiber your money can buy. If you need to get into nooks and crannies to remove stubborn polish, use a Q-tip or an orangewood stick with a cotton-swathed tip soaked in nail polish remover.

2. File and shape your nails in one direction only, parallel to the nail bed, and don't curve into the corner of the nail. Use a soft-grade file (240 grit or higher) such as OPI Long Soft File, La Cross Smooth, or Kiss Professional Butterflies.

3. Massage a light cuticle oil or moisturizer into the nail and cuticle area for a minute or two. Then soak your fingers in warm, soapy water for about five minutes to soften the cuticles. (If you like, add a few drops of your favorite essential oil. It smells nice and it moisturizes.)

4. Gently push your cuticles back with the tip of an orangewood stick. You can also use a product called Hindostone, a pumice stone shaped like an orangewood stick, which is available at most drugstores. It works beautifully and, like pumice, lasts forever.

5. Rub your hands with moisturizer, then wipe your nails with a clean cloth to get rid of residual oils on the nail and get ready for the polish. (If there is still oil or lotion on your nail, the polish can bubble.)

6. Apply a base coat to help the polish adhere. Then apply your polish. One coat is fine, but if you do apply more, make sure to let each coat dry for a few minutes in between to prevent creasing.

7. If you're in a hurry, apply a fast-drying top coat. The only drawback is that the top coat makes the top layer of polish feel dry to the touch but doesn't necessarily speed the drying process underneath. If you make sure each coat is dry before you apply another, a fast-drying top coat will work like a charm.

She trims away dry, dead skin surrounding the nail (but *not* the cuticle!), then covers the tip of an orangewood stick with cotton and pushes my cuticles back. (The one step Grace skips, which you will find at most day spas, is a paraffin wax treatment; see page 321.)

At this point, Grace massages a cuticle cream into my skin, and the heavenly hand massage continues for a couple of minutes. Then we're back to business once again, with an application of a hardening treatment, which helps strengthen the nails long term.

FINGER TIPS

▨ File in one direction only: filing back and forth causes splitting and cracking.

▨ File your nails in a shape that mirrors the shape of the nail bed.

▨ Do not file into the corners of your nails; it weakens them and can make them break more easily.

▨ A metal file is more appropriate for picking locks than for filing nails—it's too hard. Stick with a resin-coated emery board.

▨ When going to a manicurist, don't put yourself at risk of infection from someone else's germs, bacteria, or fungus (nail fungus infections are highly contagious). Bring your own manicure kit with you, or leave it with your manicurist.

▨ Two coats of polish will deepen the color and won't chip as fast as one coat, especially if you put a dab over the tip of the nail onto the underside.

▨ After nail polish dries, soak your nails in ice water to speed up the hardening process.

▨ Even if the top layer appears dry, the lower layers may not be, and any kind of pressure to the nail (even gentle tapping to see if the polish is dry) can cause creases.

▨ Be patient and wait long enough to ensure your nails are dry before touching them. Because of the glue in nail polish, it can sometimes feel dry to the touch when it isn't. Artificial nails (specifically, acrylics and silks) take 3 to 5 minutes to dry; natural nails take 5 to 10.

Grace applies a coat of ridge filler to spackle in the peaks and gulleys that make up the topography of my thumbnails. Then, she swiftly and expertly applies a base coat followed by one to two coats of polish. She caps it off with a quick-drying top coat, which allows me to put my hands back into action in 2 to 3 minutes (although Grace says I should wait 5 to 10, "to be safe").

Treating yourself to a really top-notch, professional manicure once in a while is not only good for the hands, it's a boost for the ego. Your nails will look so swell, no one will believe they're real!

The Polish

Nail trends through the decades—just like hairstyles and fashions in clothing—provide a fascinating bit of social commentary. A hundred years ago, nail powder was made of tin oxide, fragrance, and carmine coloring, the same substances used to polish horns and tortoiseshell. When rubbed on the nail with a bit of chamois cloth, it created a pinkish color. During World War I, nail enamel as we know it was developed from automotive paint. Since then, neutrals and blood reds have been the most popular shades. But as long as your nails are clean, short, and neat, almost any color can look good.

Nail polish can range in price from

CLEARING THE AIR

No portion of the beauty business contains as many hazardous chemicals as the nail industry. Getting straightforward information about these chemicals isn't always easy, however. The labels don't tell you much, and it's hard to know what to look for. The list below red-flags some potentially hazardous ingredients to avoid:

Formaldehyde, a suspected carcinogen and common allergen, can cause your eyes to water, your nose to burn, and your skin to develop dermatitis. Look for "formaldehyde-free" on the label.

Acetone, a main ingredient in many nail polish removers, may cause nausea; ear, nose, and throat irritation; dizziness; and dermatitis. Look for polish remover labeled "non-acetone."

Acrylates are ingredients ending in "crylate." They can cause nose, throat, and eye irritation, dizziness, nausea, shortness of breath, and asthma.

Acetonitrile (aka methyl cyanide) is found in many artificial nail removers; it absorbs rapidly through the skin and is extremely toxic, especially for pregnant women because it can cause birth defects. Avoid it.

Fiberglass dust. When you file or grind wraps made of fiberglass, you inhale fiberglass dust. Even though it has very few fibers, don't breathe it in.

Toluene. A chemical in spray paint, rubber cement, airplane glue, gasoline, and nail enamel, toluene acts as a thinner in nail polish, making it spreadable. But, according to the California Environmental Protection Agency, excessive exposure at certain levels and under certain circumstances can cause birth defects, such as mental retardation or a syndrome called "toluene embryopathy," characterized by reduced fetal weight, small head size, and facial deformities.

Many cosmetics companies—Revlon, Avon, Maybelline, Christian Dior, Elizabeth Arden, and Cutex—have removed toluene from their polishes. Look for polishes with the label "toluene-free."

99 cents to $19. What you're paying for is the name-brand cachet or the stylishness of the product—there is very little difference in quality. For example, Hard Candy and Urban Decay, a pioneer in opalescent heavy-metal shades, are hot brands at the moment, and the colors are extremely fashionable, which is why they can charge high-end prices.

But for most of us, the drugstore is a great place to buy polish. Revlon and Maybelline are two of the best lines for inexpensive, quality products in trendy colors. When you're shopping for polish, there are basically two guiding principles: (1) choose colors you like, and (2) buy toluene-free products (see box, above).

The Nail File

Ever since the ancient Egyptians buffed their nails with chamois skin and stained them with henna, women have attracted attention—for better or worse—with their nails. These are the highlights over the last century.

1930s

Jean Harlow's bright red talons become the look both in and out of Hollywood. Joan Crawford's style (right) becomes a popular variation, in a deeper shade with tips and half-moons left white.

1940s

The style swings back to bright, bright red. The tips are now painted, but half-moons are still exposed.

1950s

Elongated oval-shaped nails match lips (and, sometimes, clothes), in forcedly feminine shades of fire-engine red and fuchsia.

1960s

Twiggy's frosted nails usher in an era of iridescent, opalescent, psychedelic shades of pale.

1970s

Mary Quant's lacquered black cherry (and shades like "Plum Rock") usher in the disco era. At the same time, the natural, no-polish look evolves into Barbra Streisand's signature beige or coral claws.

1980s

In the gilded age, some dig gold. Alternatively, short, squared, no-nonsense nudes, tailored and businesslike, match the pin-striped "power" suit.

1990s

Fin de siècle freedom starts with the French manicure: beige polish with an opaque white tip. The style shifts and Chanel's "Vamp" starts a mania for maroon. Nail decoration gets wild with studs, stencils, and appliqués on impossibly long nails.

2000s

Anything goes: blood red, black, yellow, green, baby blue. Iridescents are back.

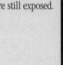

Although manicurists are obviously most at risk, if you do use polish with toluene, make sure you paint your nails in a well-ventilated space, not in an airplane cabin or subway car—it's not good for you and it's not fair to your fellow passengers. Avoid leaving the bottle open for long periods of time.

Artificial Nails

I'm not keen on artificial nails for two reasons. First, you can always spot them, just as you can easily spot a toupee. Second, the industrial-strength glues, sealants, adhesives, and chemicals involved not only can cause your real nails to suffer and leave them looking dry, cracked, and sickly but also can cause fungal infections. Once your nails start to look bad, you won't want to expose them, and then you're caught up in a cycle of acrylic addiction. Why not work on keeping your real nails strong and healthy instead? But if you must use them, here's what you need to know.

There are five types of artificial nails:

1. Wraps. These do the least damage. Made of fiberglass, linen, or silk, they're applied with a fabric mesh that is held in place by an adhesive. A sealant is put on top to make sure they stay in place.

2. Acrylics. Powder and liquid are mixed together to form a plastic paste. The paste is applied to the nail, where it hardens.

3. Porcelain. These are similar to acrylics, except that the powder contains a finely ground glasslike material.

4. Gels. Layers of resin are applied to the nail and harden when exposed to light.

NAIL CANDY

Whatever Dineh wants, Dineh gets—even if she has to make it herself. In 1995, 22-year-old premed student Dineh Mohajer launched what was to become a multimillion-dollar business. When she couldn't find a shade to match her baby blue sandals, Mohajer mixed up her own, using white polish, dye, and a bit of chemistry know-how. When she wore the polish, she was inundated with compliments, so she did what any good businesswoman would do: mixed up a batch, took it to Fred Segal in Los Angeles, and left the store with a huge order. And that's how she nailed her company, Hard Candy (sold in 1999 to Louis Vuitton Moët Hennessy), which kicked off a craze for bright, candy-colored shades ranging from lemon curd to lavender.

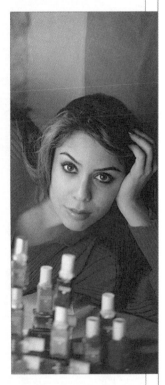

5. Tips. These plastic nail bits can cover the entire nail, but most often they're applied halfway up the nail through the tip. They're glued into place with nail glue. Acrylics, gels, or wraps are often added on top as an extra bolstering layer, then filed into shape.

Nail Kit

*If beauty is in the details, make
your well-manicured tips and toes divine.*

Although a professional manicure
or pedicure is one of life's simple
pleasures, it's easy enough to do it
yourself—with the right tools, of course. If
you have the time, give yourself the all-out
pampering treatment (see pages 299 and 307);
if not, at least keep 'em clipped and squeeze
in a quick coat of polish when you can.

The Essentials

**Natural-bristle
nailbrush.** *Nailbrushes
not only clean under
your nails but also
get rid of dead skin
around the cuticle,
which helps prevent
hangnails. Nylon-bristle
brushes are easier to
find, but the bristles
are too sharp. They
feel scratchy on the
skin and may scratch
your nails, too.*

Toothbrush. *If you
have soft nails, even
a natural-bristle
nailbrush may be too
rough. If so, scrub your
nails gently with a soft
toothbrush.*

Orangewood stick.
*This svelte wooden stick
is used to push back the
cuticle. It's been around
since Cleopatra dug her
claws into Mark Antony.*

Hindostone. *A pumice
stone shaped like an
orangewood stick; it
lasts forever, too.*

Circular buffer. *If
your nails are ridged,
this little baby will sand
them down and smooth
them out. Just don't
overdo it—once every
three to four weeks is
enough.*

Cotton washcloth.
*In a pinch, you can
use a washcloth on
wet, soapy hands to
push the cuticle back.*

Nail clippers. *Both
trim nails; fingernail
clippers cut on a curve
whereas toenail clippers
clip straight across and
help prevent ingrown
nails.*

Buff file. *Shapes your
nails. My favorite is a
four-sided cushioned
file, which is gentler
than your standard
cardboard version. Look
for a "micrograin" or
gem-dust coating, which
won't tear your nails.*

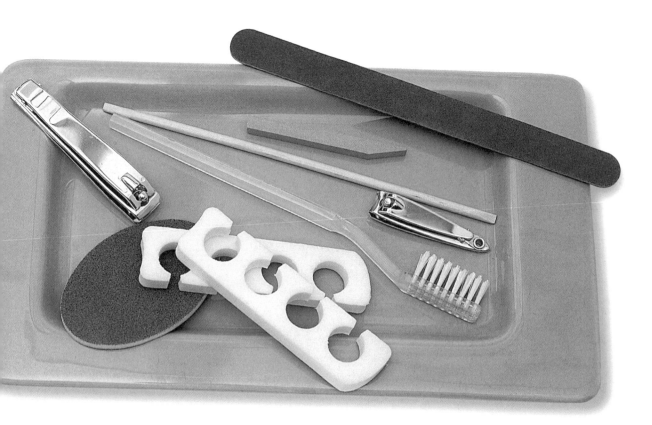

Emery board. *Use a medium-grit, resin-coated emery board, and make sure to get* *rid of it when it wears out because it will saw your nails to stumps.*

Pumice stone or lava rock; loofah or sloughing paddle. *Scrubs rough patches of dead skin and calluses from the balls and heels of the feet. Pumice (left) now comes in different grains that determine its use.*

Foam toe separator. *Ridiculous-looking apparatus for keeping toes away from each other while your polish dries.*

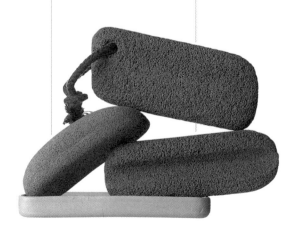

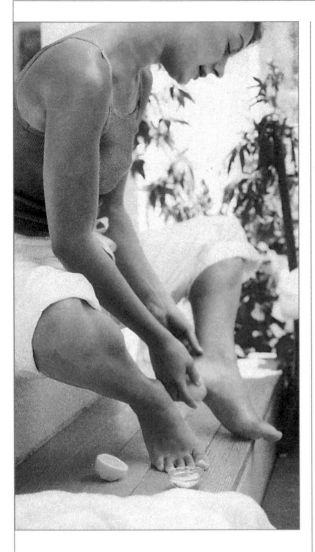

Feet

My grandfather was a podiatrist, and some of my strongest early memories involve feet. My brothers and I were sent to visit Harry, the salesman at Tru-Form shoes, several times a year; there we were fitted for "good shoes." Mine was a special case: my high arches were hard to fit, my toes were gnarled and twisted from years of ballet training, my skin was calloused and as thick as cowhide because I'd go barefoot any chance I got—I still do. My feet were far from beautiful, my shoes even less so, but I wore them while aching for a strappy sandal, a funky platform, the barest hint of a heel.

Most of us don't even want to think about our feet. We'd like our 10 little soldiers to line up straight in a row, take their marching orders, and not give us any trouble. In spite of the torture we inflict on them in high-heeled, closed-toe shoes, we want our smooth, unblemished beauties to put up, shut up, and look great in sandals. Like Cinderella's evil stepsisters, most women have had the experience of squeezing a size-8 foot into a 7½ shoe, or a 7½ into a size 6. But you can torture a foot only so long before it fights back. And the angrier it gets, the uglier it becomes, using bunions, corns, and calluses as its forms of revenge.

Since feet take so much abuse—absorbing the shock of tons of pressure from approximately 9,000 steps a day—it's really important to take good care of them or at least to show them a little love and respect once in a while.

The Classic Pedicure

Today you can tailor your toe treatments to any style you like, from "pampering" or "buff sports" pedicures to "aromatherapy" pedicures. Whatever style you choose, any good pedicure should cover the basics. It should slough off calloused skin, soothe the 7,000 nerve endings in each foot, and leave your nails trim and well groomed.

At the Salon. At the Claremont Spa in Berkeley, California, first my feet were soaked and softened in a silky, rose-petal-strewn footbath awash with fragrant essential oils and patted dry. Next, the pedicurist buffed my calluses and massaged my feet with an exfoliating slougher. She rubbed my feet with lotion and got to work clipping and filing my nails and pushing back my cuticles. Then she dipped my feet in hot paraffin wax to moisturize, soften, and exfoliate the skin.

After the paraffin hardened, she peeled it off, and then it was time for polish. It was summertime, and I was in the mood for white! When the polish dried, I was ready for my reflexology massage. (See page 308.)

Home Remedies and Recipes. Though not as luxurious, perhaps, as a spa pedicure, you can pamper your feet at home with soaks and scrubs. Here are my two favorite home remedies.

THE CITRUS SLOUGH

½ cup kosher or sea salt
Juice of ½ lemon
1–2 teaspoons olive oil

1. Mix all the ingredients together.
2. Massage into your feet.
3. Rinse with warm water. Pat dry.
4. Moisturize.

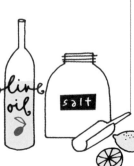

How To: pamper your pods

1. Remove old polish with cotton and clip the toenails straight across using nail clippers. To shape and smooth, file nails straight, in one direction, with an emery board. Use the shape at the nail bed as a guide for shaping the tip. (Don't trim the edges of your nails with the clipper. This can result in ingrown toenails.)

2. Fill a basin with warm water. Throw in a scoop of bath salts, kosher salt, or Epsom salts and a few drops of your favorite essential oil or bath oil. Soak your feet for 8 to 10 minutes.

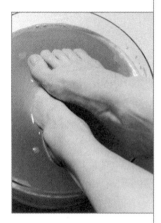

3. Apply an exfoliating body scrub or foot sloughing cream to a sloughing paddle, loofah, or wet pumice stone and scrub rough patches on the balls and heels of the feet. Use a nailbrush to scrub around and under the toenails. Rinse your feet.

4. Massage your feet with moisturizer or cuticle oil and use an orangewood stick or a Hindostone to gently push back the cuticles and dry skin. Trim any hangnails with a clipper.

5. Wash feet with soap and water to prepare for polish. Separate your toes with a foam separator so your polish won't smear. Apply your base coat, then apply polish. Let dry for 5 minutes.

Reflexology

True believers say the foot is the road map to the rest of the body.

Unlike other types of massage—Swedish, shiatsu—that are widely accepted as having therapeutic value, reflexology is a relatively unknown and misunderstood technique. Put simply, reflexology is a foot massage that can relax and rejuvenate the entire body. But even Elizabeth Willoughby, founder and director of Manhattan's Universal Reflexology Systems, agrees that "the idea lends itself to skepticism because there's no proven scientific evidence to explain how it works."

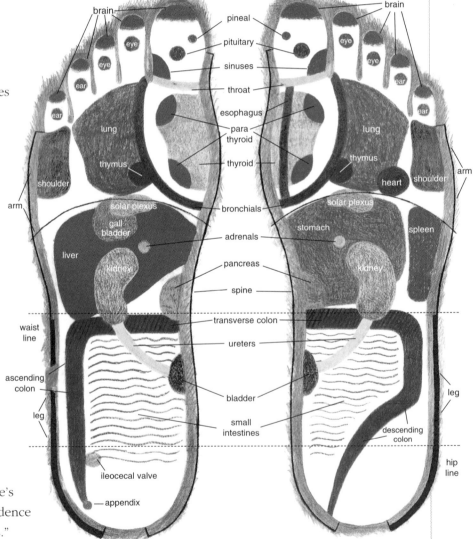

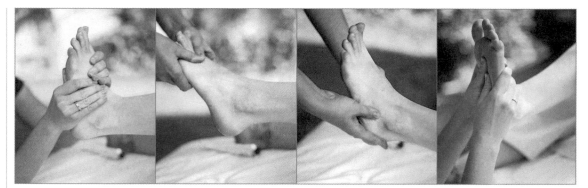

Reflexology is done on bare, not stockinged, feet; the practitioner uses a dab of cream or massage oil for softer skin.

Gently stretching the toes and rotating them in both directions loosens the toe joints.

Ankles are rocked from side to side then stretched forward to relieve tension in the lower back.

When the thumb is pressed deeply into the solar plexus point (the body's nerve center), it releases stress everywhere.

The results, based on client-practitioner experience, are strictly anecdotal. However, those anecdotal reports are pretty convincing, and I'll lend my voice to the throng singing reflexology's praises.

Like acupressure, reflexology is based on the idea that specific points in the body can be stimulated to relieve stress. But while acupressure points are located throughout the entire body (for instance, if you squeeze your inner eyebrows between thumb and forefinger, it can help relieve a tension headache), the reflexology pressure points are restricted primarily to the soles of your feet. The curves in the foot are viewed as a mirror of the curves in the spine.

Particular points on your feet correspond to different parts of the body—vital organs, muscular and skeletal structures, the glandular system—and they're connected by "a kind of nervous system which is accessed through the circulatory system," according to Willoughby. Tenderness in any particular spot on the foot, she says, may indicate "an energy imbalance in the corresponding part of the body."

According to practitioners, by massaging these points in the feet, you not only relieve tension throughout the body by stimulating an energy flow that the Chinese call *chi* but you also rid the body of toxins. The massage technique is similar to that used in acupressure, but the pressure is lighter.

The feet are the most abused part of the body. But a little therapeutic touch can go a long way. "If you use a favorite lotion or oil and give yourself a 30-second massage on each foot every night before going to bed," says Willoughby, "it will not only soften the skin, it can relax the entire body for sleep."

If you feel more ambitious, try massaging specific trigger points, using the diagram on the facing page.

THE PEPPERMINT PICK-ME-UP SOAK

A few sprigs of peppermint
A few drops of sweet almond oil

1. Combine peppermint with 1 cup water and bring to a boil. Remove from heat and let steep for 5 minutes.
2. Fill a foot basin with warm water.
3. Pour in the peppermint infusion, along with the sweet almond oil.
4. Soak for 10 minutes.

Foot Massage

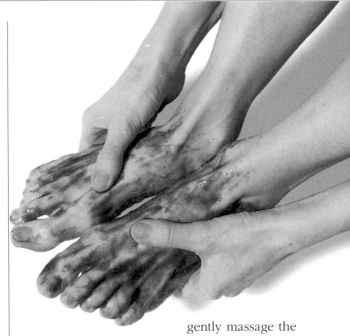

If you can perch yourself on the edge of your bathtub and bend at the waist, you can give yourself a pedicure. And if you really feel like being good to yourself, start with a foot massage.

Working one foot at a time, circle each foot around at the ankle, first in one direction, then in the reverse. Flex each foot up and down, then side to side. Curl your toes up tight into a ball, then stretch them as far apart as you can. Apply your favorite body lotion, massage cream, or foot massage lotion to each hand, then take your foot in both hands and

gently massage the lotion all over the foot and between the toes. Massage into the toenail cuticles and individually massage and rotate each toe.

With your thumb on top and your fingers underneath the arch, stroke the foot, working from the ankle toward the toes. Press and pinch along the arch and side of the foot, kneading with your thumbs and fingers. On the bottom of the foot, rotate your thumbs in rounds from the back of the heel down to the base of the toes. Gently massage down the side of each toe. Wiggle your toes gently, and shake out your hands.

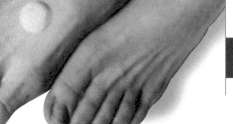

If you're pregnant, use acupressure cautiously, especially on the feet. There are pressure points on the foot that can stimulate contractions of the uterus.

warning

OH, MY ACHIN' FEET: BEST SOAKS, SLOUGHERS, AND SOFTENERS

Foot soaks feel great when your feet are achy, and they also soften the skin. Peppermint, ginger, and rosemary are the ingredients to look for: they feel tingly and stimulate circulation. When massaged into the feet, they seem to invigorate the pods, and make you feel as if you've got an extra spring in your step.

Soaks: Soak in a basin of warm water mixed with one of these products for about 8 to 10 minutes: Essentiel Elements Rosemary Bath Salts, Kniepp Bath Oils, Molton Brown Seamoss Stress Relieving Soak Therapy, Origins Ginger Salts.

Sloughers: Foot scrubs not only exfoliate feet but massage them as well. Try Bliss Scrub Super Slough, Dr. Scholl's Pedicure Essentials Salt Scrub for Feet and Legs (Dead Sea salt and olive oil), Philosophy Footnotes (pumice scrub). These body scrubs also work well as foot sloughers: Bare Escentuals Liquid Loofah, Bloom Exfoliating Body Scrub (with peppermint), Origins Ginger Body Scrub.

Softeners: Of course you don't need a special cream for your feet—your body lotion will do quite nicely. But if your feet are especially gnarly and callused, try Sally Hansen Retinol and Tea Tree Oil Foot Creme or Orjene Alpha Foot Soothing Treatment (both are available at health food stores).

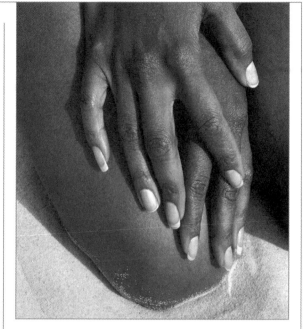

Healthy Nails

Most of us may not think of our hands and feet as key to our overall beauty. But without these frequently looked at but overlooked parts of our bodies, we would not be able to perform the everyday motions of our lives, so surely they deserve a little extra care on a regular basis. When we neglect them it shows, and when they're well cared for, we don't particularly notice them—which is as it should be.

Applying extra coats of polish or hardening treatments on top of the nails will protect them from breaking, but real strengthening has to come from within. Gelatin was the recommended miracle cure for weak nails in the old days. But if you eat a healthy diet, get enough vitamins and minerals—particularly A, C, E, F, K, biotin, iodine, selenium, and zinc—and don't abuse artificial nail products, your nails should be as strong as an eagle's talons.

rona's nail remedies

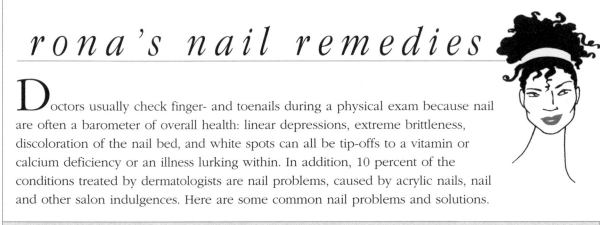

Doctors usually check finger- and toenails during a physical exam because nail
are often a barometer of overall health: linear depressions, extreme brittleness,
discoloration of the nail bed, and white spots can all be tip-offs to a vitamin or
calcium deficiency or an illness lurking within. In addition, 10 percent of the
conditions treated by dermatologists are nail problems, caused by acrylic nails, nail
and other salon indulgences. Here are some common nail problems and solutions.

PROBLEM	CAUSES	SOLUTIONS
RIDGES	*heredity*	■ Buff with a ridge sander and cream; apply ridge filler.
	damaged nail bed	■ Don't pick your cuticles, and don't jab too hard with the orangewood stick.
	frenzied manicuring	■ Be gentle.
	poor nutrition	■ Eat healthfully, and take your vitamins (see pages 16–17).
	anemia	■ If ridges are new, see your doctor. You may not be getting enough iron.
YELLOW NAILS	*fungal infection (onchomycosis)*	■ Use Dr. Scholl's over-the-counter fungal medication. ■ Soak a cotton ball in 3 percent hydrogen peroxide and dab around the nails several times a day. ■ Massage Vicks VapoRub into the nail before bed. Cover with cotton gloves (or socks). Repeat for 10 days. ■ If it doesn't clear up, see a doctor. Left untreated, the nail can separate from the nail bed. You may need a prescription antifungal medicine.
	chemicals in self-tanners, hair dye, or harsh cleansers	■ Use a hydrogen peroxide nail-bleaching product. ■ Wear rubber gloves or latex gloves when handling hair dye and harsh cleansers.
	nicotine stains	■ Stop smoking.
	top coats (most contain nitrocellulose, which turns yellow over time)	■ Give your nails a breather every once in a while—no polish, no top coat.
	heart or lung disease	■ If your nails turn yellow while you are in your 40s or 50s and none of the other causes apply, see a doctor.
HANGNAILS	*nail biting and picking*	■ Leave your hands alone! ■ Apply lavender oil or tea tree oil to the site as a softener and a deterrent.
	lack of care	■ Massage apricot oil, wheat germ oil, or cuticle cream to soften each day, then push back with an orangewood stick.

PROBLEM	CAUSES	SOLUTIONS
WEAK, BRITTLE NAILS	*overexposure to water*	■ Wear rubber or latex gloves.
	overuse of nail hardeners	■ Avoid hardeners with formaldehyde, which dries out the nails.
	yo-yo dieting	■ Eat a sensible, well-balanced diet.
	sun exposure	■ Use sunscreen on your hands *and* nails.
DRY, SPLITTING, PEELING NAILS	*peeling artificial nails*	■ When you peel the artifical nail, you can accidentally peel the real one, too, and make a big mess. Don't play with your nails, real or fake.
	filing wet nails	■ Wait until nails are dry, then file.
	using a too-hard file	■ Use a soft-grade (240 grit or higher) file.
	harsh chemicals in polish and polish remover	■ Stick with acetone-free polish remover and toluene-free, formaldehyde-free polish and polish removers.
	frequent use of antibacterial soap	■ Use antibacterial soap sparingly, and moisturize hands regularly.
WHITE SPOTS	*poking under the cuticle with sharp manicure tools*	■ Don't worry, the spots will disappear in time, but be gentle, and stop poking.
	poor nutrition	■ Eat healthfully, and take your vitamins.
HARD CUTICLES	*neglect*	■ Rub a balm or cuticle cream around the nail daily. ■ Push softened cuticles back twice weekly with an orangewood stick.
PITTED NAILS	*poor nutrition, psoriasis, smoking*	■ See a doctor.
PALE NAIL BED	*anemia*	■ Take iron supplements. ■ See a doctor.
DISCOLORED, THICKENED, CRUMBLING NAILS	*applying polish to damp nails*	■ Make sure your nails are dry before you apply anything.
	fungal infection caused when water seeps between a real and artificial nail	■ Give up the fakes until healed. See "fungal infection" above.
TORN NAILS	*daily wear and tear*	■ Cut a piece of tea bag large enough to cover the tip of the nail and extend a bit. Apply clear polish on top of the "patch," and to the nail. Tuck the ends under the nail tip. Apply another coat, then apply your color polish.

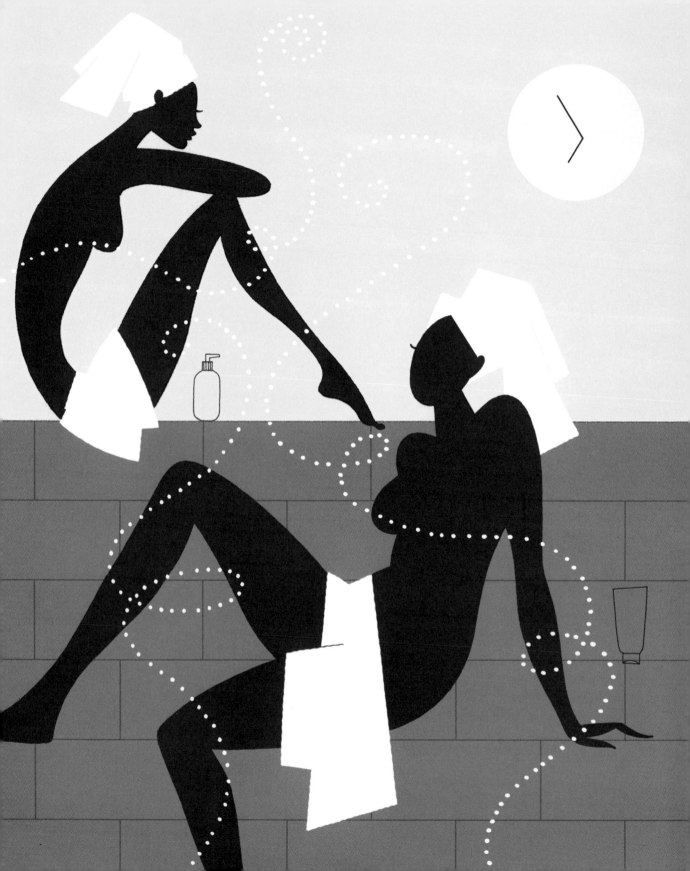

the spa

Luxury has been wrongly associated with the unattainable.

—ANDRÉE PUTMAN, *French interior designer*

At the Green Valley Spa in St. George, Utah, after a glorious morning hike through red rock canyons, I spend the rest of the day at the Relaxation Center, a soothing lair where guests de-stress as they drift from one spa treatment to another.

My afternoon of rubs, scrubs, and wraps is preceded by an Aromatic Jacuzzi Bath. For this "bath of baths," as guests call it, I am spirited into a room that looks like a scene from *A Midsummer Night's Dream.* The huge tub—surrounded by orchids, climbing vines, and a lush thicket of more exotic flora—is the size of your typical studio apartment. Scented candles flicker from the tub's wide ledge, and huge geode crystals sparkle from the forest surround. My spa attendant flicks on the bath jets and sprinkles the water with glistening oils and salts that sparkle like fairy dust. "Inhale," she says, "and relax."

"Taking the waters," or going to a spa, is a cherished European tradition that American women are beginning to appreciate, too. In Italy, trips to the *terme* (hot springs) are considered so essential to your health that these cures are often paid for by the state. In France, thermal healing is taught as a course in medical school, and the French government subsidizes spa treatments for specific ailments. According to Hannelore Leavy, executive director of Club Spa, USA, "The difference between spa culture in Europe and the United States is that in Europe spas emphasize good health, prevention of illness, and convalescence, whereas in the United States spas are heavily skewed toward beauty and fitness. But slowly the two are coming together. Europeans are exercising more, and Americans have become more interested in holistic healing."

The few spas that existed in the United States before the 1980s were either "fat farms," where a Spartan diet and rigorous exercise were de rigueur, or self-indulgent oases for the

A TASTE OF SPA

Many upscale hotel chains like the Ritz have built spas on their premises, which is an easy way to get a taste of the spa life while you're staying there on other business. A resort "spa" used to mean a few treatment rooms thrown onto the back of a hotel gym, but many of these are now state-of-the-art because they're so appealing to stressed-out, time-starved business and leisure travelers.

super-rich. Today the pleasures of hydrotherapy, hot springs, mud baths, thalassotherapy, herbal wraps, massage, and salt rubs are working their way into our holistic pursuit of good health while also appealing to our hedonistic pursuit of pleasure.

Since many of us can't afford the time or money for a typical weeklong spa vacation, day spas now offer a popular alternative—a way to de-stress in small doses. In fact, day spas are popping up everywhere, with more than 1,600 opening in 1999 alone. The spa industry is now a $14.2 billion industry, and 80 percent of that revenue comes from day spas. "Everybody's overstressed, plugged into their computers, as far away from human touch as possible," says Mary Bemis, editor in chief of *American Spa* magazine, "but it's something we all need."

A spa can restore your sense of balance and inner peace, give you take-home techniques to cope with daily stress, teach you about good nutrition, and jump-start a weight-loss or exercise program. Whether you can get away for a week, a day, or a few hours, the therapeutic benefits of a spa will make it well worth your while. This chapter will help you sort out the good from the bad and let you know what you can expect both from treatments and staff. For an annotated list of some of the best spas throughout the country, see pages 361–374.

Destination Spas

The "destination spa" is a lot like a resort; it's oriented toward an extended stay ranging from three days to a week. When you're choosing a destination spa, the first things to consider are price and locale. Prices range from $1,000 to $2,000 for a no-frills week at the Heartland or New Age Spa to $5,000 for a week of being pampered like a pasha at Canyon Ranch or the Golden Door. (Many spas also offer three- or four-day packages.)

If air travel must be factored into the price, make sure the locale is an integral part of the

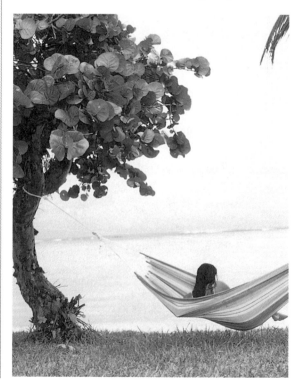

program and really enhances the experience, because if you're simply going to end up sweating indoors, you can do that anywhere. Some spa treatments play up special geographical elements like hot mineral springs or mud baths. You're likely to find seaweed and seawater treatments (thalassotherapy) in coastal regions and mud wraps in the desert. It's no surprise that California—where many treatments are enjoyed out of doors—has the most varied and trendy spa menu of any state.

Next, think about what you want to get out of a spa experience. Remember, just because a spa is top rated, it may not be the top choice for you. Some spas specialize in weight loss, some in outdoor adventure and fitness; others are more geared to pampering, beauty, and relaxation, while some have a New Age focus on wellness and spiritual rejuvenation.

Good Spa Hunting

The best recommendation, as with most things, is word of mouth from a satisfied friend, colleague, or acquaintance, but you can search for both destination and day spas by clicking onto www.spa.com and www.experiencespa.com, both highly reputable, well-researched Internet sites. Or call Spa Finders (800-255-7727), a travel agency for destination spas, which also publishes a *Spa Directory*. Club Spa USA, the Day Spa Association, will send a free directory of day spas in your area: www.clubspausa.com.

The word *spa* originated from a town in Belgium named Spa, which is known for its—guess what?—mineral springs.

For spas in Canada, click on www. spacanada.com. There are many beautiful spas up north, and the American dollar goes a long way. Or click on www.about.com, and search under "travel" and "spas." You'll find a comprehensive annotated listing by state.

If there's a particular bodycare product you love, you might start by finding out which spas use it. Call the company's toll-free number for the names of day spas in your area that use its products in their treatments. (If it's a quality product, chances are the training level of the spa staff will be, too.)

Before You Go

Some destination spas are laid back, while others resemble military academies that whip you into shape starting at the crack of dawn. You'll find evening activities at some, "lights out" at others. The food also varies tremendously, from delicious spa cuisine to the Spartan, tofu-toting, calorie-counting variety. To avoid unpleasant surprises, ask for a few sample menus ahead of time. A spa vacation is expensive; for the best possible fit—and to get your money's worth—you need to do some homework and find out as much as possible before you choose. Here are some questions you should ask.

What's included? Most spas offer packages that include room, meals, unlimited classes and lectures, use of spa facilities, and a schedule of treatments by specialists. Find out how many treatments are included and how much any extras will cost. It's smart to budget in extras like massages or a pedicure, because chances are you'll want them once you're there.

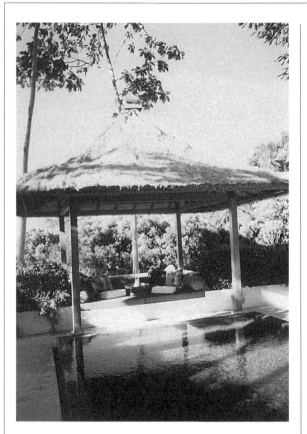

Must I book my treatments in advance?
Some spas set up orientation meetings with a staff member to book appointments when guests arrive; others prebook. If prebooking is necessary but you don't know what you want, ask the spa director for help.

When you book your spa treatments, it's important to consider not only which ones to have, but in what order. For example, hydrotherapy is terrific *before* a massage because it loosens the muscles, whereas a sauna or steam after a facial or aromatherapy treatment can irritate the skin.

What special programs are offered? For example, weight loss, healthy heart, smoke enders? Are different levels of activity available —beginner, intermediate, advanced? Can the spa put together a special program for you? Do they offer stress management through yoga and meditation? Individual fitness assessments? Are these included in the price?

What is the spa's food philosophy? Does it offer a vegetarian menu? Is it dairy-free? Is produce grown on the spa grounds? Does the menu include calorie ratings or fat content? Are there restrictions on alcohol, caffeine, sugar? What's available for snacking? Ask the spa to fax or e-mail you a sample menu. Find out whether the spa publishes a cookbook: it's often a good indication that food is a major focus. If it does, flip through it in your local bookstore.

What should I bring? Some spas issue sweat suits, like camp uniforms, to all guests. Some send a list of what to bring. Others attract a more fashion-conscious clientele. Ask whether guests dress for dinner and whether any special equipment is needed.

What facilities are available? How late are they open? Is the gym state of the art, and are there physical trainers present to show you the ropes and make sure you're using the equipment safely and efficiently? Is weight training offered? Is there a beauty salon? Are there aerobic and yoga classes? Is the spa up to speed on trendy classes you may find interesting? Can you take a midnight soak in the hot tub if you like?

Are there evening events like lectures, guest speakers, or cooking demonstrations? Find out what events are scheduled during the time of your stay and whether you'll need to reserve a spot in advance.

Day Spas

A "day spa" is a smaller facility, usually located near your home, where you can go for a day, a half day, or a single treatment. Day spas are becoming popular alternatives to "stay spas" because, let's face it, it's much easier—and more affordable— to go for a day (or an hour) than to get away for an entire week. Most independent, freestanding day spas are run by cosmetologists, fitness instructors, massage therapists, even hairstylists, who, ideally, have experience in the spa industry.

A spa is only as good as its director, who is responsible for hiring a qualified staff and overseeing training programs. Before you book an appointment, call and speak with the spa director. Ask about the spa's specialties, what types of products are used, whether it's best to take your treatments in any particular order. Make sure that he or she is courteous, informative—and accessible.

A good spa should include the following basics: private rooms for each client receiving treatments; a range of types of massage, including at least Swedish, shiatsu, and reflexology; and a range of treatments, including wraps and body polishes, hydrotherapy, facials, waxing, manicure and pedicure; cleanliness; and a fully licensed, experienced staff.

Spa Treatments

Over the centuries, the great European spas—from Montecatini to Wiesbaden— were built near the sea or near a mineral spring to cure the tired, ailing throng with "the waters."

Thalassotherapy (the use of seawater as a curative) began in France, where coastal spas pump in water directly from the sea, so that spa-goers can benefit from the therapeutic properties of the minerals. Inland spas in Europe and the United States take advantage of the health benefits of nearby mineral hot springs and lakes. The idea is the same: the therapeutic use of water—or hydrotherapy.

Hydrotherapy

In spa-speak, "hydrotherapy" refers to a deep-reaching muscle massage that takes place in an oversized tub with lots of clinical-looking knobs, hoses, and attachments. The tub is outfitted with powerful side jets and a hose (water wand) that

> **Red Alert**
>
> Both saunas and steam rooms can cause broken capillaries in the face. Before you sit in either—and especially if you go back and forth between extremes of temperature—protect your face with a light layer of moisturizer. After an aromatherapy massage or facial, avoid the sauna or steam heat for at least an hour. The mix of intense heat and essential oils can inflame the skin.

A Day in the Life of a Spa-Goer

*Here's a page torn from a spa diary—
it's typical of what you'll get at a full-service spa.*

If you've never been to a spa before, this will give you an idea of what to expect. Of course, the typical day depends on what you want, what your goals are, and how much you want to pack into your spa experience.

The road to a spa is paved with good intentions, and exercise is usually an important piece of the pavement. Some spa-goers feel compelled to try everything and end up dizzily careening from one intense aerobic workout to the next, which only leads to burnout. Don't try to do too much all at once.

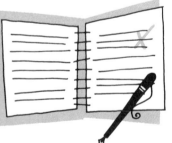

Pace yourself, and try to balance your agenda. A leisurely stretch in the morning will ease you into the day. After breakfast, you'll be ready for more vigorous activity. The overall plan that works best for most: exercise in the A.M., pampering in the P.M. Here's a typical day at a spa.

THE SCHEDULE

6:30 A.M. RISE AND SHINE. *Wrestle with the coffeemaker. Stare out the window, mug in hand, admire the always gorgeous view. (It seems as if you never face a parking lot at a spa. If you do, complain about it.)*

7:00 STRETCH CLASS. *Get the body moving, loosen the kinks, relax your mind.*

8:00 BREAKFAST. *Squeeze in as many food groups as possible—fruit, cereal, muffin, more fruit for the trail— and fuel up for an active morning.*

8:30 INTERMEDIATE-LEVEL NATURE HIKE. *Pick up the pace, and be sure to drink water on the trail. Get your heart rate up, and take big gulps of fresh air.*

10:30 AQUACIZE CLASS. *Think Esther Williams with a disco beat. Aerobic exercise in the pool, where you are weightless, has less impact on your joints. Afterward, pop into the steam room or Jacuzzi.*

12:00 LUNCH. *Main meal of the day. Ideally, there's a delicious range of food, accompanied by jugfuls of herbal tea. You're not too hungry, thanks to a healthy* breakfast and lots of activity. Remember: the more you move, the less you eat.

1:00 P.M. AROMATHERAPY FACIAL with neck and shoulder massage.

2:30 HERBAL BODY WRAP. Time to shed the snakeskin. First, drink a cup of herbal "detox" tea. Then the aesthetician mixes a blend of dried herbs with oil and massages it into the body from the neck down. Next, you're wrapped in warm, herb-infused towels, covered with blankets, and left to marinate like poultry. The herbs stimulate the circulation, exfoliate and detox the skin, and leave you feeling softly tenderized.

3:30 HYDROTHERAPY TREATMENT. Into the hydrotherapy tub, where the hydrojets untangle knotted muscles, as directed by the massage therapist. Submersed in water, the deep-tissue massage can go much deeper into the muscles, but it feels gentler than regular massage, because the water cushions the blow.

4:30 HOT PARAFFIN MANICURE AND PEDICURE starts with a relaxing reflexology massage. Then each hand and foot is dipped into a small tub of hot wax, which feels surprisingly good, and set out to dry for a few minutes. Next an attendant expertly peels the wax mitts from your hands and feet, taking all flaky bits of dry, loose skin with them. The manicure and pedicure that follow leave you free to gesticulate with prideful abandon and prance in open-toe sandals.

5:30. YOGA OR TAI CHI CLASS. This is a nice way to wind down the day. Yoga and tai chi are especially appealing because they not only provide a physical benefit but also relax the mind. The yoga class begins with 10 minutes of focused breathing through the nose (pranayama). Then you move through a series of postures that stretch the body, strengthen and firm the buttocks, torso, and limbs, and relax the neck and shoulders. The hour ends with a deep relaxation exercise to quiet the mind.

6:30 DINNER. Hearty, low-fat, healthy food with lots of vegetables. The fiber fills you up and satisfies your appetite without the calories, but make sure to get your protein. By dinnertime everyone is so "spa-brained" that dinner conversation is less than stimulating, but nobody cares because they feel so relaxed.

7:30 Choice of a lecture on relaxation techniques, a film, or organized games. Skip it and join new friends in the outdoor Jacuzzi. You consider following the warm Jacuzzi with a hot-and-cold plunge but decide against this stimulant because it's almost spa bedtime!

8:30 SWEDISH MASSAGE. What a delicious thing to do before bed. Heaven!

10:00 BEDTIME. Another cup of decaf herbal tea. Sweet dreams!

green tea

After a week of lavishing such total attention on yourself, you'll feel completely renewed (and a bit narcissistic), your skin will be preternaturally silky, and you'll have lots of energy from the fresh air and outdoor exercise. Vow to devote a small chunk of quiet time to yourself every day after you return to your routine, and see if you can bring a little bit of the spa back home with you.

the hydrotherapist (a massage therapist trained to use the hydrotub) uses to direct water toward your body's sore spots as you lie submersed in warm, frothy water.

At a spa, hydrotherapy tubs are usually located in the center of a small, tiled room with a large drain in the middle of the floor (like a French bathroom), which makes it easy for the water to wash away. At Canyon Ranch Spa in Lenox, Massachussetts, the two hydrotherapy tubs each have more than 30 jets and a giant high-pressure water wand. After the water jets have churned the water into froth, you get in, lie back, and rest on a water pillow. "The bath relaxes you physiologically," says Raya Buckley, a hydrotherapist at Canyon Ranch. "Your muscles are supported in water," she continues, "and they relax as soon as you get in." Then the hydrotherapist uses a handheld water wand to massage your entire body. Because the force of the water from the wand is so strong (although it doesn't feel that way), it can penetrate much deeper into the muscles than a more traditional massage.

"The water wand gets in around ligaments and bones, and it's great for joints," says Buckley. "It's a stimulating massage that helps muscles recover from the by-products of exercise."

THE PATHWAY TO BLISS: TREATMENT TIPS

Here are some simple tips to help you get the most out of your spa treatments.

Get there early. Rushing toward relaxation definitely won't enhance your spa experience. Arrive 10 to 15 minutes early, so you'll have time to change, sip a cup of tea, take a deep breath. If you're late, the time may be taken out of your treatment.

Go to the bathroom first. It's hard to relax into your massage or body rub when your bladder's about to burst.

Speak up. If you can't stand the smell of a massage oil or if the facial hurts, say so. Or if you have an oil that you love and want the massage therapist to use it, ask for it. Also tell your practitioner if you wear contact lenses, if your skin is sensitive, or if you have any special aches or pains.

Modesty is allowed. If you'd prefer to leave your underpants on during a massage, that's fine. It's a reasonable request, and, believe me, you're not the first to make it. Also, if you prefer a female to a male therapist, let the spa know in advance so it can accommodate you.

Linger afterward. When your masseuse tells you to take your time getting up, take her at her word. It's fine to lie there for a couple of minutes, stretch out, and absorb the good feeling. Drink lots of water.

Use of steam or sauna. Some spas make these perks available to clients before or after treatments. (If you're having a facial or body exfoliating treatment, hit the steam room *before* your treatment. Afterward, it can irritate the skin.)

Tipping. The expected tip for your spa facialist, massage therapist, manicurist, and so on ranges from 15 to 20 percent, which you can leave at the desk.

Hot and cold plunge. Scandinavians originated the use of the sauna, or dry heat, followed by an icy tumble in the snow. This combination of hot and cold is the best way to jazz up your circulation and energize and ultimately warm up your body. If you can stand it, alternating between hot (Jacuzzi or steam) and cold (plunge bath) can make you feel incredibly energetic in a brief period of time. In the gym, sit in the steam room or sauna, take a cold shower, go back to the steam or sauna, then return to the cold shower. Adapt this idea at home by taking a hot shower followed by a quick, 30-second burst of water as cold as you can stand it. Repeat. You won't believe how zippy you'll feel.

Stone Therapy

In the early 1990s, an American massage therapist named Mary Hannigan originated a massage technique incorporating the use of heated stones into a Swedish-style massage that she called La Stone Therapy. Since then, the use of stones in massage has become popular across

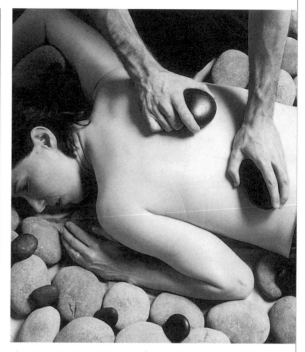

A warm stone massage relies on heat and subtle pressure to relax muscles and uncoil the kinks.

the country, and many massage therapists have adapted their own techniques using stones as massage tools.

At the Stone Spa in New York City and Los Angeles, co-owner Carla Ciuffo considers her stone massage a form of hydrotherapy, because "the stones apply warm, moist heat to the body." Ciuffo first heats up between 25 and 50 smooth basalt river rocks in 150-degree water and then uses them along with her hands and massage oil for a deep muscle massage. The combination of weight and heat not only feels incredibly soothing but is really grounding as well. "The foundation of massage," says Ciuffo, "is to give a boost to the circulatory system, encouraging the lymph to move and release metabolic waste through the blood. When you apply heat with the stones, you speed up that process."

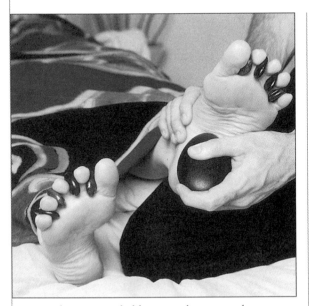

Heated stones nestled between the toes and massaged into the soles of the feet offer therapeutic benefits and bliss.

In addition, the stones, in their natural form, come in all different sizes that work into various nooks and crannies of the body. "They nestle into the palms of the hands or fit perfectly between the toes, and they're very comforting," says Ciuffo. "We all have a really childlike attraction to stones."

Wraps and Rubs

The best time to have a wrap or rub is at the change of season—winter to spring, summer to fall—which is when you're most likely to shed scaly skin like a snake.

The benefits of a wrap or rub can be any or all of the following: to exfoliate and soften the skin, stimulate the circulation, absorb excess oils, make you sweat to pull out toxins from the body, relax the muscles. Some claim that a seaweed wrap can reduce cellulite. There are as many variations on a body wrap as there are ways to marinate a chicken. The most popular recipes cooked up at spas use salt or ginseng, kitchen or Chinese herbs, seaweed or mud (aka *fango,* which is Italian for volcanic mud).

No matter what the recipe du jour, the aesthetician massages the blend into the body from the neck down. Then you are swaddled in plastic or Saran Wrap, covered with warm blankets and towels, and left to sweat out the toxins for 15 to 20 minutes. This treatment is followed by a warm shower and a rubdown with a warm moisturizer. It's a nice way to lead into a massage, if you have time for a doubleheader, because it warms the muscles.

Mud. Mud baths are as old as the pyramids, and the urge to submerge is almost as primal as the ooze itself. Wherever there are hot springs,

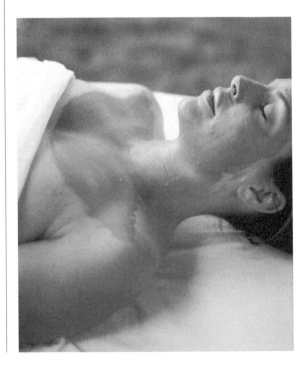

Each kind of mud has its own pedigree, depending on where it's from: mud from Sedona, Arizona, is used by Native Americans to relieve muscular aches and pains; mud from the Dead Sea is said to help psoriasis, and it's rich in potassium chloride, calcium, and magnesium chloride, which can ease arthritic and rheumatic pain. Moor mud from the bottom of inland lakes is supposed to stimulate the lymph glands and regenerate cells.

people have played in the mud, scooping up handfuls and slathering it on their bodies because it feels good. (The dirt in your backyard won't do the trick, because it isn't rich in minerals like volcanic mud or mud from hot springs.)

Europeans believe that relaxing in a warm mud bath not only softens and exfoliates the skin but also soothes tired muscles and relieves rheumatism and arthritis. There are two kinds of mud bathing. The first method is immersion in a huge tub or pool of mud at a mineral-spring spa, where one "tub" fits all (although it's heated between treatments to keep it hygienic). Sometimes, as at Calistoga Hot Springs in California, there are natural mud baths (no man-made tub or pool). The second method involves mixing powdered mud with water and then having it brushed or sponged all over your body. It is favored in smaller spas or urban areas, and the mud used in this method usually has a clay base—kaolin is a favorite—

because it absorbs the skin's oil. The mud can be combined with seaweed and seawater for a "marine mud" treatment, or with "Dead Sea mud" imported from Israel's Dead Sea, which is known for its high mineral content.

Mud and clay are said to "detoxify" and "purify" the skin. I'm not sure what these New Age terms mean, but this much I know: treatments with mud and clay make the skin smoother and tighter, remove surface debris (flakes and excess oil), feel wonderfully relaxing, and give the skin a healthy glow. California's many hot springs of mineral-rich mud and clay make it a mecca for mud bathers. The northern California town of Calistoga in Sonoma County is a spot rich in mineral springs, which makes it one of the best known for mud baths. The Glen Ivy Hot Springs Spa, a day spa outside Los Angeles known as Club Mud, is a hot-spring pool with a huge hunk of California clay sticking right up in the middle. Here's the rub: you wade into the pool, smear the reddish clay all over your body, glumph out of the pool to bake in the sun, then hit the showers to scrub it all off with a loofah.

Thalassotherapy— The Sea of Life

"Seawater is the soup of life," says Isaac Asimov. After all, life came from the ocean, and the bracing sea brine can be a powerful restorative. Seaweed and seawater are said to firm the skin, and seaweed is high in iodine and protein—both good for the skin. Not everyone can get to the sea when they need it most, but you can let the sea come to you, which is why seaweed wraps are so popular at day spas.

Algotherapy is the therapeutic use of seaweed, while thalassotherapy is the use of seawater as a curative. There are more than 3,000 types of seaweed, and each is said to have a different effect. Laminaria, or green alga, is rich in iodine and stimulates the oxygen content in the cells. Fucus, or brown algae, is rich in antioxidants and has a detoxifying effect on the body. Spirulina is a single-cell alga that is rich in protein and antioxidants. White alga, rich in calcium and magnesium, acts as an anti-inflammatory and helps to relieve water retention and stimulate the circulation.

For my seaweed wrap, Natasha (my practitioner) brushes me from neck to toe with a briny brew of white and brown-green powdered algae and seawater from Brittany. Then she wraps me in a layer of plastic and cocoons me in a heating blanket. As I lie there feeling like a human tekka makki, I ask Natasha why the heat is so intense around my hips and buttocks. "Because that's where women retain more toxins," she replies, showing a true gift for understatement. The heat allows my body to sweat out "toxins," and the seaweed will remineralize my skin, I'm told. I lie there, relaxed but sweating profusely for 45 minutes, until Natasha comes to offer me a shower with an exfoliating seaweed soap. After hosing myself down, I stand stark naked in the middle of the room while Natasha coats me in a marine green moisturizing gel.

By the time I leave, limp as a strip of seaweed, my skin feels incredibly soft, but I smell like low tide—not exactly pleasant, but it does make me feel a certain oneness with the sea. I think of what Dan Fryda, president of Spa Technologies, a manufacturer of all-natural seaweed products, has referred to as "the ecology of the ocean within." Fryda has spent 20 years researching seaweed and is an adamant believer that the source of health and beauty ebbs and flows with the sea. "Our bodies are chemically identical to seawater," says Fryda. "Every element of Mendeleyev's chart is in seawater—and in the human body. To survive in this hostile and alien land environment, we need to look back to the ocean from whence we came." In other words, we need to go with the flow.

Salt. Whether it's called a salt glow, salt rub, or salt polish, this is the ultimate spa exfoliating treatment. Some spas use coarse-grained salt, others use sugar, baking soda, even fine-grained sand mixed with oils. No matter what the abrasive, the point of the exfoliating treatment is the same: to get rid of dead skin buildup and make the skin better able to absorb moisture.

While you lie on a massage table, a practitioner rubs salt vigorously over your entire body (except for the face) using a coarse-bristle, industrial-strength brush. After lying under blankets for a while, you rinse off the salt in the shower. Back on the table, you're coated with a warm moisturizer and sent on your way with skin as soft and pliable as a baby piglet's.

Spa Massages

When a string of quickie back-rub joints ("The Great American Back-Rub") opened in New York City a few years ago offering a 10-minute massage, my initial reaction was puzzlement. Why would people want to lean on a dirty massage chair in a storefront window and subject themselves to a jock-style rubdown for the amusement of passersby? How relaxing could that be? Massage, after all, is supposed to relieve pain and stress—not cause it. As I watched the Great American Back-Rub joints close down one by one, I knew that I wasn't the only one to feel this way. To achieve the optimum effect from a massage, you need time, a highly qualified massage therapist, and a nurturing, relaxing environment.

Massage is by far the most sought-after treatment at a spa, which is not surprising, considering that modern life is the source of rampant and chronic aches and pains. Hours of daily hunching over the computer or cradling the phone on our shoulders have made us all a little tense—perfect candidates for the benefits of massage. Massage not only feels good but also has positive psychological and physiological benefits, according to studies at the University of Miami School of Medicine.

Tip Who needs "cold" cream? Squeeze some moisturizer into one palm and warm up with your other palm for a few seconds before putting on your skin. Or submerge the bottle in warm water for 10 minutes.

The skin has five million touch receptors that send messages along the spine to the brain. Simple touch, according to recent studies—a hug, a hand on the shoulder—can reduce the heart rate and lower the blood pressure. Touch also triggers the release of endorphins, the body's natural painkillers, that make you feel better and improve your mood. Prolonged touch like massage does all that—plus it can increase the metabolism, relax the muscles, improve the circulation of blood and lymph, and help the lymph system release metabolic waste. (That's why it's so important, after a massage, to drink at least a quart of water.) Massage also relieves stress by lowering levels of the stress hormone cortisol norepinephrine and triggering endorphins. Here are some massage treatments offered at most spas.

Swedish

Most massage treatments in the United States rely on this traditional method developed in the early 19th century by a Swede named Per Henrik Ling. Any massage described as "deep-tissue" is probably Swedish, as are most "sports" massages. The technique is based on a series of light to heavy strokes and kneading movements that are helped along with light oil, lotion, or cream. When the therapist uses essential oils during the massage, it is often called an aromatherapy massage.

Swedish massage is a full-body technique: the massage therapist uses the weight of his body behind his hands to reduce tension in the back, legs, arms, shoulders, and neck of the client. Though the strokes vary in length and intensity, they are smooth and flowing, not choppy like those of shiatsu. The oil lubricates the skin, which enables the massage therapist to stroke

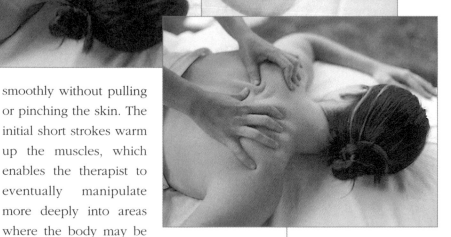

smoothly without pulling or pinching the skin. The initial short strokes warm up the muscles, which enables the therapist to eventually manipulate more deeply into areas where the body may be tense or sore.

Shiatsu

Shiatsu, probably the oldest form of massage, originated in Japan about 2000 B.C.—about the same time that acupuncture began in China. In fact, shiatsu (Japanese for "finger pressure") is often described as acupuncture without the needles. Both practices are based on the idea that there are certain pathways in the body

where energy (known in Chinese medicine as *chi*) must flow in order to feed the organs and muscles. When your *chi* gets jammed up, you need to release it by pressing on specific points in the body, which gets it circulating once again. (Reflexology is a form of shiatsu.) These "acupressure" points are based on the acupuncture points of the body.

While Swedish massage is mostly used to untangle knotted muscles, shiatsu has a broader range of therapeutic applications: to relieve nausea and constipation, to reduce stress, and so on. Unlike Swedish massage, shiatsu is administered without oil and does not involve long strokes and kneading; usually you're wearing loose clothing while it's done. The technique relies on a more rigorous form of pressure from the massage therapist's thumbs, knees, elbows, or feet. Some shiatsu is performed on a massage table; the more traditional approach is for you to lie on a mat or futon on the floor.

Your massage therapist will apply pressure gradually, aim into the center of the point, holding her finger perpendicular to the skin. The pressure should be firm but not painful. Holding an acupressure point for more than a minute causes the body to release endorphins, its natural painkillers. A good shiatsu massage will leave you feeling energized and perhaps a bit sore.

Reiki

Re means "soul" or "spirit," and *ki,* like *chi,* is the body's energy. A reiki treatment is supposed to "channel" your energy throughout your body to correct imbalances among your physical, emotional, mental, and spiritual selves. A reiki treatment is not quite a massage since it's as much hands-off as it is hands-on. In reiki, touch is used as a giant off/on switch. When the practitioner touches you, it activates your reiki; when his hands are above your body, the energy flow stops.

Watsu

Watsu is a form of underwater massage that combines water *(wa)* and shiatsu *(tsu).* It's intended to offer the physical benefit of shiatsu massage with a meditative, womblike underwater experience. The massage therapist starts by cradling you in her arms like a baby and rocking you back and forth in a pool of water while pressing points on your body and encouraging your body to flow with your breath. If you can let yourself go, you'll drift through the water to the sound of your own heartbeat while being massaged, which can be an incredibly relaxing experience. Because you are buoyed by water, the therapist is able to get in deeper between your muscles and into the acupressure points, so the physical benefits of the massage are heightened. The water also induces a dreamlike floating state that's so relaxing you may feel almost reborn.

Thai Massage

The Thai massage, an ancient technique, is an extremely athletic rubdown. Because it involves close physical contact, you're fully clothed in T-shirt and gym shorts or other loose clothing throughout the one-and-a-half-hour treatment.

The Thai takes place on a floor mat in the center of a small room. It starts with an extensive reflexology massage. The goal is to stimulate the flow of energy (called *sen*) along acupressure-like meridians throughout the body. The massage itself is a shiatsu-Swedish hybrid, where the massage therapist stretches your body into yoga poses and rocks you back and forth to loosen up your muscles and joints. The *sen* is supposed to flow up the legs, to the arms, abdomen, shoulders, and head, as your masseuse guides you into patterns of movement that resemble both physical therapy and choreographed dance. The treatment really does loosen up muscles, and you'll leave feeling energized and limber. To benefit most from Thai massage, it helps if you're flexible and uninhibited. Thai is not for the self-conscious.

Whether you can spend a week, three days, or only an hour, take a trip to a spa. You may be skeptical or hesitant about indulging yourself at first, but even one simple spa treatment 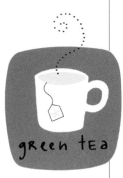 can be incredibly restorative not only because it's therapeutic but also because it feels good to know that you're taking the time to do something pleasurable for yourself.

the body time line

3000 B.C. Egyptians use the first depilatory; they apply hot wax to the skin and rip it off with gauze.

3000 B.C. Egyptian men and women of the upper classes use henna to stain their nails orange; dark nail color signifies high rank.

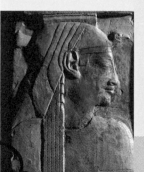

3000 B.C. In China, shiny fingernails are a sign of wealth. Fingernails are painted with beeswax, egg whites, and gum arabic.

2000 B.C. Middle Eastern women thread cotton strings between their fingers and run them quickly over their legs to catch hairs and pull them out.

2000 B.C. In the Far East, lime is combined with alkaline sulfides to remove body hair.

2000 B.C. In Babylonia, the nobility use solid gold tools to manicure their fingernails and toenails.

1000 B.C. *Ayurveda*—the science of long life—begins in India.

1000 B.C. Moses believes that bathing leads to moral purification and writes bathing rituals—Mikvah—into law for the Jews.

Fifth century B.C. The Greeks invent the shower: they stand up in the tub and wash with water poured from overhead spouts or urns held by handmaidens.

Fifth century B.C. Aromatherapy originates in Egypt. Egyptians perfect methods of oil extraction from plants and incorporate aromatic oils into their cosmetics, medicines, and religious practices.

100 B.C. Romans wash with a mix of clay, ash, and animal tallow.

First century B.C. Cleopatra cleanses with fine sand; many other Egyptians wash with essential oils.

First century A.D. The inhabitants of Pompeii are the first to make scented soap.

306. Construction of the Diocletian Baths in Rome ends. Accommodating 6,000 people in an area of more than 32½ acres, they are the largest of the imperial baths.

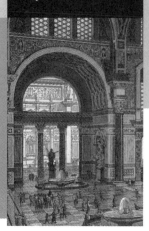

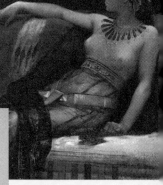

900s. The crippling practice of foot binding begins in China.

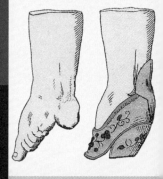

1000–1500. Medieval Christian doctrine teaches that bathing invites sin, a belief that contributes to the spread of typhus and plague throughout Europe.

1096–1291. During the Crusades, the use of essential oils in various forms is revived in Europe and remains the primary source of treatment for disease for centuries.

1400s. In England and France, common people bathe in public bathhouses, which also serve as brothels.

Late 1400s. Queen Isabella of Spain boasts that she's had only two baths in her life: at birth and before her wedding.

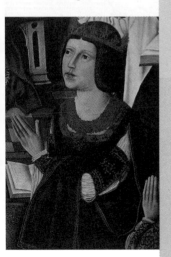

1500s. In Africa, the members of the Bantu tribe paint their faces with red clay for protection from the sun.

1500s. English bathhouses are closed by King Henry VIII because it is thought they spread disease.

1500s. Mary, Queen of Scots bathes in wine as a beautifying treatment. (Wine contains malic acid, one of the sources of the alpha-hydroxy acids used today.)

1572. Margaret of Valois sleeps on the world's first black satin sheets to show off her creamy white skin.

1600s. The European aristocracy substitute layers of perfume and cosmetics, and frequent clothing changes, for bathing. Lower classes dip into ponds and streams when they aren't too busy working to worry about it.

Late 1600s. French aristocrats literally bathed in scent. Louis XIV took on the nickname Le Roi de Parfum (the king of scent) because of his excessive predilection for the stuff.

1700s. American colonists rarely bathe; instead, they use perfumes, powders, and scented waters—some of which double as alcoholic beverages.

1700s. In America, lye-soaked cloths are applied to burn away body hair.

1750s. In America, soap-making becomes a home industry, and soaps made of ash lye and pan drippings come into use for cleansing.

1778. English women wear "chicken-skin" gloves made of a "thin, strong leather dressed with almonds and spermaceti" to bed to keep hands soft.

1800s. To keep hands soft and smooth, Europeans sleep with gloves brushed inside with a mixture of rose water, almond oil, and egg yolks. Some ladies wrap their hands in fresh meat overnight.

1800s. In France, body splashes contain vodka—the higher the proof, the better! Both vodka and white wine vinegar—known as *vinaigres de toilette*—have been used throughout history as deodorants and bactericides.

1806. Colgate & Company is founded when William Colgate opens a soap factory in upstate New York.

1827. Pears Soap, an early glycerine soap, is exported to the United States from England and sold in three-shilling pots.

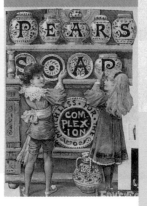

1830. The first soap in individually wrapped bars of uniform size is sold by entrepreneur B. T. Babbitt.

1837. Brothers-in-law William Procter and James Gamble combine their vocations of candlemaker and soapmaker to form the Procter & Gamble company in Cincinnati.

1851. A bathtub is installed in the White House.

1860–1900. Victorians wash with floral toilet waters.

1872. Colgate's Cashmere Bouquet is the first commercial perfumed soap.

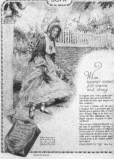

1875. Dr. Charles E. Michel of St. Louis invents the first electrolysis equipment.

the body time line

1875. When a Procter & Gamble employee accidentally beats too much air into a batch of soap, Ivory soap is born.

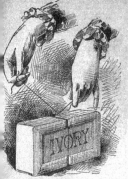

1876. John Harvey Kellogg, inventor of cornflakes, opens a sanitorium in Battle Creek, Michigan, where he treats patients with a strict dietary regimen and hydrotherapy. Years later, the story of his eccentric approach to alternative therapies inspires the popular novel and film satire, *The Road to Wellville*.

1880s. Women start sucking on violet candies to improve their breath.

1880. The Johnson Company creates Palmolive Soap entirely of vegetable oils.

1890. Simmons Liver Regulator pill is said to improve the skin—and breath.

1890. The advertising pitch for Borolyptol, an early mouthwash that was also marketed as a vaginal douche, reads, "free from poisonous or irritating effect."

1895. Lifebuoy, the first deodorant soap, is invented.

1900. English actress Lillie Langtry endorses Pears soap—one of the first celebrity product endorsements.

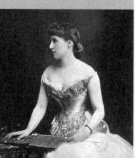

1911. Foot binding is outlawed in China.

1917. The first commercial nail polish is sold by Cutex.

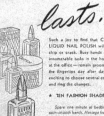

1920s. The term *aromatherapy* is coined in France by René-Maurice Gottefosse, a chemist, who burned his hand and plunged it into a nearby vat of lavender oil, which he mistook for water. The burn healed so quickly without scarring that Gottefosse decided to study the healing properties of plant oils.

1928. French perfumer Jean Patou creates Huile de Caldée, the first suntan lotion.

1930s. X rays are used to burn hair off the face and body.

1930. Koremlu, a popular depilatory cream, is found to contain rat poison.

1932. Despite warnings from the FDA, formaldehyde is a popular ingredient in antiperspirants.

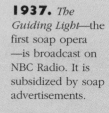

CUTEX *perfects..*

work-a-day nail beauty that *lasts!*

Such a joy to find that CUTEX LIQUID NAIL POLISH will not chip or crack. Busy hands doing innumerable tasks in the home— at the office—remain groomed to the fingertips day after day. So exciting to choose several colours and ring the changes.

★ TEN FASHION SHADES ★

Spare one minute at bedtime for satin-smooth hands. Massage fragrant, non-sticky CUTEX HAND CREAM from fingertips to wrist.
In the Cutex Series you'll find everything for the perfect manicure.

CUTEX LIQUID POLISH

1934. Elizabeth Arden opens the Maine Chance spa in Mount Vernon, Maine—the first luxury spa in the United States.

1936. Lancôme introduces Ambre Solaire, the first complete line of suntan products.

1937. *The Guiding Light*—the first soap opera —is broadcast on NBC Radio. It is subsidized by soap advertisements.

1939–1945. During World War II, soap factories supply most of the glycerine used to make nitroglycerine, the explosive ingredient in dynamite.

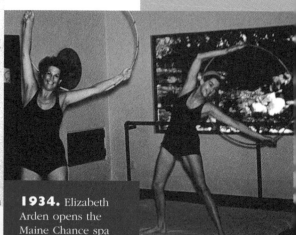

1939–1945. A wartime shortage of animal and vegetable fats leads to the use of mineral oil for fats, and synthetic soaps are born. Because these soaps deplete the skin's natural oils, emollients are added, and "cleansing bars" and "beauty bars" are created.

1939–1945. The U.S. government formulates the first sunblocks for sailors in the South Pacific. "Red Vet Pet," made of red veterinary petrolatum, is a favorite.

1948. Transparent nail top coats and undercoats, like Dura Gloss and Lustre Coat, are introduced to increase the staying power of nail polish.

1960s. Sun reflectors, baby oil, and iodine are used to maximize the tanning effect of the sun. The first UVA sunscreens are also in development, but they don't come into widespread use for 30 years.

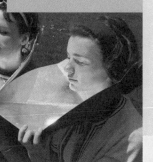

1962. Frank Gerow, a Houston plastic surgeon, performs the first breast-augmentation operation with silicone-gel implants. Because of problems arising from leaking silicone, they are outlawed in 1991.

1974. The French company Decléor develops the first comprehensive line of high-quality aromatherapy skincare products.

1975. Gillette Daisy, the first disposable razor for women, comes on the market.

1939–1945. General Douglas MacArthur forbids the "primitive" Japanese practice of shiatsu in medical treatment when U.S. forces occupy Japan, but the order is eventually overturned by President Truman.

1950. The skincare and massage treatments of Marguerite Maury, a French cosmetologist living in London, popularize aromatherapy in Britain.

1960s. The first nail extensions are made from a dental material called *kadon,* a thick paste that breaks easily and is hard to file.

1963. Crème Abricot, a nail strengthener, is created by Christian Dior.

1976. British entrepreneur Anita Roddick (below) opens The Body Shop, one of the first cosmetics and skincare companies to make political activism, animal rights, and a "cruelty-free" approach commercially appealing and profitable.

1940. Remington creates the first electric razor specifically for women.

1950s. Sally Hansen's Hard-As-Nails is the first nail hardener on the market.

1960s. California, home to numerous hot springs, becomes the nation's foremost mud- and sand-bath mecca.

1970s. The FDA and Coppertone Solar Research Center develop the Sun Protection Factor (SPF). Although not mandatory, most manufacturers adopt it for labeling.

1943. A shortage of stockings during the war leads to an increase in leg paint, the forerunner of self-tanner.

1959. Man-Tan, the first self-tanner, is marketed to men who want a rugged-looking tan.

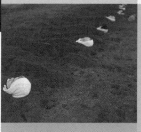

1962. Tensur Bust, the first bust cream, is launched by Clarins.

1972. Acupuncture is still relatively unknown in the United States until Nixon goes to China and James Reston, a *New York Times* correspondent covering the event, gets acupuncture treatments following emergency surgery. He writes a column singing its praises, and today millions of Americans reap the benefit.

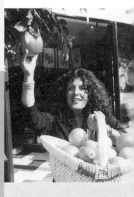

1977. French surgeon Yves-Gérard Illouz develops liposuction.

1944. PABA, one of the first UVB-absorbing chemicals, is developed and put to use in Coppertone Suntan Cream.

1960s. French physician Jean Valnet studies the antiseptic and antibacterial properties of essential oils and uses aromatherapy in his medical practice.

the body time line

1979. Bo Derek's perfect "10" launched the aerobics craze over the next decade.

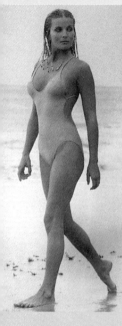

1980s. Chanel Beauté gets into the sun-protection business.

1980s. British royals Princess Diana, "Fergie," and even Prince Charles practice aromatherapy and boost its popularity.

1980s. Body-firming creams and bust creams, popular in France, make their way over to the United States.

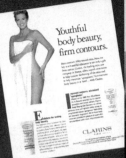

Youthful body beauty, firm contours.

CLARINS

1980s. As the risks of tanning become clearer, warning labels are now required at tanning salons.

1984. Tina Turner's great legs drive legions of women to the Thighmaster.

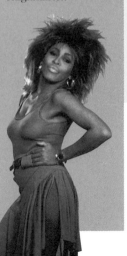

1987. According to the International Spa & Fitness Association, there are 40 day spas in the United States; less than 10 years later, there are more than 600.

1990s. Elaborate airbrushed nail designs—with or without decals—become popular.

1990. The Estée Lauder Company launches Origins, with William Lauder at the helm. Origins is the first major cosmetics company to link "natural" products with beauty and well-being.

ORIGINS

Peace of Mind
On-The-Spot Relief

1992. The FDA proposes a ban on acetone in astringents. However, it is still used as a solvent in nail polish remover.

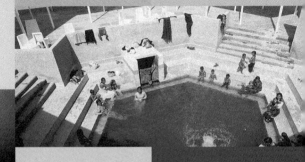

1992. Each year, more than 100 million Japanese pay a visit to a *ryokan* for a communal hot-spring bath (above).

1992. Elizabeth Arden launches its SPA line and becomes one of the first prestige companies to jump on the mind-body bandwagon.

1994. L'Oréal becomes one of the first cosmetics giants to agree to a ban on animal testing.

1995. Premed student Dineh Mohajer mixes up blue nail polish in her sink and starts Hard Candy. Four years later, she sells the company for $10 million.

1997. Americans spend $6.5 billion on vitamins this year, up from $3 billion seven years ago.

1998. Americans are creating home spas in record numbers, buying 300,000 hot tubs last year alone.

1999. Aveda is bought by Estée Lauder.

2000. Body piercings and tattoos—removable or not—become almost as mainstream as nail decals.

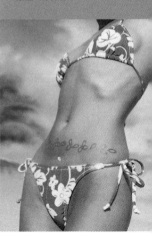

Glossary

Accutane. An acne medication that inhibits oil production. Side effects include hair loss, headaches, liver problems, extreme dryness of the skin and eyes, and birth defects.

Acetone. A solvent used in nail polish, nail polish removers, and astringents that can cause nausea, ear, nose, and throat irritation, and dermatitis.

Acetonitrile (methyl cyanide). An extremely toxic chemical found in many artificial-nail removers. Its use should be avoided, especially by pregnant women.

Acne. An inflammation caused by blockage of the oil glands, which results in blackheads and pimples.

Aesthetician. A trained professional who provides spa or salon treatments, such as facials and massages, that relax the body and clean or beautify the skin.

Age spots. See BROWN SPOTS.

Alcohol, SD (SD alcohol). Denatured ethyl alcohols found in hair- and skincare products, particularly astringents and toners. Because they can be drying to the hair and skin, people with sensitive skin should avoid using them.

Algotherapy. Therapeutic use of seaweed in spa treatments.

Allantoin. A skin-soothing, anti-inflammatory ingredient extracted from urea, comfrey, or chamomile that is used to soothe sunburned, irritated skin.

Allergen. A substance that produces an allergic reaction. Many beauty products, especially mass-market products, may contain ingredients that many people are allergic to.

Almond oil. An easily absorbed, emollient oil extracted from the seeds of sweet almonds.

Aloe vera gel. Derived from the leaves of the *Aloe barbadensis* plant, it moisturizes and soothes burns and skin irritations.

Alopecia areata. Hair loss.

Alpha-hydroxy acids (AHAs). Acid extracts from natural or synthetic sources that chemically exfoliate the top layer of skin. There are five types: citric acid, tartaric acid, malic acid, lactic acid, and glycolic acid. Also known as fruit acids.

Alum. An astringent used in antiperspirants because it prevents irritation from aluminum chloride.

Aluminum salts. Aluminum acids used in antiperspirants to stop perspiration and kill bacteria, thereby preventing body odor. Common examples include aluminum hydroxide, aluminum stearate, and aluminum caprylate. Some researchers believe that aluminum salts contribute to Alzheimer's disease.

Amino acids. Substances used by the body to build the proteins that form the base of skin, hair, and nails. Added to shampoos and conditioners, they effectively remortar cracks in the hair shaft.

Ammonium lauryl sulfate. A detergent used in shampoos and cleansers.

Ammonium thioglycolate. An active ingredient in hair relaxers (straighteners), it breaks the protein bonds that give hair its texture.

Analgesic. A substance that relieves pain.

Aniline. A colorless liquid obtained from coal tar, from which many hair colors and dyes are derived. About 1 in 100 women are allergic to it.

Animal extracts. Fat or tissue extracted from cows, sheep, and pigs that is added to skin- or haircare products with an intended rejuvenating effect.

Antifungal. Counteracts fungal infections such as athlete's foot and nail fungus.

Anti-inflammatory. Reduces swelling and inflammation. Used in skincare.

Antioxidants. Substances found in vitamins and other materials that help repair—and possibly prevent—cell damage caused by free radicals. Examples include grapeseed extract, green algae (flavonoids), lycopene (beta-carotene), ginseng, licorice, rosemary, juniper, lipoic acid, alpha-linoleic acid. The strongest known natural antioxidants are ginkgo biloba and green tea.

Antiperspirant. A substance that inhibits perspiration.

Antiseptic. A substance that kills bacteria and inhibits their growth.

Arnica. Extracts from the flowers of this plant are used to heal wounds and soothe irritated skin.

Aromatherapy. The therapeutic use of botanical oils that are distilled or cold-pressed from plants and flowers.

Ascorbic acid. Vitamin C. In cosmetics, it's considered an antioxidant and is also used as a preservative.

Ascorbyl palmitate. Fat-soluble Vitamin C.

Astringent. A substance, such as witch hazel or alcohol, that causes skin tissue to tighten.

Avobenzone (aka Parsol 1789). An ingredient in sunscreens that blocks UVA radiation.

Awapuhi. Extracted from Hawaiian white ginger and used in shampoos and massage oils, it stimulates the circulation and relieves sore muscles.

Ayurveda. An ancient science of holistic medicine that originated in India.

Azelaic acid. An oleic acid derivative used by dermatologists to treat acne.

Azulene. An anti-inflammatory extracted from chamomile and yarrow flowers, it also soothes the skin.

Babassu oil. An oil from the Brazilian babassu palm plant that is used in soaps.

Bactericidal. A substance that inhibits growth of or kills bacteria.

Bain-marie. A utensil similar to a double boiler used for heating ingredients in cosmetics manufacture.

Balm. A thick ointment, unguent, or salve that soothes the skin.

Balm of Gilead. Oil from this plant is used in ointments to soothe bruised, swollen, or irritated skin and stop itching from insect bites.

Beeswax. This wax, produced by the honeybee to build its comb, is used in lipstick, lip balm, and moisturizers.

Bentonite. A white clay used in facial masks to absorb oil from the skin, it also thickens makeup and reduces shine on the face.

Benzoic acid. A preservative used in cosmetics and foods that can be irritating to the skin.

Benzoyl peroxide. A strong disinfectant used to help kill bacteria and clear up acne. Because it can overdry skin, it should not be used for more than a week at a time.

Betaglucans. Ingredients derived from oats and shiitake mushrooms. They are used in moisturizers, shampoos, and shower gels.

Beta-hydroxy acids (BHAs). Acid extracts that chemically exfoliate the top layer of skin. They have the same effect as AHAs, but they're less irritating and come from different sources.

Bisabolol. An anti-irritant ingredient derived from chamomile that is often found in products made for people with sensitive skin.

Blackheads. Formed when oil and dead skin cells become trapped in a pore and mix with bacteria.

Botanicals. Plant-based or -derived ingredients.

Botox. A substance injected into the face to smooth wrinkles in the skin by paralyzing the underlying muscles.

Brown spots (formerly known as "liver" or "age" spots). Concentrations of melanin triggered by unprotected exposure to the sun over a long period of time.

Bunion. A protruding lump on the side of the foot caused by prolonged encasement in tight shoes.

Butylene glycol. A petroleum-based humectant and emollient that is often used in hairsprays and gels.

Calendula. An anti-inflammatory extracted from the marigold plant that is used to soothe sensitive skin and reduce puffiness.

Calluses. Hard, rough skin on the sides and soles of the feet caused by going sockless and shoeless.

Camphor. A mild antiseptic derived from the wood of the tropical camphor tree that is used to treat oily, blemish-prone skin.

Caprylic triglyceride. An emollient derived from coconut oil that is also used to disperse pigment in cosmetics.

Carbolic acid. A caustic acid used in deep facial peels performed in dermatologists' offices.

Carmine. See COCHINEAL.

Carnauba wax. A hypoallergenic wax extracted from the leaves of the Brazilian palm tree that is used to thicken foundation, mascara, lipstick, blush, and deodorant.

Castile soap. Mild, moisturizing soap made from olive oil.

Castor oil. A highly emollient oil made from the beans of the castor plant that is used to bind waxes and fragrance together, as in lipsticks.

Cellex-C. An antioxidant, antiaging skincare product with Vitamin C as its active ingredient.

Cellulite. Lumpiness found in the thighs, hips, and buttocks of many women, which is caused by fat cells trapped within the skin's connective tissue.

Ceramides. Synthetic lipids (fats) used in skin- and haircare products.

Cetyl alcohol. An emollient used in cosmetics, hair-, nail-, and skincare products.

Chamomile. An herb whose flowers and leaves are used to lighten blond hair and soothe the skin.

Cheilitis. Cracking and drying of the lips that is usually caused by a reaction to synthetic eosin dyes and perfumes in lipstick.

Citric acid. Derived from citrus fruits, it is used as a preservative, pH balancer, and astringent.

Clarifying shampoo. An acidic shampoo containing lemon juice or cider vinegar that removes the buildup of minerals, conditioners, shampoos, or styling products from the hair.

Coal-tar dyes. Derived from coal, they are used in certain FD&C dyes and in some permanent hair color. Common allergens, they cause cancer in animals.

Cochineal. A red dye obtained from the carcass of the cochineal beetle, indigenous to Latin America; extracts are used as pigment in lipstick and other color cosmetics.

Cocoa butter. An occlusive emollient derived from cocoa butter, it can clog pores.

Cocoamide DEA/MEA. A mild detergent used in shampoos and cleansers to build lather. (Shampoos that list a cocoamide before a sulfate are gentler.)

Cocoamidopropyl betaine. A mild surfactant and viscosity adjuster used in shampoo.

Collagen. A protein used in antiaging skincare products that is derived from the connective tissues of young cows (or synthetic versions). Humans also produce collagen, but so far there is no compelling scientific evidence to show that topical applications in cosmetics and skincare can penetrate the skin and affect the composition of our collagen.

Coltsfoot. A skin soother used in moisturizers, shampoos, and conditioners, it is derived from the *Tussilago farfara* plant.

Comedogenic. A substance that clogs pores.

Comedone extractor. An implement used by dermatologists to extract blackheads.

Comfrey. A skin soother that contains allantoin. It is used to treat skin irritations.

Contouring. A technique using blush and bronzing powder to better define the contours of the face.

Corns. Bumps on the top of the toes caused by toes rubbing against shoes that are too tight.

Cosmeceutical. A cosmetic that supposedly offers druglike benefits.

Cosmetics. Defined by the FDA as "articles intended to be applied to the human body for cleansing, beautifying, promoting attractiveness, or altering the appearance without affecting the body's structure or functions."

Cuticle. The skin overlapping finger- and toenails, which acts as a protective layer. Also, the outermost layer of the hair shaft.

Cyclomethicone. A silicone oil used in hair- and skincare products to impart shine and/or silkiness.

Cysteine. An amino acid that contains sulfur and is found in the protein of the hair. The bond it forms ("the cysteine bridge") strengthens the hair.

Cystic acne. Severe acne characterized by cysts. It should be treated by a dermatologist.

Cysts. Blackheads or whiteheads that have become red and swollen as a result of a deeper infection. They should be treated by a dermatologist. (See CYSTIC ACNE.)

Dandruff. A form of dermatitis caused by an overgrowth of yeast that results in dryness, itchiness, and flaking. (It can afflict oily scalps as well as dry and normal ones.)

Deionized water. Water that has been filtered and treated to remove metallic ions, kill microorganisms, and remove impurities.

Deodorant. A substance that masks offensive body odors.

Depilatory. Cream used to melt away unwanted hair with calcium or sodium thioglycolate or sulfides. (These are the same ingredients used in permanent wave and hair-relaxing solutions, but in stronger concentrations in depilatories.)

Dermatitis. Skin inflammation accompanied by redness, itchiness, dryness, or cracking.

Dermis. The inner layer of the skin.

Developer. An oxidizing agent—usually hydrogen peroxide—that allows hair dye to take hold on the hair.

Diethanolamine (DEA). A detergent, humectant, and solvent used in shampoos and shower gels.

Dihydroxyacetone (DHA). The active ingredient in self-tanners.

Dimethicone. A silicone oil used in hair- and skincare products. Adds shine to the hair and a slippery feeling to skin products.

DMDM hydantoin. A preservative used in shampoos, conditioners, and creams that can irritate the skin and may release formaldehyde.

Eczema. Red, flaky, scaly patches of dry, itchy skin that may be caused by allergic reactions.

Effleurage. A massage technique using flowing movements up and down the face and neck during a facial.

Elastin. Fibers in the skin that give it elasticity.

Electrolysis. The only permanent form of hair removal, in which electric current is used to kill hair at its root.

Emollient. An occlusive ingredient—usually a grease or an oil—that softens the skin and protects it from dryness. The emollients in moisturizers come from animal, vegetable, or mineral sources. Common ones are allantoin, cocoa butter, lanolin, squalene, castor oil, plant or vegetable oil, mineral oil, and fatty alcohols. (See individual entries for more detail.)

Emulsifier. A substance that disperses one ingredient into another in which it would not ordinarily dissolve. An emulsifier binds water with oily humectants and emollients so that the texture of a product is smooth. Common ones are beeswax, vegetable wax, TEA lauryl sulfate, cetearyl alcohol, glyceryl monostearate, stearic acid, and choleth 24. (See individual entries for more detail.)

Enzymes. Exfoliants derived from papaya, pineapple, or papain (a papaya derivative) that can help even out the skin's color and tone.

Eosin dyes. Used to give red color to cosmetics. (See CHEILITIS.)

Epidermis. The surface layer of the skin.

Epsom salts. Crystals derived from magnesium sulfate that are used in the bath to relieve common aches and pains, especially in the feet or back.

Essential oils. Essences extracted from plants that contain the scent and other therapeutic properties of the plant. (Products labeled "extract of," "essence of," or "aromatic oil of" are usually not natural oils but instead inexpensive synthetics.)

Ethylparaben. A synthetic preservative.

Evening primrose oil. Essential oil used to treat eczema, psoriasis, and dry, aging skin.

Exfoliation. The removal of dead skin cells on the skin's surface.

Extraction. The process of unclogging blackheads.

Facialist. See AESTHETICIAN.

Facial toning (facial exercise). A treatment offered by some spas. Don't buy it. Your face gets enough exercise in the natural course of a day.

Fatty acids. Used chiefly in shampoos, cleansers, and conditioners to make the skin and hair feel smooth and the hair easier to comb. Common ones include cetyl alcohol, coconut alcohol, stearyl alcohol, and oleic acid.

Fatty alcohols. Alcohols that are emollient, not drying. They are used in creams, conditioners, lotions, and shampoos. Common ones include cetyl alcohol, oleyl alcohol, lauryl alcohol, and stearyl alcohol.

FD&C dyes. Coloring agents used in cosmetics that are usually made from coal tar.

Folliculitis. An inflammation of the hair follicle that looks like a rash and is usually found in areas of the body where skin has been irritated by shaving or waxing. Also called razor bumps.

Formaldehyde. An ingredient in some nail polishes and glues, it is a known allergen and suspected carcinogen.

Free radicals. A molecule that damages normal, surrounding cells by depleting them of oxygen.

Frosting. See HIGHLIGHTING.

Fruit acid peel. A facial peel using alpha-hydroxy acid.

Fucus. Brown algae rich in antioxidants that are used in algotherapy.

Ginkgo biloba. See ANTIOXIDANTS.

Glycerine. A syrupy liquid used in skincare products for its emollient and water-retaining properties. It's good for people with oily skin.

Glyceryl cocoate. A skin-conditioning, cleansing agent derived from coconut.

Glyceryl monostearate. An emulsifier and dispersing agent.

Glycolic acid. Alpha-hydroxy acid derived from sugarcane.

Glycolic peel. A facial peel using glycolic acid.

Grapefruit seed extract. A natural preservative that is a good substitute for the parabens, but more expensive.

Gum. A resin from tropical trees and shrubs that is used as a thickener.

Halitosis. Bad breath.

Hammer toe. A deformity in which the toe is bent permanently downward.

Hemp seed oil. A rich emollient that contains fatty acids. Good for dry, aging skin.

Henna. Extracted from the *Lawsonia alba* plant, it is used to add red highlights or black color to the hair, and to condition it.

Highlighting. (1) Lighter shade or shades of hair color subtly laid onto small sections of the hair (formerly known as "frosting"). (2) The use of highlighter to "open up" the space between eyes and eyebrows, making the eyes look bigger, more open, and wide awake.

Hormone creams. Antiaging creams that contain estrogen or progesterone.

Horsetail. An herb rich in cysteine that is used to condition the hair.

Humectant. A nonoily ingredient that attracts moisture from the atmosphere, retards evaporation, and helps hold water. Common ones include glycerine, propylene glycol, sorbitol, hyaluronic acid, urea, and lactic acid.

Hyaluronic acid. A protein used in moisturizers (and also found in human skin cells) that helps hold moisture in the skin.

Hydrogen peroxide. Used as a lightener in hair color and an antibacterial in "oxygen" creams and facials.

Hydrolyzed. Broken down into smaller molecules with water.

Hydroquinine. A phenolic compound derived from benzene that is used in skin bleaches. The most tried-and-true of skin bleaches, it works by blocking the formation of melanin.

Hyperpigmentation. Dark spots on the skin.

Hypopigmentation. Light spots on the skin.

Imidazolidinyl urea. After the parabens, the most commonly used preservative in cosmetics.

Infusion. Herbs steeped in water. The resulting extract can be used as a cosmetic, a medicinal base, or a tea.

Ingrown hairs. Hairs that point in instead of growing outward and become trapped beneath the skin. They can cause folliculitis.

Iron oxides. Inert mineral compounds used to add color to cosmetics.

Isopropyl lanolate. Made from fatty acids of lanolin and an alcohol, it is used to improve penetration and spreadability of skincare products.

Isopropyl myristate. Made from myristic acid and an alcohol, it is used in skincare products to soften the skin but can be comedogenic.

Isopropyl palmitate. Made from palmitic acid and an alcohol, it is used in skincare products to soften the skin.

Jojoba oil. An excellent emollient for skin and hair that is obtained from the nut of the jojoba shrub, which is native to the North American desert.

Kalaya oil. An easily absorbed skin moisturizer that is a by-product of the Australian emu.

Kaolin. White clay widely used in facial masks. Because it takes on color really well, it's also used as a base in powder, blush, foundation, and eye shadow.

Karite. See SHEA BUTTER.

Keratin. The protein that forms the base of human skin, hair, and nails.

Keratosis pilaris (KP). A chronic, hereditary skin condition that manifests itself as swaths of hard, pimplelike bumps, without redness or irritation. KP most often appears on the backs of the upper arms, buttocks, and outer thighs.

Kojic acid. A skin lightener used in cosmetics to fade brown spots.

Lactic acid. Alpha-hydroxy acid derived from milk.

Laminaria. Green alga, rich in iodine, which is used in algotherapy.

Lanolin. A fatty secretion derived from sheep's wool. It's completely natural and easily absorbed by the skin but can cause allergic reactions and clog pores. It tends to be heavy, sticky, and greasy.

Lanolin alcohol. An emollient alcohol.

Lavender. The leaves, flowers, and oil from this plant are used in moisturizers, and haircare and body-care products. It's an antiseptic, helps clear acne, and soothes the skin.

Lecithin. An emulsifier used in lotions and creams.

Linoleic acid (aka Vitamin F). An essential fatty acid that prevents skin dryness and roughness.

Lipid barrier replacement. When the lipids that hold skin cells together in the stratum corneum get poked full of holes, water evaporates and results in dryness and sensitivity. Lipid barrier replacements such as ceramides can help remortar the wall.

Liposomes. Tiny lipid (fat) balls that deliver moisture to the skin. Because of their small molecular size, they are able to penetrate the cell wall reasonably well and are used in moisturizers.

Loofah. The skeleton of a gourd plant that's used as an exfoliating tool in the bath or shower.

Lowlights. Darker tones subtly laid into small sections of the hair.

Lubricant. An oil, cream, or other ingredient that moistens and softens skin.

Lye. A caustic ingredient (sodium hydroxide) used in hair relaxers and soaps.

Magnesium aluminum silicate. A clay.

Magnesium laureth sulfate. A surfactant used in shampoos.

Marine extracts. Mineral-rich ingredients derived from algae and/or seaweed that are used in skincare products and facial masks.

Melaleuca. See TEA TREE OIL.

Melanin. Gives pigment to the skin.

Melanoma. The deadliest form of skin cancer, it is known as a "white-collar" disease because it most often afflicts people who spend the majority of their time indoors, and then expose themselves to intense bursts of UV radiation.

Menthol. The main element in essential oil of peppermint, it is used in body-care products for its soothing properties.

Methacrylic acid. An acrylate used in nail polish that can be irritating to eyes, nose, and throat and can cause dizziness, shortness of breath, and asthma.

Methyl cyanide. See ACETONITRILE.

Methyl paraben. A preservative.

Mineral oil. A clear, odorless petroleum-based oil, it is the most commonly used oil in cosmetics. People with oily skin should avoid it.

Nanocapsules. Tiny lipid balls loaded with Vitamin E.

NaPCA (sodium PCA). A humectant and emollient.

Neroli oil. Extract from the flower of the sour orange tree; it is used in cologne, perfumes, and aromatherapy.

Niosomes. Compounds that claim to deliver moisture below the surface of the skin.

Noncomedogenic. Does not clog pores.

Novospheres. Liposomes with time-release action that supposedly moisturize the skin over a period of many hours.

Oat flour. Derived from oats, it stops itching, binds moisture, and soothes skin.

Occlusive. A substance that is impenetrable. Used as a barrier to hold in moisture.

Octyl methoxycinnamate. A sunscreen ingredient that can irritate the skin when worn for an extended period of time.

Oleic acid. An emollient and soap base derived from animal fats or vegetable oils.

PABA (para-aminobenzoic acid). A chemical sunscreen that blocks UVB rays. Its popularity has waned because it can irritate the skin.

Padimate-O. A PABA derivative.

Panthenol. One of the B vitamins used in hair conditioners, it fills in cracks in the hair shaft to strengthen the hair.

Papain. An enzyme derived from papaya that is used to exfoliate the skin.

Paraffin. Wax used at a spa to exfoliate hands and feet.

Parsol 1789 (avobenzone). An ingredient in sunscreens that blocks UVA radiation.

Pediculosis. Infestation of head lice.

Peptides. A group of two or more amino acids used in conditioners and shampoos that form a layer on the hair shaft to make the hair look thicker.

Petrolatum. A solid, waxy petroleum derivative commonly known as petroleum jelly, paraffin jelly, or Vaseline.

Petroleum products. The words "paraffin," "propylene glycol," "ozokenite," "isopropyl myristate," or anything with "butyl" or "propyl" in the name indicate that the product is made from petroleum.

pH. The measure of acidity or alkalinity of a substance, which is graded on a scale of 1 to 14. A pH 7 is neutral; below 7 is acidic; above 7 is alkaline.

Phenolic acid. A coal-tar derivative also known as carbolic acid that is used in deep phenol peels.

Phenylenediamine. A carcinogenic substance used in hair dyes, it is banned in Europe. Avoid it.

Phytotherapy. The therapeutic use of plants in skin- or haircare products.

Placenta extract. A substance used in hair- and skincare products derived from human or animal placenta.

Polyethylene glycol (PEG). A softening ingredient used in cosmetic creams.

Poly-hydroxy acids (PHAs). Similar to alpha-hydroxy acids, but from a different source, they are gentler but not as effective.

Polymers. Compounds commonly used to bind styling products to the hair and sunscreens to the skin.

Polysorbate 20. A substance used in shampoos and cleansers to build lather.

Potassium hydroxide. An alkali used in soap and shampoos.

Poultice. A warm compress applied to irritated or inflamed areas of the body.

Propellant. The primary delivery system for aerosol hairsprays and mousses. Common examples include butane, isobutane, propane, and hydrofluorocarbon.

Propylene glycol. A humectant that is good for people with oily skin.

Propylparaben. A preservative.

Proteins. Derived from synthetic and natural sources such as collagen, milk, keratin, and silk, these are found in hair conditioners and hair spritzes. They add shine and body to the hair and help smooth split ends. Common examples include hydrolyzed animal protein, hydrolyzed keratin, hydrolized soy protein, hydrolyzed whole-wheat protein, and silk amino acids.

Proteolytic. Broken down into a simpler compound so it is easier to absorb or digest, e.g., proteolytic enzymes.

Pro-vitamins. Vitamin A, B, and E derivatives used in conditioners to strengthen the hair shaft. Common examples include biotin, panthenol, and tocopherol acetate.

Quaternium ammonium compounds. Substances commonly found in hair conditioners and cream rinses. They make the hair easier to comb, give it a soft, silky feel, and reduce static, but over the long term, they may dry the hair and irritate the skin.

Quaternium 15. A synthetic preservative that can be very irritating to the skin.

Razor bumps. See FOLLICULITIS.

Resin. A sticky substance derived from tree sap and used in nail- and haircare products.

Retinoid. An antiaging product containing ingredients derived from Vitamin A.

Retinol. A Vitamin A derivative used in anti-aging skincare.

Retinyl palmitate. A Vitamin A derivative used in antiaging skincare.

Rhassoul mud. A North African clay used in face masks. In Africa, it is used for washing the hair because it absorbs oil.

Riboflavin. Vitamin B₂, an emollient and yellow coloring agent.

Rosa mosqueta oil (rose hip seed oil). An easily absorbed oil used in skincare products.

Rose water. The essence of roses diluted in water.

Royal jelly. A substance found in beehives that may retard aging.

Rutin. Vitamin P, found in buckwheat; strengthens small capillaries in the skin and may help prevent broken capillaries.

Salicylic acid. An antibacterial, skin-softening ingredient that comes from willow bark. A main ingredient in beta-hydroxy acids, it helps exfoliate dry, flaky skin and prevent and heal blemishes.

Saponification. The process of making soap.

Sclerotherapy. The process of eradicating spider veins by injecting them with saline solution. It is performed in a dermatologist's office.

Seaweed. A mineral-rich plant used in facial masks and other skincare products.

Sebaceous glands. Oil-producing glands attached to the hair follicles.

Sebum. The oil secreted onto the skin from the sebaceous glands.

Shea butter (karite). A buttery emollient from the fruit of the African karite nut tree. An extremely effective ingredient in moisturizers, shampoos, and conditioners.

Shelf life. The amount of time a product will remain fresh after it is opened.

Silica. A mineral used in face and body powders and facial masks to absorb oil and make them feel slippery.

Silicones. Inert, nonreactive substances derived from silica or sand, they are popular in hair-styling aids and, at one time, were used in breast implants. They are the words with a "-cone" ending on ingredients labels: for example, dimethicone, cyclomethicone.

Silk amino acids. Used in hairsprays and as a hair and skin conditioner.

Sodium cocoate. An alkali used in soap.

Sodium hydroxide. Lye used in hair relaxers and soaps.

Sodium lactate. A pH adjuster.

Sodium laurel sulfate. One of the most ubiquitous—and most irritating—of all detergents, it is widely used in bubble baths, shampoos, cleansers, and shower gels. It's less irritating when combined with cocoamidopropyl betaine or sodium lauroyl sarcosinate, as it often is in shampoos.

Sodium laureth sulfate. A detergent used in cleansers and shampoos that is gentler than sodium lauryl sulfate.

Sodium lauryl sulfate. A harsh detergent used in cleansers and shampoos.

Sodium PCA. A humectant and emollient.

Sodium tallowate. Lard used to make soap.

Sorbitol. An alcohol used in cosmetics as a humectant.

Spirulina. Algae rich in proteins and antioxidants that are used in algotherapy.

Squalene. A rich emollient that penetrates extremely well into the skin. It is derived from shark liver oil and is also found in olive oil and wheat germ oil.

Stearic acid. A fatty acid used as a cosmetic base and emollient.

Stearyl alcohol. An emollient emulsifier.

Stratum corneum. The uppermost layer of the skin.

Subcutaneous. Under the skin.

Sugaring. A method of hair removal similar to waxing, but the depilatory used is a mixture of sugar and honey. It is more expensive and time-consuming than waxing, but gentler and less painful.

Sulfur. An element used in antiacne products.

Sun Protection Factor (SPF). The number tells you the amount of time it will take your skin to burn with sunscreen compared to the amount of time before you'd burn with no sunscreen. (In other words, an SPF of 8 means you can stay in the sun 8 times as long as you could with no protection on your skin before your skin begins to burn.)

Superoxide dismutase. An enzyme used in skincare products.

Surfactants. Detergents that act on the hair or skin to emulsify, lift, and remove dirt. Usually more than one is present in a product because they need buffering. Common examples include ammonium laureth sulfate, ammonium lauryl sulfate, cocoamide MEA, cocoamidopropyl betaine, cocoamphodiacetate, sodium laurel sulfate, sodium lauryl sulfate, sodium laureth sulfate, and sodium lauroyl sarcosinate.

Sweet almond oil. This soothing, highly absorptive oil from the kernel of the almond is a very effective moisturizer for the skin and hair.

Talc. A powder ground from magnesium silicate that is used in bath and face powders and other powder-based cosmetics. Talc should not be inhaled over a prolonged period of time because it can irritate the lungs.

***Tapotement*.** A gentle, tapping movement on the face made during a facial massage to stimulate circulation.

TEA lauryl sulfate. A popular emulsifying ingredient in moisturizers and shampoos, it is also a detergent that can be drying to skin and hair.

Tea tree oil. Also known as melaleuca, it is extracted from the leaves of the Australian tea tree for its antiseptic, antibacterial uses.

Texturizer. A substance used to keep the consistency of a cosmetic smooth.

Thalassotherapy. The therapeutic use of seawater in bath and body care.

Thioglycolate. The sulfur-based chemical used in traditional permanent wave solutions. Avoid using it if possible.

Titanium dioxide ("micronized"). A full-spectrum sunscreen, which means that it protects the skin from both UVA and UVB rays. It is also used to give opacity to face powder, eye shadow, and foundation.

Tocopherol. Vitamin E. Especially useful in treating burns, abrasions, and other skin problems.

Tocopherol acetate. Vitamin E.

Toilet water. A less expensive, less potent version of perfume that is diluted by the addition of alcohol.

Toluene. A toxic solvent used in nail polish, it is slowly being taken off the market because it can cause liver damage and may also cause cancer.

Top coat. A clear protective coating of polish used on top of nail polish to prevent chipping.

Tretinoin. A Vitamin A derivative that is the active ingredient in antiaging prescription drugs such as Retin-A and Renova.

Trichologist. A hairstylist specially trained to treat problems of the hair and scalp.

Trichotillomania. An obsessive-compulsive-related disorder characterized by repetitive hair pulling.

Triclosan. An antibacterial ingredient found in antibacterial soaps. It's too harsh for use on the face but can be used on hands. (Use a moisturizer to counteract the drying effect.)

Tyrosine. A protein used by the body to produce melanin.

Urea. An antiseptic used in deodorants and antiperspirants, mouthwashes, moisturizers, and shampoos.

UV light (ultraviolet). Rays from the sun (UVA and UVB) that penetrate the skin and cause premature aging and skin cancer.

Walnut extract. Used for brown coloring in brunette shampoos and hair products.

Waxing. A method of removing unwanted hair using hot or cold wax.

Wheat germ oil. From the germ of the wheat plant, it is rich in Vitamin E and often used in nail creams.

Witch hazel. An astringent derived from the twigs of the *Hamamelis virginiana* plant.

Xanthan gum. A stabilizer that keeps cosmetic ingredients from separating and helps maintain a consistent texture.

Zinc oxide. An opaque, full-spectrum sunscreen also used to give opacity to face powder and foundation.

Zinc pyrithione. A strong antidandruff ingredient that is both a bactericide and fungicide. It can be irritating to the skin.

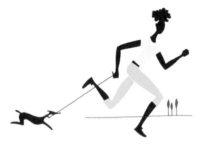

Cosmetic Surgery

In a memorable scene from *The First Wives Club,* a film about women who triumph over middle age, Elise (Goldie Hawn), a 45-year-old film star, leans her cushiony, collagen-inflated lips across an elegant restaurant table and whispers in her friends' ears, "Yes, I've had some work done." She then gives pals Annie (Diane Keaton) and Brenda (Bette Midler) what she obviously considers a wake-up call. "It's the nineties," she says with growing impatience. "Plastic surgery is like brushing your teeth."

Nowadays, cosmetic surgery is marketed so well that it sounds cute, stylish, and almost irresistible—just like the cosmetic surgeons themselves, most of whom (at least the ones I've interviewed) are extremely handsome, suave, youthful-looking members of their own Dorian Gray club. Once the exclusive province of wealthy film stars and socialites who would jet off to South America and come back from "vacation" looking "refreshed," cosmetic surgery is now more accessible, acceptable, and safer than ever.

But no matter how glib the hype, surgery, elective or not, is still surgery. I've already outlined some drawbacks in chapter 4: the benefits are temporary, not permanent, and there is no such thing as "preventive" maintenance, no matter what some doctors will try to tell you. Even the best face-lift will last 8 to 12 years, maximum. So starting early with this game only means you'll play it longer and go more rounds. And as with all surgeries, there is pain, there are side effects, and there are risks—ranging from loss of sensation in the affected area to a tragically botched face. Perhaps most important of all to remember, the surgeon may be able to reconfigure your *face,* but he can't "fix" your *life.* You can smooth out wrinkles in your skin, but that doesn't mean that your marriage will straighten out, too.

If you are considering surgery, I recommend two good books written by women who have gone through it: *Lift,* by Joan Kron, and *Welcome to Your Face Lift,* by Helen Bransford. I advise you to think carefully about what you're doing—and why—before you do it. Then, if you really feel that cosmetic surgery is for you, read on and follow these steps for the safest, best way to get what you want.

Find the Best Doctor

"People spend more time researching their car repairs than their surgery," says Dr. Richard A. Marfuggi, a board-certified plastic surgeon at Manhattan's Cabrini Hospital. Don't make that mistake: whether you'll end up looking like a well-rested, younger version of yourself or a startled doe in the headlights depends on the skill of the doctor you choose. So take the time to research your practitioner thoroughly and make a good decision. Cosmetic surgery is no place to cut corners with either your time or your money.

The best way to find a good surgeon is through a personal referral, as you would for any other medical professional. Many veterans of plastic surgery still prefer not to talk about it, but if you know someone who's had work done on her face and she looks good and had a positive experience, ask her to refer you to her doctor.

For the procedures covered in this appendix, you will need either a plastic surgeon or a cosmetic surgeon. A plastic surgeon has a broader training and can perform both reconstructive and cosmetic surgery. A cosmetic surgeon specializes exclusively in surgery to enhance your appearance and as a result may have more experience in the specific procedure you want.

Look for a doctor with board certification from the American Board of Medical Specialties (ABMS) and specialty training; a current affiliation with a good hospital; and experience in your particular surgery. If you choose a plastic surgeon, make sure he is "board-certified in plastic surgery" by the American Board of Plastic Surgery (ABPS) in the area of his specialty (a board-certified ophthalmologist trained in eye lifts, for example, or an ear, nose, and throat specialist who knows how to do nose jobs), along with a subspecialty in plastic surgery for the area.

Many plastic surgeons and cosmetic surgeons have subspecialties: you want to find a practitioner who specializes in the precise surgery you plan to undergo and has performed it hundreds, if not thousands, of times.

The American Society of Plastic Surgeons (800-635-0635; www.plasticsurgery.org), which represents 97 percent of all doctors certified by the American Board of Plastic Surgery, will give you the names and credentials of reputable surgeons in your area who specialize in your

procedure. The American Academy of Facial Plastic and Reconstructive Surgery also runs a toll-free hot line that will help you find board-certified surgeons in your region who specialize in facial plastic surgery (800-332-3223). So does the American Society for Aesthetic Plastic Surgery (888-272-7711). Or ask your primary-care doctor or dermatologist for a recommendation.

Before you actually have your surgery, check up on your doctor to make sure all his qualifications are current and that his reputation is solid. Your state licensing board can verify if his medical license is current. The Office of Professional Misconduct can assure you he hasn't gotten himself into trouble. The ABMS (800-776-2378; www.certifieddoctor.org) will verify that the doctor is board-certified, and the medical staff office of the hospital he's affiliated

TRUST YOUR INSTINCTS

Throughout the process of finding a doctor, follow your instincts. Watch out for demagoguery—a character trait that runs high in a field where someone plays Pygmalion to countless Galateas. On the other hand, don't go looking for a bargain: top surgeons usually won't slash their prices—they don't have to. (Many are booked a year in advance.) So if a doctor offers to drop his price from $4,000 to $1,500, don't take that as a good sign: he may need you more than you need him. And be suspicious of salesmanship. (The friendly nurse who talks a patient into an additional procedure often gets a commission from the doctor.) As you head through this maze, just remember that you're in the driver's seat: if you don't feel comfortable with a particular doctor for whatever reason, don't use him!

with can verify that his affiliation is current. Don't feel funny about conducting your own private investigation.

Schedule a Consultation

Once you have a short list of names, schedule a few consultations and shop around. Go in armed with lots of good questions. You'll want to know what the doctor thinks is the best procedure for you, and what the risks and benefits are for each of the procedures being considered.

On the first visit, ask about the doctor's qualifications and about the procedures themselves.

Is the doctor board-certified? What is he certified in? By which board? Ask about his specific credentials in cosmetic surgery, where he got his training, how much he had, what his subspecialty is, and how long he has been performing the procedure you're considering.

How many times does he perform this surgery in an average week?

Where will the surgery be performed? (Many procedures can now be performed in the doctor's office, but if so, it's especially important to ask about backup emergency arrangements.) What types of equipment will be used?

Is he affiliated with a hospital? Which one? (A doctor's hospital affiliation is one measure of his professional standing; besides, you need to know this information in the event of an emergency.)

Where will the incisions be made? Will there be any scars? Where? (Even Tina Turner, who presumably could afford any surgeon she wanted, ended up without any hair in front of her ears because of incisions that were improperly made during her face-lift.)

What are the possible complications of this procedure? What are the side effects? (Look for an honest answer here, not a gloss-over. If the doctor says that the surgery is quick, easy, and there are never any problems, be suspicious. All surgeries have risks, and you have a right to know what those risks are.)

What if I don't like what's done? Will he fix it at no extra charge?

Are before and after photos of patients available? Can I speak with other patients who've had my surgery?

Will I need special postoperative care? Some people arrange for special nurses or check into special hotels (see page 354) after surgery, because they need extra support for a while.

How long will I be swollen or bruised?

When can I reappear comfortably in public? When can I go back to work? (Part of this depends, of course, on your lifestyle, how much "work" you've had done, and how discreet you want to be about the procedure.)

What can I do to aid my healing and minimize recuperation time?

When will I have to come back and have the procedure done again?

After you've narrowed your choices, go for a second consultation to get into more specific aesthetic concerns. Some surgeons use computer-imaging machines to show you what you can expect from the operation; others literally draw on your photograph. One approach is not necessarily better than the other. What is important is that the doctor work *with* you to determine what would be best for your face. Most of us wouldn't mind having a nose like Sharon Stone's, but obviously most of us don't have a face like hers to go with it. Choose a doctor who is willing to guide you by virtue of his expertise, but who ultimately seems comfortable letting *you* choose what is best for you. "Would you let your doctor buy your clothes for you? Or select your hairstyle?" asks Dr. Zachary Zerut, a clinical assistant professor of plastic surgery at Albert Einstein Medical Center in Manhattan. "Then why let him choose your nose?"

Choose Your Procedure

Successful cosmetic surgery won't make a dramatic change in your looks. The old-time face-lift that rendered women flat-faced and void of expression is, thankfully, almost obsolete. If it looks like cosmetic surgery, it's bad cosmetic surgery—period. The new techniques yield a subtle result: ideally, people won't be able to quite figure out what's different about you. They'll say you look rested or ask if you've been on vacation. Or they'll ask for the name of your hairstylist or whether you've changed your makeup. If you are thinking about more than one procedure, it makes sense to have both done at the same time to avoid doubling your recovery time. Besides, when you've been through it once, you might not have the nerve to go back. Here are the basic choices.

Face-Lift

The face-lift (aka prosopexy) is a procedure that tightens the skin of the neck and the bottom half of the face, from the top of the cheeks down; it was first performed around the turn of the century in Europe. Someone with droopiness in the middle of the face, around the nasolabial folds, is a person who may consider a face-lift. To get a crude approximation of what a face-lift will accomplish, place your fingers in front of your ears and pull out and up.

In the old days, a face-lift consisted of simply removing "excess" skin and tightening the skin that remained. Today's procedures include removing fatty tissue from the lower neck and chin and tightening the muscles of the neck. This procedure yields a more natural-looking, longer-lasting lift. Each surgeon has his own favorite face-lifting technique. Basically, an S-shaped incision is made in front of the ears and back into the hairline. The facial skin is then separated from the muscle and tissue below with surgical tools (a technique called "undermining"), the excess skin is cut off, and the remainder is pulled back and stitched down.

The operation is usually performed under general anesthesia and can last from three to four hours. For the first two to three days after surgery, you'll need to be monitored closely by your doctor, and you'll look worse before you look better, because of the swelling, bruising, and tissue trauma. (Don't look in the mirror: it's a traumatic sight!) You'll be on painkillers and a liquid diet for two to three days. Bandages are removed two days after surgery, and you'll look pretty swollen and beaten up for a couple of weeks. (Some doctors advise their patients to sleep with their face in a sling for a month to protect the healing tissues from bumps in the night.) Because face-lifts don't remove fine lines and wrinkles, they are often eventually followed by a peel.

If you want work done anywhere else on your face—forehead, chin, eyelids, nose—it can be tacked onto a face-lift and done at the same time, but the pricing is strictly à la carte.

Preparation. Try to be well rested and in the best possible health before the surgery. Avoid aspirin and Vitamin E for three to four weeks before surgery. Aspirin thins the blood and can cause bleeding after surgery; Vitamin E interferes with clotting and can also cause bleeding.

Healing. Two to six weeks.

Downside. Potential problems include loss of feeling due to nerve damage, possible scarring at the incisions, possible infection, and difficult psychological adjustment due to disappointment or simply adjusting to the change. Surgeons must be extremely careful not to cut any nerves or arteries or pull the skin too tight. When blood vessels are severed, hematomas (sacs of blood that collect below the skin's surface) can form—and do, in 10 percent of cases, but these are easily removed. A cut nerve, on the other hand, can lead to a temporary or permanent "droop," numbness, or facial paralysis. When the blood supply to part of the skin is cut off—caused by a severed artery, a hematoma, or skin that's pulled excessively tight—the skin dies, leaving scar tissue. Face-lifts are not permanent and generally need to be repeated every 8 to 12 years, depending on the individual.

Mini Lift

The "mini lift" is an abbreviated version of a face-lift; it is the recommended procedure for patients whose skin looks flaccid in the cheek and jowl area but not in the neck. A "mini lift" is often performed on women in their early 40s instead of a full lift, because their skin is still reasonably resilient and not yet showing full signs of aging. The "mini lift" is also sometimes recommended as a follow-up a year after a full face-lift, if the skin wasn't stretched tightly enough in the first place or if the doctor didn't want to overdo it the first time. An incision is made in the hair of the temple and extends in front of the ear. The skin is "undermined" and pulled back, and the excess is cut off.

Preparation. See "Face-Lift."

Healing. Two to six weeks.

Downside. See "Face-Lift."

Cheek (Malar) Implants

Women with high cheekbones age well, because the cheekbone helps to anchor skin that would otherwise sag and fold around the middle of the face. For this reason, and because of the influence of glamorous celebrity role models with good bone structure—Faye Dunaway, Anjelica Huston, Keith Carradine, Michelle Pfeiffer, Brad Pitt, Arsenio Hall—cheek implants are gaining in popularity. The implants themselves are made of a hard rubber or plastic that resembles a dental retainer without the wire. They are inserted through an incision inside your mouth or through a cut made during a face-lift. Cheek implants can make a round face more angular and widen a long, narrow face into an oval.

Preparation. See "Face-Lift."

Healing. Up to 10 days, with residual sensitivity lasting up to eight weeks.

Downside. The swelling and bruising last 7 to 10 days, and the area around the implant remains sensitive for six to eight weeks. If your face is asymmetrical going into surgery, you'll come out with high cheekbones—but they'll still be asymmetrical.

Chin Implants

In the infancy of this procedure, living bone or cartilage was grafted over the chin to build up a weak or receding chin. Now that the technique has grown more sophisticated, doctors use the same rubber or plastic used in cheek implants. The chin implant is inserted through an incision in the skin under the chin or through a cut inside the lower lip. The latter, obviously, doesn't leave a scar, but some doctors believe there's a greater risk of infection that way.

Preparation. See "Face-Lift."

Healing. Up to 10 days, with residual sensitivity lasting up to eight weeks.

Downside. Sometimes the implant shifts as it heals and appears crooked. Occasionally, implants can erode the bone of the chin, and you'll end up worse off than when you started, with a receding chin and damage to your own bone.

Eyelid Surgery

The eye area is often the first part of the face to show signs of aging. Blepharoplasty, or an eye lift, can remove puffiness under the eyes or tighten and smooth sagging skin folds on the upper eyelid. It can remove excess, sagging eyelid skin, excess eyelid fat, lower-lid puffiness, and certain types of dark circles. It cannot dissolve wrinkles or smile lines under the eyes (that's left for a peel or laser surgery).

Unlike a face-lift, surgery on the puffy lower lids is usually a one-shot deal: once the offending fat is removed, it's gone forever. (Your body possesses only a certain number of fat cells: once they are removed, they are gone permanently, which is one reason why liposuction is so appealing to many women.) The sagging skin on the upper lid, however, once tightened, can sag again, so it's not unusual to have repeat surgery on the upper eyelids.

Blepharoplasty on both the upper and the lower lids is done under local anesthesia. For the traditional lower-lid lift, the doctor makes an incision beneath the lash line. He removes excess fat, cuts the excess skin, then pulls the remaining skin toward the lower lid and stitches it there, leaving a tiny scar. For people in their 20s and 30s with lower-lid puffiness, a doctor can perform a "subconjunctival" blepharoplasty, which means he makes the incision through the inner eyelid (no scar) without pulling or cutting skin, because the skin is still elastic enough to snap back on its own. For an upper-lid blepharoplasty, the doctor makes an incision in an existing fold of the upper eyelid, removes the excess skin and fat that cause the heavy-liddedness, then stitches it up with fine sutures.

Preparation. See "Face-Lift."

Healing. Swelling and bruising will last for five days, maybe longer, depending on how well your body heals and how rigorously you apply ice packs.

Downside. If the doctor removes too much skin, you'll get that perpetually wide-eyed, startled-doe look. In extreme cases, you won't be able to close your eyes completely, and your vision could even be impaired (corneal ulceration). And unless your doctor uses a laser or cuts inside the lower lid, you'll have a tiny scar.

Nose Surgery

The vast majority of "nose jobs" (aka rhinoplasty) are performed on teenage girls. Doctors do occasionally perform them on 45-year-olds in conjunction with face-lifts, but as you age, they get harder to perform because the skin thickens, becomes less flexible, and won't easily shrink down over the new nose as it should. But it's certainly not impossible to be a candidate for a nose job at a later age; just ask your doctor about it.

In a traditional nose job, the surgeon's goal is to make a large nose look smaller. Unfortunately, many rhinoplasties still result in the "pinched" Michael Jackson look. But nowadays, many surgeons actually *add* cartilage, which is harvested from the ear, to mold the nose into a more natural shape that better suits your face.

Most doctors go up through the nostrils to work inside the nose. A fairly recent advance is the "open rhinoplasty," where the skin is lifted back off the nose (this leaves a small scar), allowing the surgeon to see exactly what he's working with and to reconfigure the cartilage with sutures.

Don't be surprised if the surgeon suggests a chin implant along with a nose job if he feels it will help to better proportion the face—which it often does. You'd be surprised at how cosmetics alterations start to add up once you get started.

Preparation. See "Face-Lift."

Healing. Ninety percent of the swelling is gone in two weeks. The remainder may take six months or more.

Forehead Lift/Brow Lift

The goal here is to smooth forehead lines and vertical "scowl" lines above the nose. With the old "coronal" brow lift, the scalp was cut across the hairline, from ear to ear. The skin would be pulled up and the excess cut, then stitched down. Although the resulting scar would be hidden by hair, you could end up with nerve damage or numbness above the scar and bald spots in the area of the cut.

The new, improved version is an endoscopic brow lift, which involves much less actual cutting. Instead of making the long incision along the hairline, the doctor makes several tiny cuts behind the hairline. He inserts an endoscope—a tiny camera and lights mounted in fiber-optic tubes—into the incision on the end of a surgical probe. The endoscope guides the doctor's progress by transmitting an image on a small screen as he delves beneath the skin and separates the muscles behind the brow from the bone. In some cases, he'll snip the procerus muscle between the brows so that you will never squint again (no squinting, no wrinkles). (See "Botox," page 81.) Then he pulls up the muscles, tissues, and skin, and anchors them down inside the tiny cuts without cutting the skin.

Preparation. See "Face-lift."

Healing. Up to three weeks.

Downside. It can change the shape of the eyes, making them appear wider.

Recovery

Celebrities may rent a cottage at the Bel-Air Hotel in Beverly Hills or a suite at the Beverly Prescott after their surgeries. Those not quite ready to "face" family or friends after cosmetic surgery can check into any number of plastic surgery hideouts—a select group of pricey hotels that are set up as recovery houses—with private nurses. But most real people recuperate at home. After surgery, have a family member or friend available to stay with you, and *don't* look in the mirror for a week after a face-lift. Give yourself some time to adjust to the change and attend to your physical recovery.

Depending on the surgery, you may want to spend a night in the hospital. Consider hiring a private nurse, if you can afford it, because having one will make you feel more comfortable and secure. She'll take your temperature, check your blood pressure, and help you get up and walk to the bathroom. She'll check your bandages for bleeding and infection and ice your face continuously—which you'll need to do for the first few days that you're home. You may feel out of it because of painkillers, but you'll need to be careful not to move your face and neck muscles too much.

For your recovery to go as quickly and smoothly as possible, follow your doctor's instructions to the letter. If he says to use an ice pack three times a day, once is not enough. If he tells you not to bounce around, stay away from your kick-boxing class! And don't supplement your painkillers with anything other than what the doctor orders, or you risk serious complications.

Before you leave the hospital, talk to your doctor about how often you should ice your face and when you can wash your hair and wear makeup (see "Mineral Makeup," page 77). Invest in a good pair of wraparound sunglasses and a wide-brimmed hat. Expect to sleep on your back and eat soft food, such as oatmeal, yogurt, mashed potatoes, and broth, for a while. Take it easy and baby yourself for a few weeks. Don't downplay what you've just been through! Surgery is surgery, after all.

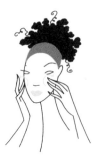

Insider Shopping

Here are just a few of the hot spots where makeup artists and hairstylists shop. If you can't make it to the stores, give them a call or check out their Websites. Some will send catalogs on request, and they'll all ship anywhere.

CHICAGO

TERRAIN NATURAL SOLUTIONS
2542 North Halsted Street
Chicago, IL 60614
773-549-0888
800-837-7246
www.terrainpersonalcare.com

Cozy and welcoming, this old-fashioned European-style apothecary sells Terrain brand hair, skin, and body products as well as other botanical-based lines. Hair treatments available.

LOS ANGELES

APOTHIA AT FRED SEGAL
8118 Melrose Avenue
Los Angeles, CA 90046
877-APOTHIA

Apothia ("apothecary" mixed with "utopia") is stocked with the latest gems and must-haves. Kiehl's, L'Occitane, Molton Brown, Aesop, Fresh, Hard Candy, Stila, Urban Decay, Creed, Comptoir Sud Pacifique, Bumble and bumble, Fudge, Philip B., and Phyto are among the selections.

FRED SEGAL SCENTIMENTS
AND ESSENTIALS
500 Broadway
Santa Monica, CA 90401
310-394-8509

Three stores in one: Studio 500 is devoted to cosmetics, Scentiments houses fragrance, candles, and bath and body, and Essentials has skin- and haircare.

They carry hard-to-find specialty lines like Stila, Kiehl's, Molton Brown, Bumble and bumble, L'Artisan, and Peter Thomas Roth.

MEMPHIS

ZOE
4564 Poplar Avenue
Memphis, TN 38117
901-821-9900

An "oasis in the desert," Zoe supplies Memphis with chic products that are hard to find elsewhere in the city. Zoe's cosmetic, fragrance, and skincare lines include Agraria, Annick Goutal, Creed, Darphin, Nars, Diptyque candles, Fresh, Kiehl's, Le Clerc, L'Occitane, M.D. Formulations, Paula Dorf, Philosophy, and Quelques Fleurs. Plus, Zoe offers her own specialty cosmetic line—ZoeFace.

NEW HOPE, PENNSYLVANIA

SCARLETT COSMETICS
129 South Main Street
New Hope, PA 18938
www.scarlettcos.com

Scarlett carries a carefully selected, genuinely interesting range of products, with an emphasis on all-out glamour and great skincare. Scarlett's funky Website offers fun and trendy products: Arcona Alchemy, Blue Funk, Cow Girl, Erbe, Fudge, Gummi Bear fragrance, Molton Brown, Peter Thomas Roth, Two Girls, Zazou—plus Scarlett's own line of cosmetics.

NEW YORK CITY

AEDES DE VENUSTAS
15 Christopher Street
New York, NY 10014
212-206-8674
888-233-3715
www.aedes.com

One of the best-edited shops in the world, this is a great place to find obscure but irresistible body products. Its fragrance lines include traditional scents and formulas dating back to the 17th century as well as custom blends created for royalty and celebrities (like Grace Kelly's wedding scent, Fleurissimo). Aedes de Venustas also carries Aesop, Agraria, Atro, Creed, Czech & Speak, Diptyque, Fresh, Jurlique, Nicolai, and Sundari.

ALCONE
235 West 19th Street
New York, NY 10011
212-633-0551
800-466-7446
www.alconeco.com

A professional theatrical line, Alcone is very reasonably priced. Best buys include cream blush (Ben Nye's "Color Wheel," $9) and makeup sponges ($2.50 for eight). Alcone's products include: Fast Lash, Super Matte Anti-shine, Hardware Nail Polish, and Precut Deluxe Sponge. The New York City shop and catalog also carry Ben Nye, R.C.M.A., Visiora, and William Tuttle.

APTHORP PHARMACY
2201 Broadway
New York, NY 10024
212-877-3480
800-775-3582

Opened in 1910, this old-fashioned European-style apothecary is a great uptown source for quality bath and body products, plus innovative lines like B. Kamins. Apthorp's haircare lines include J. F. Lazartigue, MOP, Phyto, and Terax.

HENRI BENDEL
712 Fifth Avenue
New York, NY 10019
800-HBENDEL

An intimate boutique known for its cutting-edge makeup artists' lines. Free weekly makeup artist events, led by industry professionals, showcase products and vendors.

C. O. BIGELOW APOTHECARIES
414 Sixth Avenue
New York, NY 10011
800-793-5433
www.bigelowchemists.com

This downtown makeup mecca always carries top bath and body lines; plus, it has a comprehensive homeopathic pharmacy. Believe its slogan: "If you can't get it anywhere else, try Bigelow."

COSMETICS PLUS
1201 Third Avenue
New York, NY 10021
212-628-5600
212-319-2120 (corporate office)
www.cosmeticsplus.com

Multiple locations in New York City. Reasonable prices on a bounty of products and brands for tweens on up.

FACE STOCKHOLM
110 Prince Street
New York, NY 10012
212-966-9110
888-334-FACE
www.facestockholm.com

Founded by a mother-daughter team from Sweden, it has inviting, high-quality makeup and skincare products. Call for other locations in NYC or to receive a mail-order catalog.

FRESH
57 Spring Street
New York, NY 10012
212-925-0099
800-FRESH20
www.fresh.com

There are more than 300 vegetable-based soaps to choose from plus skin- and body care, fragrances, and makeup. Environmentally friendly products made from all-natural ingredients (like milk, honey, and soy) appeal to smart, conscientious shoppers. Other locations are at 1061 Madison Avenue in New York and 121 Newbury Street in Boston.

KIEHL'S
109 Third Avenue
New York, NY
212-677-3171

Founded more than 100 years ago, this old-style apothecary is the source for great skin- and haircare products. Sales staff will give generous free samples to take home and test.

L'OCCITANE
10 East 39th Street
New York, NY 10016
212-343-0109
www.loccitane.com

All-natural products created with traditional Provençal techniques.

M·A·C
14 Christopher Street
New York, NY
212-243-4150

Beloved mecca for industry professionals. Hip and knowledgeable makeup artists offer customers professional advice.

PASTEUR PHARMACY
806 Lexington Avenue
New York, NY 10021
212-838-2500

Prices are good on salon lines like Bumble and bumble and Goldwell and specialty lines like Terax and Molton Brown.

MAKE UP FOR EVER
409 West Broadway
New York, NY 10012
212-941-9337

For everything from daily cosmetic needs to theatrical performance, Make Up For Ever has wild, extreme colors and custom-blended foundations. Boutiques are located around the country including in Atlanta, Boston, Chicago, Los Angeles, and Philadelphia.

RAY'S BEAUTY SUPPLY
721 Eighth Avenue
New York, NY 10036
212-757-0175

Here you can find everything you could ever need for your hair, from salon shampoos to styling paraphernalia.

RICKY'S
718 Broadway
New York, NY 10003
212-979-5232

Discounts on many name brands, and it doesn't get trendier than this. They ship phone orders anywhere.

SALLY BEAUTY SUPPLY
800-ASK-SALLY

With more than 2,250 stores nationwide and more than 5,000 professional hair, skin, and nail products, Sally Beauty Supply is one of the largest distributors of professional beauty supplies in the world. Just call to find the location nearest you.

SEPHORA
636 Fifth Avenue
New York, NY 10020
212-245-1633
www.sephora.com

The second largest beauty retailer in Europe, Sephora's growing list of U.S. stores artfully display three worlds of beauty: fragrance, color, and well-being.

SAN FRANCISCO

BENEFIT COSMETICS
2117 Fillmore Street
San Francisco, CA 94115
415-567-0242
800-781-2336
www.benefitcosmetics.com

Beauty is fun—BeneFit makes sure of it. Products like Bye-bye blemish cream, Thigh Hopes exfoliating body wash, and Honey Snap Out of It Scrub are good for a laugh and for your skin. Its sassy Website is worth the visit.

M·A·C COSMETICS
1833 Union Street
San Francisco, CA
415-771-6113

See New York City listing for details.

LONDON

BOOTS
Multiple locations around London
www.boots.co.uk

A cheap source of beauty bounty.

CRABTREE & EVELYN
6 Kensington Church Street
London, W8
020-7937-9335
www.crabtree-evelyn.com

Inspired by the early English home apothecary, when the family garden played an important role in the home, Crabtree & Evelyn bath, body, and haircare products celebrate country living.

LUSH
Units 7 & 11, The Piazza
Covent Garden, London, WC2E8RA
020-7240-4570
888-733-5874
www.lushcanada.com
www.lush.co.uk

If you can't get to its cute little shop in Covent Garden, where the bath and body products are hand-made while you wait, you can order through its Website or by phone.

NEAL'S YARD REMEDIES
15 Neal's Yard
Covent Garden, London, WC2
020-7379-7222

Top-notch aromatherapy line and an impressive selection of organically grown herbs. Great place to shop for vegetarian and vegan products.

NELSONS PHARMACY
73 Duke Street
London, W1
020-7629-3118

The bright staff at this pharmacy answer questions and fill homeopathic prescriptions.

SPACE NK APOTHECARY
4 Thomas Neal Centre
37 Earlham Street
London, WC3
020-7379-7030

Covent Garden shop packed with the coolest products and clients. The place to go for the latest trends in cosmetics.

PARIS

GUERLAIN
68 avenue des Champs-Elysées, 8th
Paris
01-45-62-52-57

A Parisian gem on the world famous Champs-Elysées. Certain royally inspired fragrances, along with traditional Guerlain cosmetics and body products, are sold only in the boutique.

L'ARTISAN PARFUMEUR
24 boulevard Raspail, 7th
Paris
01-42-22-23-32

If you love the distinctive scent of vanilla, a stop at L'Artisan is a must.

L'OCCITANE
55 rue St. Louis-en-l'Ile, 4th
Paris
01-40-46-81-71

More than 20 stores in or near Paris, featuring fragrance and bath and body care. See New York City listing for details.

LORA LUNE
22 rue du Bourg-Tibourg, 4th
Paris
01-48-04-31-24

Want to purchase just a slab of soap, a pinch of bath salts, or a jug of lotion? Not a problem—here, in one of Paris's newest boutiques, you pay by weight.

MAKE UP FOR EVER
5 rue La Boétie, 8th
Paris
01-42-66-01-60

Don't be fooled by the English name—this place is 100 percent French. See the New York City listing for details.

MONOPRIX
97 rue de Provence, 9th
Paris
01-45-48-18-08

Stop by one of the 30 Paris locations for affordable basics.

PRISUNIC
109 rue La Boétie, 8th
Paris
01-42-25-27-46

Great department store deals. A total of 21 stores around the city.

SEPHORA
70 avenue des Champs-Elysées, 8th
Paris
01-53-93-22-50

See the New York City listing for details.

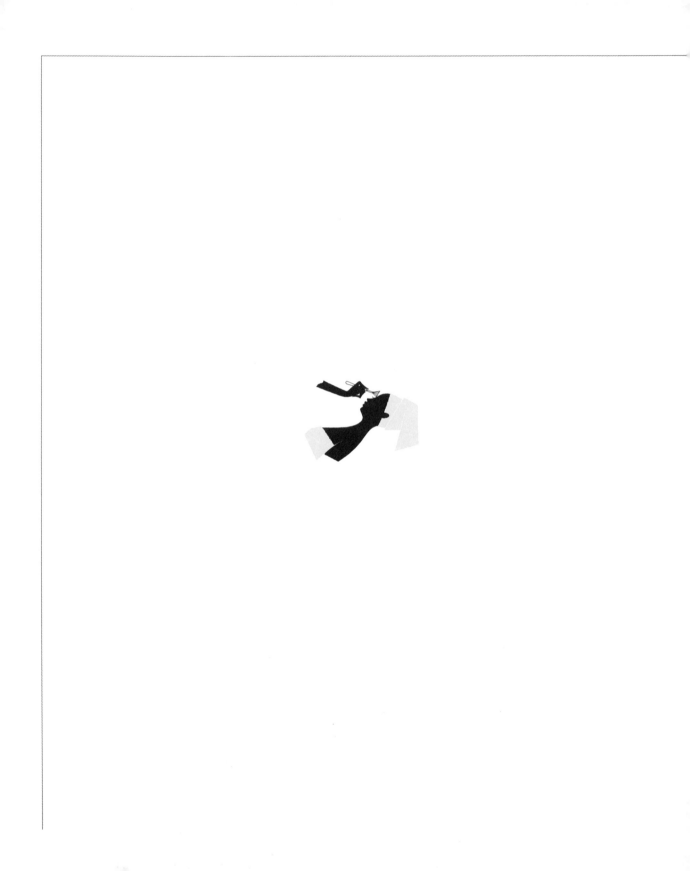

Day Spas

Here's where to find some of the best facials, massages, manicures, pedicures, and body treatments out there, at a location near you.

ASPEN, COLORADO

THE ASPEN CLUB
1450 Crystal Lake Road
Aspen, CO 81611
970-925-8900
www.aspenclub.com

The rugged Rockies have become a palace for pampering. The majestic setting is the perfect place to rejuvenate the body. Choose from the SpaAspen, HealthFitness, Sports Medicine, or WellBeing centers.

ATLANTA

JOLIE THE DAY SPA
3619 Piedmont Road
Atlanta, GA 30305
404-266-0060
www.joliethedayspa.com

Traditional spa with skilled staff. Hour-and-a-half seaweed or Cypress Clay treatments for $90. A sister of Jolie the Day Spa in Bethesda, Maryland, and Raleigh, North Carolina.

THE SPA ON PACES
3209 Paces Ferry Place
Atlanta, GA 30305
404-237-7712
www.homegrownorganics.com

Owner Maria Heckscher's line of organic products, the Homegrown Organic Collection, is used in the spa. Beauty and nature are celebrated in this southern spa experience.

BOSTON

BELLA SANTE: The Spa on Newbury
38 Newbury Street
Boston, MA 02116
617-424-9930
www.bellasante.com

East meets West in historic Boston. The Newbury Street Escape is two hours of bliss—facial treatment, sea salt body buff, and revitalizing spa massage. Acupuncture and acupressure treatments available.

L'ELEGANCE
105 Newbury Street
Boston, MA 02116
617-262-5587

Intensive microglide facials treat fine lines, wrinkles, sun damage, and acne.

CALISTOGA, CALIFORNIA

There are lots of small places to take the mud in this small, northern California town. Here's the protocol at any of the spots below: soak in the mud, take a mineral-water shower, follow it with a whirlpool bath and a stint in the steam.

DR. WILKINSON'S RESORT
1507 Lincoln Avenue
Calistoga, CA 94515
707-942-4102

CALISTOGA VILLAGE INN AND SPA
1880 Lincoln Avenue
Calistoga, CA 94515
707-942-0991

CALISTOGA HOT SPRINGS
1006 Washington Street
Calistoga, CA 94515
707-942-6269

CHICAGO

AMERICAN WHOLEHEALTH
990 West Fullerton Street, Suite 300
Chicago, IL 60614
773-296-6700
www.americanwholehealth.com

Physician-supervised wellness facility.

CHANNING'S DAY SPA
54 East Oak Street
Chicago, IL 60611
312-280-1994
800-280-1995
www.channings.com

Quaint Victorian digs give Channing's a homey feeling; aromatherapy facial, massage, and pedicure with foot scrub are star treatments.

TIFFANI KIM INSTITUTE
310 West Superior Street
Chicago, IL 60610
312-943-8777
www.tiffanikiminstitute.com

The detox seaweed wrap is the one to go for.

URBAN OASIS
12 West Maple
Chicago, IL 60610
312-587-3500
www.urban-oasis.com

Here in the Midwest, the Southwest meets the Far East—go for the fango mud wrap or the shiatsu massage.

CINCINNATI, OHIO

MITCHELL'S SALON AND DAY SPA
8118 Montgomery Road
Cincinnati, OH 45236
513-793-0900

The "Seventh Heaven" treatment includes an exfoliating body massage with pedicure, facial, and reflexology—the works!

CONNECTICUT

ADAM BRODERICK IMAGE GROUP
89 Danbury Road
Ridgefield, CT 06877
203-431-3994
800-438-3834
www.adambroderick.com

Traditional and specialized spa treatments. Ask about the Bindi herbal body treatment using medicinal Indian herbs and the Shirodhara meditative massage.

NOELLE SPA FOR BEAUTY AND WELLNESS
High Ridge Road
Stamford, CT 06905
203-322-3445

Holistic, serene, clean, soothing. Its founder, the late Noelle DiCaprio, was a pioneer in holistic spa treatments.

DALLAS

THE GREENHOUSE DAY SPA
5560 West Lovers Lane
Dallas, TX 75209
214-654-9800
www.thegreenhousespa.com

State-of-the-art treatments including laser facials and hair removal. Branches located in California, Colorado, Michigan, Minnesota, New York, and Texas.

ORIGINS FEEL-GOOD SPA
Suite 612
North Park Center
Dallas, TX 75225
214-265-7116
800-ORIGINS
www.origins.com

Go for the facial or massage.

PHILADELPHIA AREA

SPA BIBA
261 Old York Road
Jenkintown, PA 19046
215-576-7000

A cozy spa with a lavender-scented mud massage that will warm you to the bone.

LOS ANGELES AREA

THE ARCONA STUDIO
12030 Riverside Drive
Valley Village, CA 91607
818-506-5192

Try Arcona's contouring facial with an incredible massage; your fine lines totally disappear for hours.

BEVERLY HOT SPRINGS
308 North Oxford Avenue
Los Angeles, CA 90004
323-734-7000
www.beverlyhotsprings.com

Built on top of a mineral spring, this is where to go for a mineral-pool soak, shiatsu massage, or body scrub. Separate-sex facilities.

MARIANA CHICET NATURAL
EUROPEAN SKINCARE
8238 West Third Street
Los Angeles, CA 90048
323-651-0979
800-995-4490

Chicet is an extremely attentive, knowledgeable aesthetician. She makes her own products, and they're fantastic.

SONYA DAKAR
8309 Beverly Boulevard
Los Angeles, CA 90048
323-655-3061
877-727-6692 (warehouse)
www.sonyadakar.com

If she's good enough for Cameron Diaz and Drew Barrymore, she'll do for you. The cost of a facial includes follow-up treatment.

THE FACE PLACE
8701 Santa Monica Boulevard
West Hollywood, CA 90069
310-855-1150
877-587-6723

The name says it all: this is the face place. Forget pampering, this is a serious facial as part of an ongoing skincare process.

GLEN IVY HOT SPRINGS
25000 Glen Ivy Road
Corona, CA 91719
909-277-3529
800-454-8772
www.glenivy.com

World-renowned red-clay mud baths detoxify and revitalize. Relax in one of the 15 mineral spas or try a deep-cleansing facial using Glen Ivy's product line.

TERRI LAWTON SKIN CARE
AND AGE MANAGEMENT
9725 South Santa Monica Boulevard
Beverly Hills, CA 90210
310-276-8044

East meets West meets Euro skincare. Terri will help coax a glow out of your skin.

MICHAELJOHN SALON AND SPA
414 North Camden Drive
Beverly Hills, CA 90210
310-278-8333

Another star-studded client roster. Try the facial with a warm azulene mask for dry skin.

OLE HENRIKSEN OF DENMARK FACE/BODY
8622 Sunset Boulevard, Suite A
Los Angeles, CA 90069
310-854-7700
800-327-0331
www.olehenriksen.com

Celebrity central. The lavender hydration facial is a delight!

THIBIANT
449 North Canyon
Beverly Hills, CA 90210
310-278-7565
800-825-2517
www.thibiant.com

The matriarch of European-style facials. Stick with the basic version. It works!

BURKE WILLIAMS DAY SPA
1460 Fourth Street
Santa Monica, CA 90401
310-587-3366
www.burkewilliamsspa.com

Its specialty: Hunter's Retreat—water treatment with body exfoliation and massage.

MIAMI AREA

AGUA AT DELANO HOTEL
1685 Collins Avenue
Miami Beach, FL 33139
800-949-7414

This is an ultrachic Madonna haunt. Try its heated honey-and-sesame-oil massage.

THE BILTMORE HOTEL AND SPA
1200 Anastasia Avenue
Coral Gables, FL 33134
305-445-1926
www.biltmorehotel.com

Ask for facialist Martha Elisa Estinosa, one of the best in Miami.

MINNEAPOLIS

JUUT SALONSPA
2945 Hennepin Avenue South
Minneapolis, MN 55408
612-827-9200

An Aveda concept spa offering hair- and scalp care, massage, manicures, pedicures, and more.

NEW YORK CITY

ALLURE DAY SPA AND HAIR DESIGN
139 East 55th Street, Ground Floor
New York, NY 10022
212-644-5500
www.alluredayspa.com

This midtown spa covers the basics plus. Specialized body treatments include algae body-exfoliating peel and anticellulite body therm wrap.

CATHERINE ATZEN
856 Lexington Avenue
New York, NY 10021
212-517-2400
800-468-4362
www.atzen.com

Patented lymphobiology treatment—a massage of the lymph nodes that helps rid the skin of excess water and toxins. Great antiacne gel.

AVEDA INSTITUTE
233 Spring Street
New York, NY 10013
212-807-1492
www.aveda.com

Minneapolis headquarters aside, this is the center-piece of the Aveda empire. Go for an aromatherapy facial or the botanical arm and hand treatment (exfoliation with warm paraffin).

AVON CENTRE SPA AND SALON
Trump Tower
725 Fifth Avenue
New York, NY 10022
212-577-AVON
888-577-AVON

One-stop shopping, and the services are consistently good. Highlights: celeb colorist Brad Johns; "eyebrow boutique" run by eyebrow guru Eliza Petrescu. Plush, glitzy, glamorous—nothing at all like the Avon lady!

AWAY SPA AND GYM
541 Lexington Avenue, Fourth Floor
New York, NY 10022
212-407-2970
www.wellbridge.com

Signature treatments, day package including a Javanese lulure, a beautifying ritual that cleanses, exfoliates, and leaves skin soft and scented with jasmine. Hot stone massage.

ELLA BACHE SPA
8 West 36th Street
New York, NY 10018
212-279-8562
800-922-2430

Some like them hot, some like them cold—Ella Bache has both. Cold waxing helps with circulation; the azulene warm green wax is great with sensitive skin. Traditional French facials are customized to individual skin types, but they are extraction-free.

MARIO BADESCU
320 East 52nd Street
New York, NY 10022
212-758-1065
800-BADESCU
www.badescu.com

Eastern European–style salon with a luxurious hour-and-a-quarter facial that incorporates Badescu's own products.

DORIT BAXTER
47 West 57th Street, Third Floor
New York, NY 10019
212-371-4542
www.doritbaxter.com

Specializes in Dead Sea mineral treatments. Ten varieties of facials to choose from.

BLISS
568 Broadway, Second Floor
New York, NY 10012
212-219-8970
888-243-8825
www.blissworld.com

Oxygen facials, hip, friendly. Fashion-model haven. Two spas in New York City with one on the way in London.

CARAPAN
5 West 16th Street
New York, NY 10011
212-633-6220
www.carapan.com

New Mexico–style New Age in the heart of New York City. Offers good body massage.

ERBE
196 Prince Street
New York, NY 10012
212-966-1445
800-432-ERBE

Excellent, tiny space with plant-based Italian-style treatments. Herbal facial and aromatherapy massage.

ETTIA HOLISTIC DAY SPA
239 West 72nd Street
New York, NY 10023
212-362-7109
www.ettia.com

Chi facial, with Taoist healing massage. East meets West. Small, no-frills New Age gestalt, but Ettia really knows her stuff.

> FACIAL DYNAMICS
> 129 East 80th Street
> New York, NY 10021
> 212-794-2961
> 877-237-9040

This intimate Upper East Side pampering palace is run by June Meyer, a one-woman show featuring an hour-and-a-half facial with Essensa (plant-based) products. Manicurist Nina Novy (Nails by Nina) is in the next room.

> HAVEN
> 150 Mercer Street
> New York, NY 10012
> 212-343-3515

Tiny Soho spot; go for the "80 minutes in Haven" and "for your eyes only" facial treatments.

> GEORGETTE KLINGER
> 501 Madison Avenue
> New York, NY 10022
> 212-838-3200
> 800-KLINGER

Specializes in facial treatments using products produced at the Georgette Klinger Laboratories. Including New York City, there are eight main branches around the country: Beverly Hills; Chicago; Costa Mesa, Cal.; Dallas; Palm Beach; Short Hills, N.J.; and Washington, D.C.

> PAUL LABRECQUE SALON AND SPA
> Reebok Sports Center
> 160 Columbus Avenue
> New York, NY 10023
> 212-595-0099
> 888-PL-SALON
> www.paullabrecque.com

Fashion hangout with full hair-salon and spa services. Spa offers Rolfing body techniques as well as aromatherapy facials.

> LING
> 12 East 16th Street
> New York, NY 10003
> 212-989-8833
> 888-415-LING
> www.ling-skincare.com

Incorporates principles of Chinese medicine. Straightforward, no-nonsense. Ling's own line of skincare products is available in her three New York City locations.

> DR. MARGOLIN'S WELLNESS SPA
> 166 Fifth Avenue, Second Floor
> New York, NY 10010
> 212-675-9355
> www.drmargolins.com

The place to go for massage—the Cagnina-Margolin deep-tissue, deep-muscle massage is a therapeutic massage developed by Sam Cagnina and Dr. Margolin to rejuvenate, relax, and support the spine.

> ORIGINS FEEL-GOOD SPA
> CHELSEA PIERS SPORTS COMPLEX
> Pier 60, Second Floor
> West 23rd Street
> New York, NY 10011
> 212-336-6780
> www.origins.com

Natural-style treatments—using Origins products, of course. Young, athletic, energetic staff, and reliable treatments.

> PREMA NOLITA
> 252 Elizabeth Street
> New York, NY 10012
> 212-226-3972

Holistic skincare, including the pricey but wonderful Anne Semonin products. All products are made from plant, flower, herb, and essential oil extracts.

THE PENINSULA HOTEL
700 Fifth Avenue, 21st Floor
New York, NY 10019
212-903-3910

Soothing in spite of its large size; the aromatherapy facial and deep-cleaning facial are always popular.

REPECHAGE
115 East 57th Street
New York, NY 10022
212-319-1770
800-284-5044
www.repechage.com

Owner Lydia Safadi is a big believer in the powers of seaweed. Try the four-layer facial for dehydrated skin.

JANET SARTIN
500 Park Avenue
New York, NY 10022
212-751-5858
800-321-1779
www.sartin.com

Everyone loves her cosmetics and her deep-cleansing facials.

ELENA SCHELL
330 West 58th Street, #304
New York, NY 10019
212-245-2170

She'll make your acne go away with her Elena Schell natural facial products specially designed to treat blemished skin.

SCOTT J. SALON & SPA
257 Columbus Avenue
New York, NY 10023
212-769-0107
www.scottj.com

Hair salon with day spa downstairs. Small, but good for the basics: waxing, manicure, pedicure.

SOHO INTEGRATIVE HEALTH
62 Crosby Street
New York, NY 10012
212-431-1600

Created by dermatologist Lori Polis, here you can combine state-of-the-art pampering treatments with a visit with the doc.

SOHO SANCTUARY
119 Mercer Street
New York, NY 10012
212-334-5550

Dr. Hauschka holistic facials; come early and sit in the steam, or take a yoga class.

STONE SPA
104 West 14th Street, Second Floor
New York, NY 10011
212-741-8881
www.stonespa.com

A light-filled, warm, and welcoming temple of tranquillity. The stone massage—a Swedish-shiatsu hybrid in which the therapist uses heated basalt river rocks to noogie into the tight spots—is pure, unadulterated bliss.

TEJ AYURVEDIC SKINCARE CLINIC
162 West 56th Street, Suite 204
New York, NY 10019
212-581-8136

Pratima Raichpur, founder, is a doctor of Naturopathy. She uses ancient ayurvedic principles, and her products are all-natural, homemade, and based on essential oils and herbs.

W HOTEL AWAY SPA AND GYM
541 Lexington Avenue, Fourth Floor
New York, NY 10022
212-407-2970

Escape the hustle of Manhattan with a hot stone massage and charismatic staff.

PORTLAND, OREGON

FACES UNLIMITED
25–7 Northwest 23rd Place
Portland, OR 97210
503-227-7366
800-835-4998
www.facesunlimited.com

Try the antiaging Guinot Paris Hydradermie facial.

SYLVIE DAY SPA
1706 Northwest Glisan
Portland, OR 97209
503-222-5054
www.sylviedayspa.com

Gentle facial with steamed towels and plant-based
FloraSpa products.

SAN FRANCISCO AREA

CAT MURPHY'S SKIN CARE SALON
561 Bridgeway, Suites 1 and 2
Sausalito, CA 94965
415-332-4296
800-869-8705
www.catmurphysskincare.com

Specialized treatments for sun-damaged skin and pre-
and postsurgery.

CLAREMONT RESORT AND SPA
41 Tunnel Road
Berkeley, CA 94705
800-555-7266
510-843-3000
www.claremontresort.com

The spa underwent a total renovation in fall 2000 and
now features state-of-the-art treatments, breathtaking
views, and grounds that would make Jay Gatsby feel
right at home.

OSMOSIS ENZYME BATHS
209 Bohemian Highway
Freestone, CA 95472
707-823-8231
www.osmosis.com

Incredibly relaxing, Japanese-style heat treatments in
a redwood tub full of organic rice bran, cedar, and
plant enzymes imported from Japan.

SPA RADIANCE
3061 Fillmore Street
San Francisco, CA 94123
415-346-6281
www.sparadiance.com

European skincare, facial treatments, body massages,
scrubs, reflexology and bronzing. The popular "So
You've Got a Problem" facial removes acne and is followed by a deep-cleansing mask.

SEATTLE

JAROSLAVA DAY SPA
1413 Fourth Avenue
Seattle, WA 98101
206-623-3336

Traditional European day spa. Plush facial bed, with
Decléor aromatherapy products.

KATE'S DAY SPA
2713 East Madison
Seattle, WA 98112
206-322-3350

Casual, T-shirted, attentive staff; heavenly facial
includes arm, neck, face, and hand massage.

UMMELINA INTERNATIONAL DAY SPA
1525 Fourth Avenue
Seattle, WA 98101
206-624-1370

Try the stress-busting aromatherapy hydro-massage.

St. Louis, Missouri, Area

THE FACE & THE BODY DAY SPA
7736 Forsythe Boulevard
Clayton, MO 63105
314-725-8975
www.faceandbodyspa.com

Traditional European facials catering to women and men.

SALON ST. LOUIS
3012 South Grand Street
St. Louis, MO 63116
314-771-8820

Gentle, extraction-free facial using Aveda products.

Washington, D.C., Area

JOLIE THE DAY SPA
7200 Wisconsin Avenue
Bethesda, MD 20814
301-986-9293
www.joliethedayspa.com

Great place to get a massage—therapeutic, deep tissue, or aromatherapy. Sister to the Jolie The Day Spas in Atlanta and Raleigh.

Manicures and Pedicures

Los Angeles

HANDS-ON
243 South Beverly Drive
Los Angeles, CA 90212
310-860-0137
www.hands-online.com

Clean, clean, clean!

JEANNIE NAIL CARE
8036 West Third Street
Los Angeles, CA 90038
323-651-5268

They do all the basics but specialize in nail art—and you may spot Jennifer Lopez at the next table.

New York City

GARREN NEW YORK (AT HENRI BENDEL)
712 Fifth Avenue, Third Floor
New York, NY 10019
212-841-9400

Manicurist Grace Koniecko is, hands down, the best.

HELENA RUBINSTEIN BEAUTY GALLERY
135 Spring Street
New York, NY 10012
212-343-9963

Helena Rubinstein has changed with the times—swanky and hip, all the latest trends are here.

THE J. SISTERS INTERNATIONAL SALON
35 West 57th Street
New York, NY 10019
212-750-2485

Seven Brazilian sisters run this Vanderbilt townhouse salon, focusing on intense nail-care treatment—no rushing clients here! The Padilha sisters' celebrity clientele includes Gwyneth Paltrow, Naomi Campbell, and Kate Moss.

NAILS BY NINA
129 East 80th Street
New York, NY 10021
212-288-8130

In the same suite as Facial Dynamics Day Spa.

OSCAR BOND SALON & SPA
42 Wooster Street
New York, NY 10013
212-334-3777
www.oscarbondsalon.com

Relaxing aromatherapy manicure and pedicure, including paraffin dip (my favorite). Ask for nail technician Beatrice Najera.

RESCUE NAIL SPA
21 Cleveland Place
New York, NY 10012
212-431-3805

A downtown haven that features aromatherapy manicures and pedicures. They're a little pricey, but a worthwhile indulgence.

JIN SOON NATURAL HAND & FOOT SPA
56 East Fourth Street
New York, NY 10003
212-473-2047

Until she opened this soothing shop, Jin Soon was the manicurist on countless photo shoots. She specializes in all-natural treatments for hands and feet.

PARIS

INSTITUT DE BEAUTÉ YVES SAINT LAURENT
32 rue du Faubourg-St.-Honoré, 8th
Paris
01-49-24-99-66

Indulge in the pure luxury of a French spa. An hour-long pedicure with Mr. Ho will put the bounce back in your step and add a long-lasting sparkle to your toes.

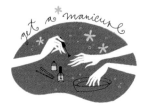

Destination Spas

ARIZONA

CANYON RANCH TUCSON
8600 East Rockcliff Road
Tucson, AZ 85750
520-749-9000
800-742-9000
www.canyonranch.com

Roadrunners and coyotes are part of the southwestern appeal of this Sonoran Desert resort. The 60,000-square-foot spa complex has it all—even a yoga dome.

MIRAVAL
5000 East Via Estancia Miraval
Catalina, AZ 85739
520-825-4000
800-232-3969
www.miravalresort.com

Achieving "life in balance" is the theme of this Santa Catalina Mountain resort. Hiking, Pilates, tai chi, and yoga help create balance. The spa offers hot stone massages, hydrotherapy, and more.

THE PHOENICIAN
6000 East Camelback Road
Scottsdale, AZ 85251
602-941-8200

A luxury spa in the desert, with a wellness center that features desert flora—sage, aloe vera, jojoba—in spa treatments.

CALIFORNIA

CAL-A-VIE
2249 Somerset Road
Vista, CA 92084 (40 miles south of San Diego)
760-945-2055
www.cal-a-vie.com

Tranquil setting offers unpretentious luxury. Mediterranean-style cottages accommodate only 22 guests total. The seven-day Euro plan includes 16 treatments plus an individualized fitness program.

GOLDEN DOOR
777 Deersprings Road
San Marcus, CA 92069
760-744-5777
800-424-0777
www.goldendoor.com

Modeled after Japanese *honjin*; individual attention is paramount. Sprawling acres of gardens, trails, and orchards create an isolated, serene getaway. Extensive spa treatments.

THE LODGE AT SKYLONDA
16350 Skyline Boulevard
Woodside, CA 94062
650-851-6625
www.skylondalodge.com

Hiking in the redwoods is the centerpiece, along with a serene ambience and sumptuous cuisine.

THE OAKS AT OJAI
122 East Ojai Avenue
Ojai, CA 93023
805-646-5573
800-753-6257
www.oaksspa.com

Reasonably priced fitness package with quality spa treatments to revitalize and energize guests in a non-intimidating environment.

SONOMA MISSION INN AND SPA
18140 Highway 12
Boyes Hot Springs, CA 95416
707-938-9000
800-862-4945
www.sonomamissioninn.com

Located in the heart of California's wine country, the spa is situated above 135-degree thermal mineral springs. Climb into an outdoor hot artesian mineral pool and soak in the healing water.

TWO BUNCH PALMS
67425 Two Bunch Palms Trail
Desert Hot Springs, CA 92240
(110 miles from Los Angeles)
760-329-8791
800-472-4334
www.twobunchpalms.com

Film-industry hot spot. You'll have a good time—as well as a good facial—if you ask for one of the twin sisters "Sunrise" or "Loveland."

CANADA

MOUNTAIN TREK FITNESS RESORT AND SPA
Ainsworth, B.C.
800-661-5161
www.hiking.com

A mind-body program, featuring hiking, hiking, and more hiking, in the fabulous Kootenay Mountains. No treatments except massage, and you'll need it.

COLORADO

THE PEAKS AT TELLURIDE
136 Country Club Drive
Telluride, CO 81435
800-SPA-KIVA

New Age orientation in world-class digs, with emphasis on total rejuvenation of mind-body-spirit. State-of-the-art gym, pools, and treatments.

THE SPA AT THE BROADMOOR HOTEL
1 Lake Avenue
Colorado Springs, CO 80906
719-634-7711
800-634-7711
www.broadmoor.com

Native Colorado Rocky Mountain flora and fauna are incorporated into spa treatments. The one-of-a-kind Broadmoor Falls Shower and Spray uses temperature-controlled mountain water in a traditional Swiss shower.

CONNECTICUT

THE SPA AT NORWICH INN
607 West Thames Street
Norwich, CT 06360
860-886-2401
800-ASK-4-SPA
www.norwichinnandspa.com

Everything from Swedish massage to ayurvedic facials and wraps. Popular treatments include the antiaging facial, the hot stone massage, and the vitality vitamin wrap.

FLORIDA

PGA NATIONAL RESORT & SPA
450 Avenue of the Champions
Palm Beach Gardens, FL 33418
561-627-3111
800-843-7725
www.pgaresort.com

Golfer's heaven. The Waters of the World outdoor mineral pools use age-old water-healing therapy. The full-service spa offers more than 100 services.

THE SPA AT DORAL
8755 Northwest 36th Street
Miami, FL 33178
305-592-2000
800-71-DORAL
www.doralgolf.com

European-style spa catering to relaxation as well as fitness. Lush gardens and spacious facilities add to the total spa experience.

SPA INTERNAZIONALE AT FISHER ISLAND
1 Fisher Island Drive
Fisher Island, FL 33109
305-535-6030
800-537-3708

The only way to reach this island getaway is by ferry or helicopter. Like the peacocks that roam the island, you'll want to strut your stuff after a thermal mineral kur mud treatment.

ILLINOIS

HEARTLAND SPA
1237 East 1600 North Road
Gilman, IL 60938
815-683-2182
800-545-4853
www.heartlandspa.com

Get back to the basics at this quaint yet contemporary farm environment. Healthy living and quality treatments.

MASSACHUSETTS

CANYON RANCH IN THE BERKSHIRES
165 Kemble Street
Lenox, MA 01240
413-637-4100
800-742-9000
www.canyonranch.com

World-class 100,000-square-foot spa complex bundled in the charm of New England and the beauty of the Berkshires. Hydrotherapy is a specialty.

MEXICO

LAS ROCAS RESORT & SPA
Playas de Rosarito
Baja California, Mexico
888-527-7622

A seaside resort and spa, 25 miles south of Tijuana. Go for the spa—Basalt Rock Massage and Exfoliating Salt Glow are favorites—and take the family on vacation.

RANCHO LA PUERTA
Baja California, Mexico
800-443-7565
www.rancholapuerta.com

A hiking spa, run by the founders of the Golden Door, which features nine gyms, four tennis courts, three pools, a meditation center, delicious organic vegetarian cuisine (grown on premises), and enough wraps and facials to keep you very happy.

NEW MEXICO

TEN THOUSAND WAVES
3451 Hyde Park Road
Santa Fe, NM 87504
505-982-9304

An aquatic adventure—communal teak tub, waterfall tub, waterfall spills, baths—even aquatic massages. More than 100 massage therapists create the team of specialists.

NEW YORK

GURNEY'S INN RESORT SPA
290 Old Montauk Highway
Montauk, NY 11954
631-668-2345
www.gurneys-inn.com

On the beach at the outermost tip of Long Island. Ask about the thalassotherapy.

NEW AGE HEALTH SPA
Route 55
Neversink, NY 12765
914-985-7600
800-682-4348
www.newagespa.com

The scenic Catskills with seasonal opportunities set the stage for varied packages at this no-frills spa. New Age practices and well-rounded spa treatments —hydrotherapy, ayurvedic therapy, and colonic irrigation.

TENNESSEE

TENNESSEE FITNESS SPA
299 Natural Bridge Park Road
Waynesboro, TN 38435
931-722-5549
www.tfspa.com

An extremely inexpensive weeklong spa experience, with weight loss and fitness as focal points.

TEXAS

THE GREENHOUSE
1171 107th Street
Grand Prairie, TX 75050
817-640-4000

Personalized daily agendas, attentive staff, and top-of-the-line treatments.

LAKE AUSTIN SPA RESORT
1705 South Quinlan Park Road
Austin, TX 78732
512-372-7360
800-847-5637
www.lakeaustin.com

Healthy, mouthwatering cuisine is just an appetizer to the full courseload of fitness and relaxation regimes.

UTAH

GREEN VALLEY SPA
1871 West Canyon View Drive
St. George, UT 84770
435-628-8060
800-237-1068
www.greenvalleyspa.com

The spa soaks in the gorgeous surroundings using desert botanicals in its complete line of all-natural skincare products. Perhaps the only spa to offer a Native American program of spa treatments.

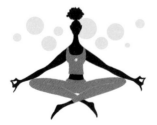

Hair Salons

Y ou may not have heard of some of these spots, but you will have heard of the glamorous women who frequent them.

LOS ANGELES AREA

BIGOUDI INTERNATIONAL SALON
21720 Ventura Boulevard
Woodland Hills, CA 91364
818-887-3627

Cut and color, $50 and up.

SALLY HERSHBERGER AT JOHN FRIEDA
8440 Melrose Place
Los Angeles, CA 90069
323-653-4040

Sally Hershberger put the tousle in Meg Ryan's hair. Her specialty: beautiful, lived-in looks.

HAIR AMERICA (AT THE ART LUNA SALON)
827 Hilldale Avenue
West Hollywood, CA 90069
310-247-9092

At Luna's celeb-studded salon, you may find yourself being shampooed next to Daryl Hannah. But this adjunct to Luna's main salon caters to young women and teens at more affordable prices. Single-process hair color costs $45 to $65; cuts run from $30 to $65 (at the main salon, these begin at $100).

LATHER BEAUTY SHOP
727 North Fairfax Avenue
Los Angeles, CA 90048
323-658-8585

A perch for fledgling film stars and MTV players. Cuts for men, $50; women, $60 and up. For classic cuts, ask for Jay Diola.

PRIVÉ
8458 Melrose Place
Los Angeles, CA 90069
323-651-5045

Laurent D. does Hollywood's 'dos. Located on a quiet, tree-lined street, Privé is a small, private salon full of celebrities.

SHAMPOO BY NEZI
310 North Florence
Los Angeles, CA 90048
323-653-2275

The Nezi brothers will blow out your curly hair in 10 minutes (literally), without using flat irons or truckloads of straightening goop, for about $45.

NEW YORK CITY

JEAN-CLAUDE BIGUINE
230 Park Avenue
New York, NY 10169
212-867-8534
www.biguine.com

Jean-Claude Biguine's chic French chain now has five New York City locations.

BUMBLE AND BUMBLE
146 East 56th Street
New York, NY 10022
212-521-6500
800-7-BUMBLE
www.bumbleandbumble.com

Chic razor cuts and super-stylish headbands. Cut, $75 and up; color, $81 and up; highlights, $140 and up.

DEVACHAN
Soho Salon
588 Broadway
New York, NY 10012
212-274-8686

When they say natural products, they mean it. Specialty: curly hair.

FRÉDÉRIC FEKKAI BEAUTÉ DE
PROVENCE
15 East 57th Street
New York, NY 10022
212-753-9500
800-F-FEKKAI

Full-service chichi salon and spa. Cut, $80 and up; color, $85 and up; highlights, $150 and up.

GARREN NEW YORK (AT HENRI BENDEL)
712 Fifth Avenue, Third Floor
New York, NY 10019
212-841-9400

Small and exclusive, Garren New York offers a relaxing and private salon experience. Cut, $100-plus; color, $100-plus.

MARK GARRISON
820 Madison Avenue
New York, NY 10021
212-570-2455
www.markgarrison.com

Laid back, especially for Madison Avenue. Mark's southern upbringing and Madison Avenue address result in creative styling in a hospitable atmosphere. Bicoastal stylist Philip B. flies in regularly to offer his all-natural oil treatments.

STEPHEN KNOLL
625 Madison Avenue
New York, NY 10022
212-421-0100
800-728-7822

Stephen and his stylists offer lots of individual attention. The salon is fashioned with the look and feel of a private home. Cut, $100 to $350; color, $85 and up; highlights, $225 and up.

LEPINE NEW YORK
667 Madison Avenue
New York, NY 10021
212-355-4247
888-750-4247
www.lepinehair.com

France-born owner Kim Lepine specializes in the personal touch. Colorist Arlene Bradley can clean up anyone else's mess.

LOCKS 'N' CHOPS
365 West 34th Street
New York, NY 10001
212-244-2306

Unisex salon specializing in African American hairstyling using all-natural products. Cut, $20 and up; color, $40 and up.

LOUIS LICARI COLOR GROUP
693 Fifth Avenue
New York, NY 10023
212-517-8084

Louis is the "master blonder."

PIERRE MICHEL
131 East 57th Street
New York, NY 10022
212-593-1460

Giselle gives great highlights.

LISA MITCHELL SALON
90 Rivington Street
New York, NY 10002
212-982-0085

Queen of relaxing and hair weaves—but pricey.

OUIDAD SALON
846 Seventh Avenue
New York, NY 10019
212-333-7577
800-677-HAIR
www.ouidad.com

Curly hair cuts, treatments, and products.

RUTHERFORD/LISSETTE HAIR, INC.
8 Beach Street, Second Floor
New York, NY 10013
212-965-8992

Lissette Martinez, a gentle color genius, was the colorist at Barney's Roger Thompson Salon for years until she teamed up with London-born Rutherford, who does the cuts. Color, $85 and up; cut, $125.

SALON AKS
694 Madison Avenue
New York, NY 10021
212-888-0707
www.salonaks.com

The three owners—formerly with Frédéric Fekkai—have created an unintimidating salon where the cuts and color are primo. Ask for Kathleen Flynn-Hui for any kind of color treatment. The salon's Website provides valuable hair-treatment advice for women undergoing chemotherapy.

SNIP 'N' SIP
204 Waverly Place
New York, NY 10014
212-242-3880

The owner trained under the fashionista hair guru Orlando Pita. Cuts start at $55.

San Francisco

ALBANESE HAIR SALON
323 Geary Street, Suite 306
San Francisco, CA 94102
415-397-7969
www.albanesehairsalon.com

Small, intimate salon overlooking Union Square. Fabulous highlights. Cut, $75 and up; color, $80 and up; highlights, $125 and up.

Cheap Treats

Many top salons around the country offer discounted or free treatments on staff training nights, when experienced assistants are supervised by master stylists. Services are usually booked two weeks to a month in advance. The following salons offer discounted services as of this writing, but not all services are available at all times, and some salons require phone consultations first, so call ahead and find out. Expect to be wait-listed for an appointment.

AVEDA INSTITUTE
233 Spring Street
New York, NY 10013
212-807-1492

AVEDA INSTITUTE
400 Central Avenue, SE
Minneapolis, MN 55414
612-331-1400

The Aveda Institute centers in both Minneapolis and New York City function as educational centers as well as spa/salons. Aveda's founder, Horst Rechelbacher, offers workshops and seminars on everything from skincare to makeup application and massage. You can get haircuts for $9, coloring starting at $18, and facials go for $15 if you're willing to be treated by a trainee.

ATLANTA

VIDAL SASSOON
Lenox Square
3393 Peachtree Road, NE
Atlanta, GA 30326
404-237-7870 (main salon)
404-233-9518 (training program)

Call in advance for a phone consultation to be an assistant model. Cut, $10 to $13; color or perm, $20 and up.

BOSTON

SALON MARIO RUSSO
9 Newbury Street
Boston, MA 02116
617-424-6676

Training sessions held two or three nights a week. Cut, $15; color, $20 and up.

CHICAGO

MAXINE
712 North Rush Street
Chicago, IL 60611
312-751-9338

Cut, free; color or perm, $25.

SANTA MONICA

VIDAL SASSOON ACADEMY
321 Santa Monica Boulevard
Santa Monica, CA 90401
310-255-0011
www.vidalsassoon.uk.co

Cut, $15; color, $32 and up.

MIAMI

EGO TRIP SALON
1623 Michigan Avenue
Miami Beach, FL 33139
305-672-0871

Student training program, $40 by appointment only for women's cuts. Stylists, $65 for a woman's cut; color, $50 and up. It carries Bumble and bumble, Fudge. Relaxed, tranquil environment.

STELLA SALON
404 Washington Avenue
Miami Beach, FL 33139
305-532-0024

Training cuts on Wednesday for $15; styling, $45; color, $60 and up. Stella's top stylists are Jonny Levy and Gian Luca Mandelli.

NEW YORK

BUMBLE AND BUMBLE
146 East 56th Street
New York, NY 10022
212-521-6580, extension 265

Cut and color free for selected styling models—plus a $50 gift certificate.

JACQUES DESSANGE
505 Park Avenue
New York, NY 10022
212-750-3007

Classes on Sundays and Mondays. Cut, $15; color, $20.

JOHN FRIEDA
30 East 76th Street
New York, NY 10021
212-744-9856

Classes held on Wednesday nights and every other Tuesday. Cut, $25; color, $25 to $40.

PAUL LABRECQUE SALON AND SPA
Reebok Sports Center
160 Columbus Avenue
New York, NY 10023
212-595-0099
888-PL-SALON
www.paullabrecque.com

Call to request an appointment as a styling model. Cut, $10; color, $20.

SAN FRANCISCO

VIDAL SASSOON
359 Sutter Street
San Francisco, CA 94108
415-397-5105
www.vidalsassoon.co.uk

Cut, $16; color or perm, $15 to $25. Regular salon prices; cut, $59 to $93; color, $65 and up.

SCOTTSDALE, ARIZONA

VIDAL SASSOON
6961 East Fifth Avenue
Scottsdale, AZ 85251
480-949-3337
www.vidalsassoon.co.uk

Training programs offer cuts for $14 to $17; color or perm, $16 to $25. Regular stylists cost $50 and up; color, $40 and up; perms, $50 and up.

SEATTLE

PHASE 3
99 Blanchard Street
Seattle, WA 98121
206-728-9933
www.garymanuel.com

A training salon for Gary Manuel Salon. Cut, $20 to $28; color, $40 and up. Training stylists have been handpicked by Gary.

WASHINGTON, D.C., AREA

VIDAL SASSOON
Tyson Galleria
1855 G International Drive
McLean, VA 22102
703-448-9884
www.vidalsassoon.co.uk

Student training classes: cut, $10; color or perm, $15 and up.

WICHITA

ERIC FISHER SALON
306 North Rock Road
Wichita, KS 67206
316-681-0077
877-9-EFSALON

Free cuts as part of stylist workshops every Tuesday night.

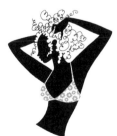

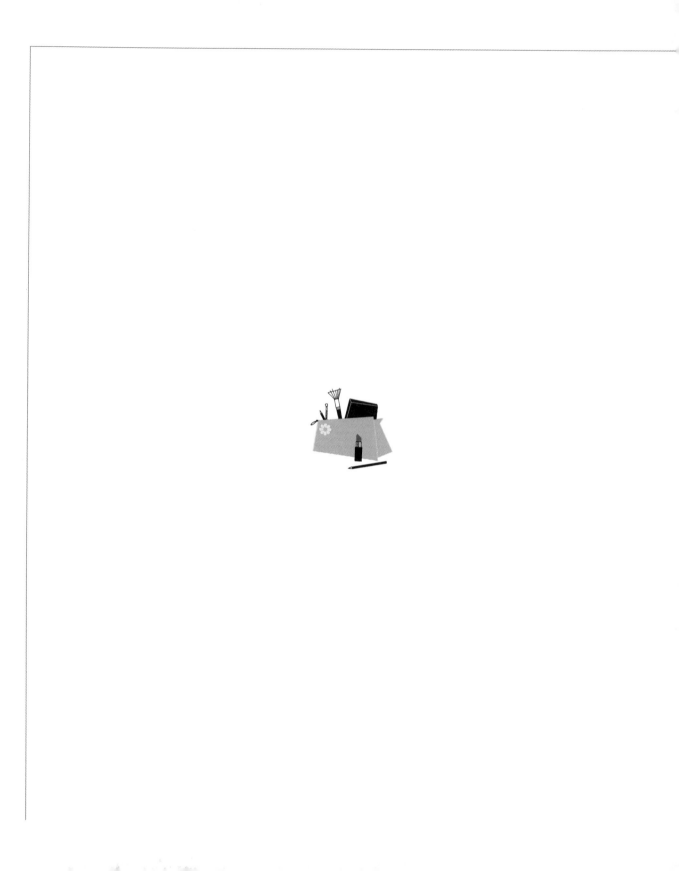

Recommended Reading

Ackerman, Diane. *A Natural History of the Senses.* Random House, 1990.

Aucoin, Kevyn. *Face Forward.* Little, Brown and Company, 2000.

Austen, Jane. *Emma.* Penguin, 1997.

Banner, Lois W. *American Beauty.* University of Chicago Press, 1984.

Beling, Stephanie. *Power Foods.* HarperCollins, 1998.

Bransford, Helen. *Welcome to Your Facelift: What to Expect Before, During, and After Cosmetic Surgery.* Doubleday, 1998.

Brinton, D.G., and G.H. Napheys. *Personal Beauty.* Applewood, 1994.

Brody, Jane. *The New York Times Book of Women's Health.* Lebhar-Freedman, 2000.

Brown, Bobbi, and Annmarie Iversen. *Teenage Beauty.* Cliff Street Books, 2000.

Carper, Jean. *Miracle Cures: Dramatic New Scientific Discoveries Revealing the Healing Powers of Herbs, Vitamins, and Other Natural Remedies.* HarperCollins, 1998.

Cash, Thomas F. *What Do You See When You Look in the Mirror: Helping Yourself to a Positive Body Image.* Bantam, 1995.

Castleman, Michael. *Nature's Cures.* Bantam, 1997.

Catalano, Julie, and Robert L. Rowan. *The Women's Pharmacy.* Dell, 2000.

Classen, Constance, David Howes, and Anthony Synnott. *Aroma: The Cultural History of Smell.* Routledge, 1994.

Croutier, Alev Lytle. *Taking the Waters.* Abbeville Press, 1992.

Crute, Sheree. *Health and Healing for African-Americans: Straight Talk from More than 150 Black Doctors on Our Top Health Concerns.* Rodale, 1997.

Fraser, Kennedy. *Ornament and Silence: Essays on Women's Lives.* Alfred A. Knopf, 1996.

Friedman, Rita. *Bodylove: Learning to Like Our Looks and Ourselves.* Harper & Row, 1988.

Gray, Henry. *Gray's Anatomy.* Running Press, 1999.

Hales, Dianne. *How Gender Science Is Redefining What Makes Us Female.* Bantam Books, 1999.

Hampton, Aubrey. *What's in Your Cosmetics?* Odonian Press, 1995.

Kron, Joan. *Lift: Wanting, Fearing & Having a Facelift.* Viking Penguin, 1998.

Lamott, Anne. *Bird by Bird.* Pantheon, 1994.

Lavabre, Marcel. *The Aromatherapy Workbook.* Inner Traditions, 1996.

Leigh, Michelle Dominique. *The Japanese Way of Beauty.* Birch Lane Press, 1992.

Love, Susan M., with Karen Lindsey. *Dr. Susan Love's Breast Book.* Perseus Publishing, 1990.

Mittleman, Stu. *Slow Burn.* HarperResource, 2000.

Munro, Alice. *Lives of Girls and Women.* Dutton, 1994.

Nelson, Miriam. *Strong Women Stay Young.* Bantam Books, 1998.

Norman, Laura, and Thomas Cowan. *Feet First: A Guide to Reflexology.* Fireside, 1988.

Norris, Gloria, ed. *The Seasons of Women.* Norton, 1996.

Northrup, Christiane. *Women's Bodies, Women's Wisdom.* Bantam, 1998.

Null, Gary. *The Complete Guide to Health and Nutrition.* Dell, 1984.

Phillips, Katharine A. *The Broken Mirror: Understanding and Treating Body Dysmorphic Disorder.* Oxford University Press, 1996.

Raichur, Pratima, and Marian Cohn. *Absolute Beauty.* HarperCollins, 1999.

Sachs, Melanie. *Ayurvedic Beauty Care.* Lotus Press, 1994.

Sieber, Roy, and Frank Herreman, eds. *Hair in African Art and Culture.* Museum for African Art, 2000.

Stacey, Michelle. *Consumed: Why Americans Love, Hate, and Fear Food.* Touchstone, 1995.

Suskind, Patrick. *Perfume.* Alfred A. Knopf, 1987.

Tisdale, Sallie. *Talk Dirty to Me: An Intimate Philosophy of Sex.* Doubleday, 1994.

Tisserand, Robert B. *The Art of Aromatherapy: The Healing and Beautifying Properties of the Essential Oils of Flowers and Herbs.* Destiny Books, 1987.

Villarosa, Linda, ed. *Body & Soul: The Black Women's Guide to Physical Health and Emotional Well-Being.* Harper Perennial, 1994.

Weil, Andrew. *Eight Weeks to Optimum Health: A Proven Program for Taking Full Advantage of Your Body's Natural Healing Power.* Alfred A. Knopf, 1997.

Weinberg, Norma Pasekoff. *Henna: From Head to Toe!* Storey Books, 1999.

Werbach, Melvyn. *Healing with Food.* HarperCollins, 1993.

Winter, Ruth. *A Consumer's Dictionary of Cosmetic Ingredients.* Crown, 1989.

Worwood, Valerie Ann. *The Complete Book of Essential Oils & Aromatherapy.* New World Library, 1991.

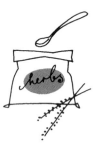

Organizations

American Academy of Dermatology
P.O. Box 4014
930 North Meachum Road
Schaumburg, IL 60168
847-330-0230
Fax: 847-330-0050
www.aad.org

American Electrology Association
106 Oak Ridge Road
Trumbull, CT 06611
203-374-6667
www.electrology.com

American Society of Plastic and
Reconstructive Surgeons
444 East Algonquin Road
Arlington Heights, IL 60005
847-228-9900
www.plasticsurgery.com

International Assocation of Trichologists
Kalamazoo, MI
Fax: 616-372-3224

International Guild of Professional Electrologists
308 North Main Street, Suite A
High Point, NC 27262
800-830-3247
Fax: 336-841-5187

Look Good, Feel Better
800-395-LOOK

Beauty professionals who help cancer patients with techniques to deal with the side effects of chemotherapy and radiation.

National Alopecia Areata Foundation
710 C Street, Suite 11
San Rafael, CA 94910
415-456-4644

Support groups, referral, and helpful information on hair loss.

haircolorist.com; haircolorhow2.com

A source of names of certified colorists in your area. Log on to find hair-color case histories with how-to instructions.

www.fda.gov

The official FDA Website offers answers to some of the most frequently asked cosmetics-related questions, plus the latest results of FDA safety testing.

Cosmetic, Toiletry, and Fragrance Association
www.ctfa.org

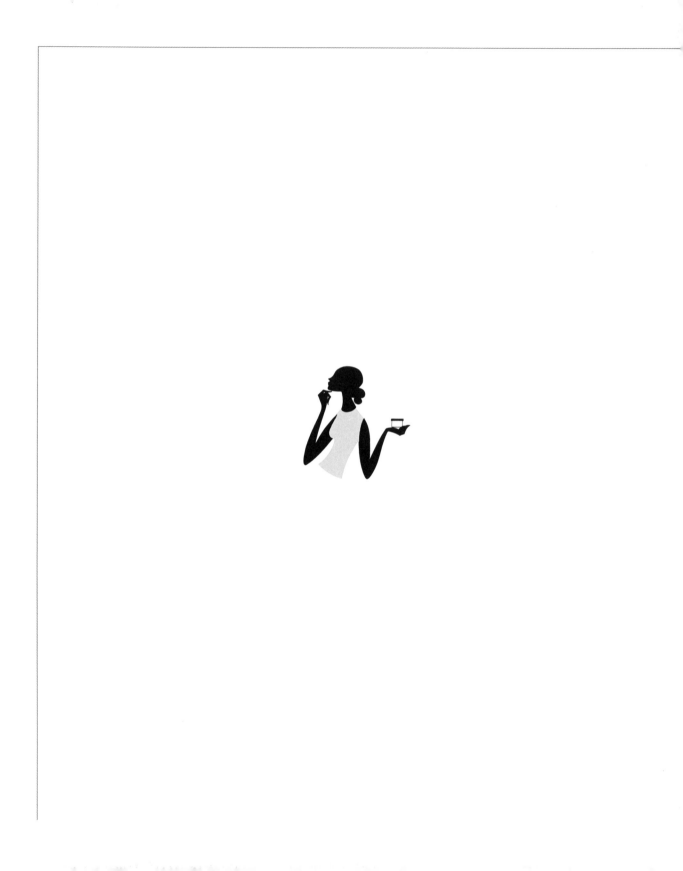

Acknowledgments

Tremendous thanks to my editor, Ruth Sullivan, the most passionate, dedicated, and talented editor a writer could ever hope for; whose contribution to this book is immeasurable and invaluable; who never let her sky-high standards slip and who always brought out the best in me.

Thanks to my photographer, Deborah Jaffe, and illustrator, Anja Kroencke, whose outstanding talents made an amazing contribution to this book. To my agent, Kris Dahl, whose good humor, barbed wit, and unwavering support mean the world to me.

Special thanks to Peter Workman, a publishing visionary, who saw the potential in this project early on. Thanks to Paul Hanson and Elizabeth Johnsboen, for their incredible art direction; Tracey Keevan and Peggy Boulos, for research assistance; Giema Tsakuginow and Kara Mia Vigilia, for photo research; and Rosie Schaap, for excellent camaraderie and editorial know-how.

My boundless gratitude to everyone at Workman, Artisan, and Algonquin who contributed so much talent and support, and made me feel so much at home that I almost never left: Bruce Harris, Carolan Workman, Andrew Mandel, Elisabeth Scharlatt, Ann Bramson, Joni Miller, Elizabeth Gaynor, Ina Weisser, Janet Harris, Antonia Fusco, Katherine Dietrich, Kim Shannon, Kim Cox, Steve Andrews, Anthony Cacioppo, Greg Galati, Barbie Altorfer, Lydia Buechler, Patty Berg, Dusty Fisher, Patty Bozza, Jenny Mandel, Mary Wilkinson, Saundra Pearson, Suzanne Rafer, Mike Murphy, Irene Demchyshyn, Malcolm Felder, Judy Hirsch, Barbara Peragine, Paul Gamarello, Lela Moore, Amy Hayworth, Wayne Kirn.

I have also benefited from the expertise of many generous people over the course of writing this book. Thanks to all of you for graciously answering my intrusive questions.

To the good doctors I've interviewed along the way: Diane Berson, Lori Polis, Patricia Wexler, Ellen Gendler, Richard Noodleman, Alan Hirsch, Sara Colby, Mark Rubin, Thomas Romo, and many others.

To the talented hairstylists: Mark Garrison, Philip B, Mark Garrison Salon; Ouidad, Ouidad Salon; Vidal Sassoon; Frédéric Fekkai, Beaute de Provence; Lorraine Massey, Devachan; Kim Lepine, Arlene Bradley, Kim Lepine Salon; Michael Brimhall; Kathleen Flynn-Hui, Danielle Petrulli, Angelique Flynn, Alex Huang, Kao Hui, Alain Pinon, Susanna Romano, AKS Salon; Horst Rechelbacher, Aveda; Ademolle Mandella, Locks 'n' Chops; Wendy Bond, Oscar Bond Salon; Lissette Martinez, Rutherford/Lissette; Michael Gordon, Bumble and bumble; Patrick Ales, Phytotherapy; Young Hee Kim, Young Hee Salon; Bret Stange, Larissa Fortuno, Randy Farrell-Forstein, Lauren Lavelle, Michelle B.

To the incredible makeup artists: Kevyn Aucoin, Sue Devitt, Sue Devitt Studio; Carol Shaw, Lorac; Liz Michael; Laura Mercier, Laura Mercier Classique; Hagan Linss, M.A.C.; Suzette Rodriguez, Gigi Hale; Jenine Lobell, Stila; Geri Cusenza, Trucco; Bobbi Brown, Bobbi Brown

Essentials; Frank Toscan, François Nars, Nars; Shu Uemura; Thierry, YSL; Hiromi Ando; Brian Kim; Stephanie Parent; David Tabola.

Thanks to the beautiful women who took time out of their busy lives to model for this book: Patty Berg, Angela Crimaudo, Cameron Howell, Giema Tsakuginow, Margot Herrera, Pat Upton, Kim Walker, Rosie Schaap, Luisa Oviedo Dlugacz, Marjorie Lee, Ellen Wright, Leah Jaffe, Lucy Simon, Julie Simon, Mary Lynn Blanks Supino, Jenny Wonderling, Catharine Long, Brenna Berger, Marion C. Long, Andra Olenik, Linda Romero, Michele Barker, Elizabeth Aubrey, Peggy Boulos, Susan Jaffe, Robinne Lee, Lacey Angioletti, Molly MacDonald, Heather Thorne, Suzanne Achtemeier Shapiro, Lara Meyerratken, Leah Wonski.

And to Aida Thibiant, Laura Peck Fennema, Donna Karan, Norma Kamali, Bethann Hardison, Elena Schell, Marcia Kilgore, Tammy Ha, Jamie Morse Heidegger, Colette Malouf, Eliza Petrescu, Kim Marshall, Daniel Horton, Mark Potter, Mary Bemis, Nikki Gersten, Nancy Hathaway, Dael Orlandersmith, Chris Molinari, Alison Mazzola, Leslie Stevens, Michele Feeney, Alison Moore, and Janet Hulstrand. Thanks to the New York Society Library, a great place to work. To good friends: Sheri Duxin, who loves to play with powder and paint almost as much as I do, and Anne Simmons, who doesn't. And to my cousin Leslie Roth, a soulmate in style.

And to the countless others who shall remain unnamed—you know who you are, and I thank you.

Photo Credits

All photographs are by Deborah Jaffe unless noted below.

Page 5 *(right, top and bottom):* The Advertising Archives

Page 12 *(clockwise from left):* Franklin D. Roosevelt Library, The Advertising Archives, The Advertising Archives

Page 35: Evan Agostini/Liaison Agency

Page 52: Lauren Greenfield/Corbis Sygma

Page 53: Courtesy of Yves Saint Laurent

Pages 68–69: Susan Sarandon, Steve Sands/Corbis Outline; Candice Bergen, Photofest; Diane Keaton, Photofest; Dayle Haddon, Theo Westenberger/Liaison Agency; Vanessa Redgrave, Conna-Kipa/Stava/Corbis Sygma; Judith Jamison, Jack Mitchell/Corbis Outline; Lauren Hutton, Photofest

Page 100: Courtesy of the American Cancer Society

Page 104: Courtesy of Shu Uemura

Page 106: Jerry Hall, Ian Jones/Liaison Agency; Halle Berry, Evan Agostini/Liaison Agency; Jennifer Lopez, Darlene Hammond/Archive Photos; Joan Chen, Photofest

Page 107: Dayle Haddon, Theo Westenberger/Liaison Agency; Winona Ryder, Thomas Lau/Corbis Outline; Alek Wek, Gerald Forster/Corbis Outline; Drew Barrymore, Gerardo Somoza/Corbis Outline

Page 108: Bobbi Brown, Deborah Feingold/Corbis Outline

Page 109: Iman, Cori Wells Braun/Corbis Outline; Laura Mercier, courtesy of Susan Magrino Agency; Carol Shaw, George Lange/Corbis Outline; Frank Toscan, Alexis Duclos/Liaison Agency

Page 110: François Nars, Kafka/Liaison Agency; Shu Uemura, courtesy of Shu Uemura; Jenine Lobell, courtesy of Stila Cosmetics; Sue Devitt, courtesy of Sue Devitt Studio; Geri Cusenza, courtesy of Sebastian International, Inc.

Page 117 *(right):* Evan Agostini/Liaison Agency

Page 125: Hulton Getty/Archive Photos

Page 131 *(top):* The Advertising Archives

Page 133: 1910s, Archive Photos; 1920s, 1930s, 1940s, 1950s, Photofest; 1960s, The Advertising Archives; 1970s, 1980s, Photofest; 1990s, Frank Trapper/Corbis Sygma; 2000s, Kwaku Alston/Corbis Outline

Page 143: 1920s, 1930s, 1940s, 1950s, Photofest; 1960s, Bettman/CORBIS; 1970s, AP/Wide World Photos; 1980s, Jeff Slocomb/Corbis Outline; 1990s, Kelly Jordan/Corbis Sygma; 2000s, Frank Trapper/ Corbis Sygma

Pages 174–180: 4000 B.C., Fulvio Roiter/CORBIS; Second century A.D., The Granger Collection; Third century A.D., Giraudon/Art Resource, NY; 1550, Victoria & Albert Museum, London/Art Resource, NY; 1603, Scala/Art Resource, NY; Late 1600s–1700s, The Granger Collection; 1900, Curt Teich Postcard Archives; 1902, The Advertising Archives; 1909, Bettmann/CORBIS; 1913, The Advertising Archives; 1914, The Advertising Archives; 1923, The Advertising Archives; 1932, Bettmann/CORBIS; 1935, Inge Morath/Magnum Photos; 1937, The Advertising Archives; 1940s, Bettmann/CORBIS; 1952, The Advertising Archives; 1954, The Advertising Archives; 1963, Bettmann/CORBIS; 1967, The Advertising Archives; 1974 (Lauren Hutton), Photofest; 1974 (Beverly Johnson), Dirck Halstead/Liaison Agency; 1985, The Advertising Archives; 1990, Deborah Feingold/Corbis Outline; 1991, Terry Ashe/Archive Photos; 1995 (Vamp), The Advertising Archives; 1995 (RuPaul), Victor Malafronte/Archive Photos; 1997, Mitchell Gerber/CORBIS

Page 188: The Advertising Archives

Page 209 *(top to bottom):* Evan Agostini/Liaison Agency, A. Uzzle/Liaison Agency, Kelly Jordan/ Corbis Sygma, Pierre Vauthey/Corbis Sygma

Page 220 *(bottom right):* Bob Roth

Page 221: Alix Malka/Corbis Sygma

Page 232 *(left):* Chabassier/M.P.A./Liaison Agency

Page 233: (Nancy Kwan) courtesy of Fishman Creative Associates

Page 234 *(top):* Underwood & Underwood/CORBIS

Page 241: Horst Rechelbacher, courtesy of Aveda

Page 242: Michael Gordon, courtesy of Bumble and bumble; Lorraine Massey, courtesy of Devachan; Frédéric Fekkai, Gerardo Somoza/Corbis Outline; Jami Morse Heidegger, courtesy of Behrman Communications; Jherri Redding, courtesy of Nexxus

Page 243: Ouidad, courtesy of Ouidad; Philip Berkowitz, courtesy of Philip B Inc.; Patrick Ales, courtesy of Phytotherathrie; Geri Cusenza, courtesy of Sebastian International, Inc.

Page 245: *(top)* Evan Agostini/Liaison Agency; *(bottom)* Steve Sands/Corbis Outline

Page 261: Allen Kirschen

Pages 262–266: 4000 B.C., Erich Lessing/Art Resource, NY; 1370–1352 B.C., The Granger Collection; 35 B.C., Giraudon/Art Resource, NY; 17th and 18th centuries, The Granger Collection; 1780s, The Granger Collection; 1840s and 1850s, The Granger Collection; 1880s, The Advertising Archives; 1902, Archive Photos; 1906, The Granger Collection; 1907, Archive Photos; 1917, Bettmann/CORBIS; 1920, Bettmann/CORBIS; 1930, Photofest; 1931, The Granger Collection; 1939, courtesy of Gamsberg Macmillan Publishers (Pty) Ltd., Windhoek, Namibia; 1940 (Rita Hayworth), Photofest; 1940 (Veronica Lake), Photofest; Late 1940s, courtesy of Carita; 1941, The Granger Collection; 1950s, Archive Photos; 1952, Photofest; 1953, Phil Burchman/Archive Photos; 1954, Photofest; 1955, The Advertising Archives; 1960s (Supremes), Archive Photos; 1960s (Twiggy), Popperfoto/Archive Photos; 1963, London Daily Express/Archive Photos; 1967 *(Hair)*, Archive Photos; 1967 (Angela Davis), Bettmann/CORBIS; 1970s, Photofest; 1974, Photos International/Archive Photos; 1975, RUOGM Hairstyles Drawing, P.O. Box 1203, Ibadan, Nigeria/Museum for African Art, NY; 1976 (Dorothy Hamill), Photofest; 1976 (punk rock), Vednio/Liaison Agency; 1979, Photofest; 1980, Andy Schwartz/Corbis Outline; 1981, Photofest; 1988, Neal Preston/Corbis Outline; 1994, Barry King/Liaison Agency; Late 1990s, Steve Sands/Corbis Outline; 1999, Jeff Slocomb/Corbis Outline; 2000, Lugura or Kuguru, Tanzania/*Joyce Marie Sims,* photo by Jerry L. Thompson/Museum for African Art, NY

Page 281: courtesy of Burt's Bees

Page 286: *(top and bottom)* New York Public Library/The Picture Collection; *(center right)* Victoria & Albert Museum, London/Art Resource, NY

Page 297: Catherine Leuthold/nonstock

Page 302: 1930s, Photofest; 1940s, Archive Photos; 1950s, 1960s, 1970s, The Advertising Archives; 1980s, Holger Maass/nonstock; 1990s, Francis Hammond/nonstock; 2000s, Macduff Everton/CORBIS

Page 303: Mojgan Azimi/Corbis Outline

Page 308: courtesy of Universal Reflexology

Page 311 *(right):* Lucien Clergue/Stone

Page 323: courtesy of Stone Spa

Page 324 *(left):* courtesy of Stone Spa

Pages 330–334: 3000 B.C., Werner Forman/Art Resource, NY; 100 B.C., Giraudon/Art Resource, NY; A.D. 306, The Granger Collection; 900s, illustration reprinted from *Shoes* (Workman Publishing Co.); Late 1400s, The Granger Collection; 1827, The Advertising Archives; 1872, The Advertising Archives; 1875, The Advertising Archives; 1900, The Granger Collection; 1917, The Advertising Archives; 1934, Eve Johnson/Archive Photos; 1939–1945, Hulton Getty/Archive Photos; 1948, Bettmann/CORBIS; 1960s, Trip/A. Ghazzal; 1976, Andrew Buurman/ESP/Liaison Agency; 1979, Archive Photos; 1980s, The Advertising Archives; 1984, Tony Costa/Corbis Outline; 1987, Joe Viesti/Viesti Associates, Inc.; 1990, courtesy of Origins; 1992, Trip/H. Rogers

Index